Cognition and mood
interactions

DATE DUE

			PRINTED IN U.S.A.

COGNITION AND MOOD INTERACTIONS

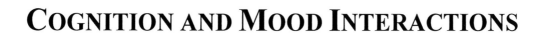

COGNITION AND MOOD INTERACTIONS

MIAO-KUN SUN
EDITOR

Nova Biomedical Books
New York

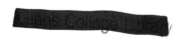

Library of Congress Cataloging-in-Publication Data
Cognition and mood interactions / Miao-Kun Sun, editor.
     p.   cm.

Includes index.
ISBN 1-59454-229-5 (hardcover)
1. Cognition disorders. 2. Affective disorders. 3. Dementia--Pathophysiology. 4. Depression, Mental--Pathophysiology. 5. Neurobehavioral disorders. 6. Neuropsychiatry. I. Sun, Miao-Kun.
RC554.C64C645   2004
616.8--dc22   2004024014

Published by Nova Science Publishers, Inc. ✤*New York*

Contents

Contributors[1]

Daniel L. Alkon, M.D., Blânchette Rockefeller Neurosciences Institute, 9601 Medical Center Dr., Johns Hopkins Academic and Research Bldg., Rockville, MD 20850 USA [33]

Chad E. Beyer, Depression and Anxiety Research, Neuroscience Discovery Research, Wyeth Research, Princeton, NJ 08543-8000, USA [19]

J. Douglas Bremner*, Departments of Psychiatry and Behavioral Sciences, Emory Center for Positron Emission Tomography, Emory University School of Medicine, 1364 Clifton Road, Atlanta, GA 30322, USA, E-mail: jdbremn@emory.edu [149]

Safa Elgamal, Dept of Psychiatry and Behavioral Neurosciences, McMaster University, Canada [117]

Paul R. Gard*, School of Pharmacy and Biomolecular Sciences, University of Brighton, Brighton BN2 4GJ, UK, Tel: +44 1273 642084, Fax: +44 01273 679333 E-mail: p.r.gard@brighton.ac.uk [71]

Robert Gerlai*, Department of Psychology, University of Hawai'I, 2430 Campus Road, Honolulu, HI 96822 USA, E-mail: robert_gerlai@yahoo.com [89]

Utpal Goswami, Department of Psychiatry, Darlington Memorial Hospital (CDDPS NHS Trust), Hollyhurst Road, Darlington, DL3 8HX, UK [1]

Reinhard Heun*, Department of Psychiatry, University of Bonn, Sigmund Freud Street 25, D-53105, Bonn, Germany, E-mail: heun@uni-bonn.de [1]

Robert F. Kennison, Leonard Davis School of Gerontology, Andrus Gerontology Center, University of Southern California, Los Angeles, CA, USA [161]

Noriyuki Kitayama, Departments of Psychiatry and Behavioral Sciences, Emory University School of Medicine [149]

Glenda M. MacQueen*, Department of Psychiatry and Behavioral Neurosciences, McMaster University Medical Centre, 1200 Main St. W., Hamilton, ON, Canada L8N 3Z5, Tel: 905 525 9140, Fax: 905 304 5376, E-mail: macqueng@mcmaster.ca [117]

Elena Mariani, Sezione di Gerontologia e Geriatria, Dipartimento di Medicina Clinica e Sperimentale, Università degli Studi di Perugia, Perugia, Italy [105]

---

[1] The contributors are listed alphabetically. The numbers in brackets are the opening page numbers of the contributors' chapters. *: Corresponding authors.

Patrizia Mecocci, Sezione di Gerontologia e Geriatria, Dipartimento di Medicina Clinica e Sperimentale, Università degli Studi di Perugia, Perugia, Italy [105]

Antonio Metastasio, Sezione di Gerontologia e Geriatria, Dipartimento di Medicina Clinica e Sperimentale, Università degli Studi di Perugia, Perugia, Italy [105]

M. Cristina Polidori*, Institute of Physiological Chemistry I, Heinrich-Heine University, Dusseldorf, Germany, E-mail: polidori@uni-duesseldorf.de [105]

Lee E. Schechter*, Depression and Anxiety Research, Neuroscience Discovery Research, Wyeth Research, CN 8000, Princeton, NJ 08543-8000, USA, Tel: 732 274 4060, Fax: 732 274 4755, E-mail: schechl@wyeth.com [19]

Miao-Kun Sun*, Ph.D., Blânchette Rockefeller Neurosciences Institute, 9601 Medical Center Dr., Johns Hopkins Academic and Research Bldg. Room 319, Rockville, MD 20850 USA, Tel: 301 294 7181, Fax: 301 294 7007, E-mail: mksun@brni-jhu.org [33]

Marta Weinstock*, Department of Pharmacology, Hebrew University Faculty of Medicine, Jerusalem 91120, Israel, Tel.: 972-2-6758731, Fax: 972-2-6758741, E-mail: martar@cc.huji.ac.il [185]

Katsuhiko Yanagisawa*, Department of Dementia Research, National Institute for Longevity Sciences, Obu, Japan, E-mail: katuhiko@nils.go.jp [137]

ElizabethM. Zelinski*, Leonard Davis School of Gerontology, Andrus Gerontology Center, University of Southern California, Los Angeles, CA 90089-0191, USA, E-mail: zelinski@rcf.usc.edu [161]

Abbreviations

5HIAA	=	5-hydroxy-indoleacetic acid
5HT	=	5-Hydroxytryptamine (serotonin)
Aβ	=	amyloid β peptide
AAMI	=	age-associated memory impairment
ACC	=	Anterior cingulate cortex
ACE	=	Angiotensin Converting Enzyme
ACh	=	Acetylcholine
AChE	=	Acetylcholinesterase
ACTH	=	Adrenocorticotropic hormone
AD	=	Alzheimer's disease
ADHD	=	attention deficit hyperactivity disorder
AIF	=	apoptosis-inducing factor
AMPA	=	α-amino-3-hydroxy-5-methyl-4-isoxazoleproprionate
AMPT	=	alpha-methyl-para-tyrosine
AP-5	=	D-2-amino-5-phosphopentanoic acid
AP-7	=	D-2-amino-7-phosphoheptanoic acid
APA	=	American Psychiatric Association
APOE	=	apolipoprotein-E
APP	=	amyloid precursor protein
APTD	=	acute phenylalanine/tyrosine depletion
AT$_1$	=	Angiotensin Receptor Subtype 1
AT$_2$	=	Angiotensin Receptor Subtype 2
AT$_4$	=	Angiotensin Receptor Subtype 4
ATD	=	acute tryptophan depletion
BDNF	=	Brain-derived neurotrophic factor
cAMP	=	Cyclic AMP
CGP39653	=	(±)-(E)-2-amino-4-propyl-5-phosphonopentenoic acid
CGS19755	=	[(±)-2-carboxypiperidin-4-yl]methyl-4-yl]phosphonic acid
CNQX	=	6-cyano-7-nitroquinoxaline-2,3-dione
CNS	=	central nervous system
CPP	=	[3-[(±)-carboxypiperazin-4-yl]prop-1-yl]-phosphonic acid

CPP-ene	=	[3-[(±)-2-carboxypeprazin-4-yl]-propen-1-yl]-phosphonic acid
CREB	=	cAMP response-element binding protein
CRH	=	Corticotropin-releasing hormone
CSF	=	cerebrospinal fluid
D2	=	dopamine D2 receptor
DA	=	Dopamine
CSF	=	Cerebrospinal fluid
DNQX	=	6,7-dinitroquinoxaline-2,3-dione
DSM IV	=	Diagnostic and Statistical Manual of Mental Disorders, fourth revision
ECS	=	Electroconvulsive shock
EPSCs	=	Excitatory postsynaptic currents
ES cell	=	Embryonic Stem cell
GABA	=	γ-amino butyric acid
GR	=	Glucocorticoid receptors
HA-966	=	3-amino-1-phenylglycine
HPA	=	Hypothalamo-pituitary-adrenal axis
ICD 10	=	International Classification of Diseases, tenth revision
i.c.v.	=	Intracerebroventricular
iGluR	=	ionotropic glutamate receptor
IRAP	=	Insulin-Regulated Amino Peptidase
LC	=	Locus coeruleus
LTD	=	long-term depression
LTP	=	long-term potentiation
MAO	=	monoamine oxidase
MAPK	=	Mitogen Activated Protein Kinase
MCI	=	Mild cognitive impairment
MDD	=	Major depressive disorder
mGluR	=	metabotropic glutamate receptor
MK-801	=	(+)-5-methyl-10,11-dihydro-5H-dibenzo[a,d]cyclohepten-5,10-imine; dizocilpine
MR	=	Mineralocorticoid receptors
MRI	=	magnetic resonance imaging
MTL	=	Medial temporal lobe
NA	=	Noradrenaline
NAA	=	N-acetyl-aspartate
NFTs	=	Neurofibrillary tangles
NIMH	=	National Institute of Mental Health
NKA	=	Neurokinin A
NKB	=	Neurokinin B
NMDA	=	N-Methyl-D-aspartate
NPs	=	Neuritic plaques
NPY	=	Neuropeptide Y
NR	=	NMDA receptor

NTF	=	neuro-fibrillary tangle
PCP	=	phencyclidine
PD	=	Parkinson's disease
PET	=	Positron emission tomography
PFC	=	Prefrontal cortex
NRI	=	Selective NA reuptake inhibitors
PS	=	presenilin
PSD	=	postsynaptic density
PTST	=	posttraumatic stress disorder
PVN	=	Paraventricular nucleus
rCBF	=	Regional cerebral blood flow
SERT	=	Serotonin transporter
SNRI	=	serotonin/norepinephrine reuptake inhibitor
SP	=	Substance P
SSRI	=	Selective serotonin reuptake inhibitors
Tg	=	transgenic
TCA	=	Tricyclic antidepressant
UFC	=	urinary free cortisol
VTA	=	ventral tegmental area
WHO	=	World Health Organisation
YAC	=	yeast artificial chromosome

In: Cognition and Mood Interactions
Editor: Miao-Kun Sun, pp. 1-18

ISBN 1-59454-229-5
2005 © Nova Science Publishers, Inc.

Chapter I

Fundamentals of Dementia and Depression

Reinhard Heun* and Utpal Goswami[#]

Department of Psychiatry, University of Bonn, Germany and
[#]Department of Psychiatry, Darlington Memorial Hospital, Darlington, UK

This chapter describes the definitions, classification, aetiology, epidemiology, symptoms, course, and comorbidity of dementia and depression. The two clinical syndromes could be independent psychiatric disorders. They may also be the consequences of various physical and medical disorders. Dementia is an organic psychiatric syndrome, fundamentally consisting of characteristic memory disturbance and other neurocognitive deficits, often persistent and severe enough to severely affect the patient's life. Depression is characterised by depressed mood and loss of interest or pleasure in most daily activities over a period of time. Apart from these *core symptoms*, a number of *additional* depressive symptoms are recognized. Depression is often the main clinical component of an underlying mood disorder. However, a number of depressive symptoms can also be present in other psychiatric disorders such as schizophrenia, obsessive-compulsive disorders, dysthymia, anxiety disorders and others. Several major medical disorders that adversely influence brain functions can *secondarily* lead to clinical depression. The clinical profiles of these disorders have significant differences, *as well as similarities*, that may potentially lead to diagnostic confusion. The *course* is often the best clinical discriminator. Dementia is caused by many different disorders with often well-defined aetiologies and pathologies. In contrast, depression may be the consequence of many disorders, but its aetiology and neurobiology remain imprecise.

1. Introduction

Dementia and depression are clinical syndromes of diverse and uncertain aetiologies, and *not* discreet disease entities or specific psychiatric disorders. However, depression as well as dementia can be part of several other psychiatric disorders. Not infrequently, they also may be the consequence of many physical and medical disorders (Roberts at al., 1997).

Dementia is a psychiatric syndrome consisting of multiple neurocognitive deficits, which are persistent and severe enough to affect the patient's life. Dementia is a core feature of different psychiatric and medical disorders, which directly or indirectly affect the brain function. Dementia of Alzheimer type and different types of vascular dementia are among the clinically relevant and most frequently encountered disorders in this group.

Depression is a well-known and universally experienced mood. If it is disproportionate to the demands of the situation and/or unduly persistent over a period of time, it may be considered as pathological. Depression is a symptom of several underlying medical and/or psychiatric conditions as well. As a clinical syndrome, Depression is characterised by certain *core symptoms:* depressed mood and loss of interest or of pleasure in most daily activities. In addition to these core symptoms, some people complain of having variable experience of loss or increase of appetite, weight and sleep disturbances. These are known as endogenous or biological or vegetative symptoms of depression, classically seen in endogenous or melancholic depression. Other important and characteristic features include decreased (or increased) psychomotor activity, lack of energy, altered sexual drive, feelings of worthlessness or guilt, difficulties in thinking and concentrating, difficulties in making decisions, recurrent thoughts of death or suicidal ideations, plans or attempts (APA, 1994).

Often depression is the core feature of a major depressive episode, unipolar or bipolar. However, some depressive symptoms can also be present in other psychiatric disorders such as schizophrenia, obsessive-compulsive disorders, and anxiety disorders. Additionally, all major medical disorders that affect the brain can secondarily lead to depression.

In the following paragraphs, we will describe the symptoms, courses, usual definitions, common classification, aetiology, epidemiology and comorbidities of dementia and depression. We will comprehensively highlight different and common features of both syndromes. This description will focus on the most common classification systems, the International Classification of Diseases, Tenth Revision, published by the World Health Organisation (ICD 10) (WHO, 1991) and the Diagnostic and Statistical Manual of Mental Disorders, fourth revision, published by the American Psychiatric Association (DSM IV) (APA, 1994).

2. Symptoms in Dementia and Depression

2.1. Symptoms of Dementia

The essential characteristics of dementia are the developments of multiple cognitive deficits such as memory impairment, aphasia, apraxia, agnosia and disturbances in executive functioning (APA 1991; WHO, 1994). To qualify for dementia according to ICD 10 or DSM-IV criteria, the symptoms have to be severe enough to cause impairment in occupational or social life. They also have to represent a decline from previously higher level of social or occupational functioning.

The most frequent and diagnostically relevant symptom of dementia is memory impairment. It is also usually one of its earliest symptoms. Memory impairment includes the inability of a subject to learn new material and the increased forgetting of previously learned material. Usually both symptoms i.e., problems in acquiring new data and accessing previously learned material co-occur (Au et al. 2003, Heun et al 1998). However, it can be extremely difficult to assess forgetting in subjects who have severe problems learning. During their day-to day life, subjects may frequently lose their valuables such as wallets and keys; they may forget items during cooking or leave hot meals on the stove. In the early stages of dementia, patients usually forget things they have learned most recently. Items, which are stored in long-term memory such as previous occupation, previous life-events, names of family members, refer to autobiographic memory, and may be remembered until the later stages of the disorder (Dorrego et al., 1998, Frommholt et al., 2003). Memory is usually tested by asking to learn and later recall different types of information such as word lists or lists of pictures. Asking for immediate or delayed recall or recognition of items is used to test retrieval (e.g. Burkart et al., 1998). In advanced stages subjects may become extremely disorientated even in very familiar areas such as neighbourhoods or their own home. In the most severe stages of dementia even the most important and over-learned items of autobiographic memory such as learned occupation, names of children or even the own birth date or name may be forgotten. The memory deficits of demented patient correlate quite well with atrophy of the hippocampus (Heun et al. 1997).

Aphasia, the deterioration of language functions, manifests itself by difficulties naming known objects or persons. The speech of individuals with aphasia becomes vague, precise descriptions of items are replaced by more generalised expressions or even by naming them as things (Moreaud et al. 2001). In later stages of dementia the comprehension of spoken and written language may be severely compromised or may even be lost. In the final stages of dementia, patients may become mute and may produce only words that they heard shortly before (echolalia) or they might repeat sounds or words over and over (palilalia, Hier et al. 1985). Language is usually examined by asking patients to name items, body parts and by asking them to follow simple and complex commands and to repeat words and sentences.

Apraxia is the impairment or the inability to execute complex motor activities in spite of the presence of intact motor abilities and sensory functions (Smith et al. 2001). Apraxia is more common in severe dementia (Kramer and Duffy 1996). Apraxia may impair abilities of daily living such as cooking, dressing and writing. In later stages demented subjects may be impaired in their ability to perform more simple tasks such as filling a cup, combing hair or even waving goodbye.

Agnosia refers to the failure to recognise or identify objects even though the subject may have perfectly intact sensory functions (Kramer and Duffy 1996). Even though people see a chair or a pair of scissors they might not recognise its function and may have problems using it. In later stages patients may even be unable to recognise their own personal reflection in a mirror.

Executive functioning refers to the ability for abstract thinking, for planning, initiating, sequencing, monitoring and stopping complex behaviours. Demented patients may have problems performing these tasks and will be severely impaired in situations, which require the adequate processing of complex information (e.g. Rainville at al. 2002). Subjects may also have a reduced ability to generate and process non-verbal information and to perform related executive functions and complex motor activities. Usually, the ability of abstract thinking is assessed by interpreting similarities and differences between related words or concepts (e.g. stairs and ladders) and by interpreting complex images, stories and proverbs. It is helpful to ask the patient or even better an informant, about the ability of the patient to perform complex activities such as planning the day or managing their own budget (Kiosses et al. 2001, Potkin 2002).

To qualify for a diagnosis of dementia, the cognitive deficits should be severe enough to cause significant impairment in social or occupational functioning and have to represent a decline from previous levels.

2.2. Symptoms of Depression

Depression is a syndrome that consists of the concurrent presence of several symptoms, according to ICD 10 and DSM-IV the most important being: depressed mood most of the day, diminished interest in activities most of the day, significant weight loss, not dieting or weight gain or decrease or increase of appetite nearly every day, insomnia or hypersomnia, psychomotor agitation or retardation, fatigue or loss of energy, feelings of worthlessness or inappropriate guilt, diminished ability to concentrate or think and recurrent thoughts of death or recurrent suicidal ideations. These clinical features of depression may be classified in different categories (APA 1994):

Mood disturbances include sadness, feeling depressed, feeling unhappy, feeling empty, worried and irritable. It has been held traditionally that the mood is qualitatively different in endogenous depression as compared to normally felt sadness. Diurnal variation of mood is well known; the depressed subjects may experience a difference in the severity of depression though the day, with early morning worsening and a slight but definite improvement later in the day. The mood is not influenced by reassurance or in company of friends.

Cognitive symptoms include loss of interest, difficulty concentrating, lack of self-esteem, negative thoughts, indecisiveness, feelings of guilt, feelings of suicidal thoughts, hallucinations and delusions.

Behavioural symptoms cover psychomotor retardation or agitation, crying, social withdrawal, personal dependency and suicidal behaviour.

Somatic symptoms include sleep disturbances such as insomnia or hypersomnia, chronic fatigue, decreased or increased appetite, change of weight such as weight gain or weight loss, increased feelings of pain, gastro-intestinal problems and decreased libido.

In general, patients only suffer from some but not all symptoms during different disease episodes (Seretti et al. 2002).

2.3. Overlap and Differences of Symptoms in Both Disorders

There is a large overlap of symptoms in dementia and depression. In both disorders there may be lack of drive, lack of interest, slowing of mental processes and reduction of mental activities as well as a reduction in concentration. Both disorders have in common that there is a regular decline from normality to clinical relevance and further on to severe episodes of dementia or depression. The clinical distinction between both disorders is made by the discrimination whether cognitive deficit or changes in mood are the core and clinically most relevant features of the disorder. However, in the elderly where co-morbidity and lack of opportunities to be active are frequent this is quite difficult to assess (Tractenberg et al. 2003). In summary, all symptoms, which are found in dementia, can also be found in severe depression. Consequently, symptomatic differences between dementia and depression are not categorical, but refer to the severity, the relevance and clinical presentation of the symptoms by the patient. The course of the disease and the time course of symptom presentations are usually different and allow the distinction of both disorders (see below).

3. Course of Dementia and Depression

3.1. Course of the Dementias

Dementia is usually a syndrome affecting the elderly. The term dementia historically implied a progressive or irreversible course of cognitive deterioration. The current definition of dementia however, is more based on the pattern of cognitive decline and the deterioration in comparison to a previous level of functioning (ICD 10, DSM IV). The course of dementia usually depends on the underlying aetiology (Hachinski et al. 1975). However, in general, most disorders severely affecting the brain lead to a stepwise or more chronic progressive deterioration of cognitive functions. There might be some improvement by specific anti-dementia drugs, however, these effects are usually temporary and in general cognitive deficits during dementia are chronically progressing. However, specific aetiologies such as a dementia caused by an acute episode of hypoxia or following an accident, might be stable and static over many years (Tabaddor et al. 1984). In Alzheimer's disease, which is the most common type of dementia, the course is usually chronically progressive and clinical changes might be even very small and nearly insidious over short periods of times. Vascular dementia more often has a more abrupt or stepwise and fluctuating course characterised by the changes in functioning (Hachinski et al. 1975). However, even the course of vascular dementia as well as its neuropathology might vary considerably between individuals (Jellinger 2002, Roman 2002).

3.2. Courses of Depressive Disorders

Major depression usually starts at around the mid-twenties, but depressive disorders may also occur at any age of a patient's life (Ernst and Angst 1995). The course of the depression is very variable. People may have isolated periods of depression, which are separated by many years of perfect health. Others may suffer various clusters of episodes (Dew et al. 1997).

A single depressive episode may last between several days to several years or in rare events, even for decades. However, most patients' depressive episodes last for a few weeks or months and after that the patients slowly regain partial or complete health.

The definition of major depressive episode as well as its diagnostic specifications depends very much on the course of the presence of symptoms (see below). In case the depression is recurrent, the course again is very variable. In a reasonable number of patients episodes during earlier years are more severe and longer than those during later life (Ernst and Angst 1995). The healthy intervals between the episodes may be shorter in the early years of the disorder, however, in some patients it is the other way round. The number of prior episodes is a strong predictor of the development of later major depressive episodes (Barkow et al. 2003). About 60% of subjects who experience one depressive episode are most likely to experience a second one in their later life classifying for the diagnosis of recurrent depressive disorder. If you already had two depressive episodes, then the chance to have a third is even higher and so on.

A single depressive episode may end in full remission with patients regaining complete mental health. However, many patients only have partial remission such as suffering some depressive symptoms over a prolonged period (Kessling 2004). Follow-up studies suggest that several months after a diagnosis of major depressive episode about 50% of individuals still have symptoms that meet criteria for full depression (e.g. Storosum et al 2004). Others have only some minor symptoms without meeting the full criteria for a major depression. The rest of possibly 40% will have no depression any more. The more severe a depression is the longer it takes to regain full remission and the more likely it is to relapse (Kessling 2004). The course of depression may be influenced to some extent by the presence of psychosocial problems, chronic medical conditions or substance abuse (Nanko and Demura 1993).

3.3. Similarities and Differences of Disease Course

The course in dementia may be fluctuating to a minor extent depending on the underlying aetiology. However, in most cases the cognitive deficits deteriorate slowly and gradually. Major improvements during an untreated, naturalistic course of the dementia are rare. In contrast, the course in depression is much more variable, usually a depressive episode, even untreated, will end in improvement and even complete remission. Subjects may have different episodes over their lifetime with complete remission in between. However, in some patients there is persistence of their depressive symptoms, but only extremely rarely there is a chronic progressive course leading to slow deterioration over years or during lifetime.

In depression in which the underlying medical cause of the disease is unknown in most cases, the course is a very important specifier of different types of the disease. In contrast, the classification of dementia depends much more on the underlying aetiology. In summary, there is little overlap between the courses of dementias and depressions. The course is one of the most important characteristics to distinguish dementia and depression.

4. Definitions of Dementia and Depression

4.1. Definition of Dementia

To classify for a diagnosis of dementia, the above-mentioned symptoms and cognitive deficits must be sufficiently severe to cause impairment in occupational or social functioning. They usually represent a significant decline from previous better or higher levels of cognitive functioning. The course of dementia usually implies a progressive and irreversible course of the disease. DSM-IV and ICD-10 (APA 1994, WHO 1991) define dementia as the development of cognitive deficits from previously better and more adequate level. It does not give any information about the course. However, the main types of dementia are chronic, progressive, such as Alzheimer's disease or vascular dementia.

4.2. Definition of Depression

A major depressive episode is defined by the coexistence of a number of symptoms, usually 5, at the same time for most of the day over at least 2 weeks.

According to DSM IV criteria, five symptoms must be present. Depressed mood most of the day, nearly every day, markedly diminished interest or pleasure in many activities, significant weight loss or weight gain, i.e. over 5% of body weight in a month, insomnia or hypersomnia nearly every day, psychomotor agitation or retardation, fatigue or loss of energy, feelings of worthlessness or excessive inappropriate guilt, diminished ability to think or concentrate or indecisiveness nearly every day and recurrent thoughts of death.

The symptoms should be severe and persistent enough to cause clinical significant distress or impairment in social occupation or other important areas of life, they should not be substance induced or the consequence of a general medical condition, they are not better accounted for by bereavement (DSM-IV, APA 1994).

4.3. Overlap and Differences of Definitions

Both dementia and depression are defined by the presence of a number of symptoms. Dementia requires a deterioration of cognition from previous cognitive functioning and also requires some persistence of this deterioration. In dementia it is required that the severity of the symptoms is severe enough to affect a social functioning and activities of daily living. This type of thinking also applies to depression where the symptoms should be significantly different from what people usually experience in their life. However, even though this is often the case with major depressive disorders, this is not a requirement of the definition of major depression.

5. Classification and Aetiology of Depression and Dementia

5.1. Classification and Aetiologies of the Dementias

The differential diagnosis of dementia includes delirium, amnestic disorder, and mental retardation. Delirium is characterised by disturbances in consciousness and attention and has a fluctuating clinical course depending on the underlying brain disorder (Edwards 2003). Amnestic disorder is characterised by memory impairment without impairment of other cognitive functions. Mental retardation is characterised by the fact that cognitive deficits have developed early in life without major reduction of performance during later life.

Severe cognitive deficits may also appear in schizophrenia, however, the age of onset of schizophrenia is much earlier and there is usually a history of paranoid symptoms such as hallucinations (McBride et al. 2002). Major depressive disorder may also be associated with complaints of memory impairment, difficulty in thinking and concentrating. There may be some problems in elderly subjects who differentiate in both disorder, but there is also a high comorbidity (see below).

Apart from these clinically relevant discriminations of dementia from other disorders the classification of the dementias refers to its aetiology (see below). Alzheimer's disease and vascular dementia are the most prevalent in the elderly and will therefore be discussed, other dementing disorders including dementia of Lewy Body type, dementia in Parkinson's disease, Pick's disease, Chorea Huntington, Amyotrophic Lateral Sclerosis, dementia in Human Immune Deficiency Virus Infection, dementia after intracerebral haemorrhages and the many other causes of dementia cannot be presented for lack of space. An overview is given by Heun (1997).

5.2. Alzheimer's Disease

Dementia of the Alzheimer type is a chronic neurodegenerative disorder in which the neuro-degeneration in the early stage affects the hippocampus and parietal lobes of the neocortex (Henderson and Finch 1989). These areas are most important for memory. Consequently, memory disturbance is usually one of the earliest symptoms of dementia of the Alzheimer type. Patients with Alzheimer's disease usually suffer loss of brain volume, which histopathologically is reflected in a loss of neurites, dendrites and neuronal cells. Other hallmarks are extracellular deposits of beta-amyloid peptides and intracellular deposits of neurofibrillary tangles (Selkoe 2000). Alzheimer's disease usually is classified according to its onset. Patients with early onset Alzheimer's disease frequently have mutations in specific genes such as the amyloid precursor protein gene and the preseniline 1 and preseniline 2 genes on chromosomes 21, 14 and 1, respectively. The aetiology of the late onset type of Alzheimer's disease is less clear and there are usually several susceptibility genes to be involved in the aetiology (Finckh 2003). Late onset Alzheimer's disease shows a significant family aggregation (Heun et al. 2001). Diagnostic criteria for the dementia of the Alzheimer's type are the development of cognitive deficits including memory impairment such as impaired ability to learn new information as well as at least one additional cognitive symptom such as aphasia, apraxia, agnosia or disturbance in executive functioning such as planning, organisation, sequencing and abstract thinking. These cognitive deficits in memory and in other areas should be sufficiently severe to cause social or occupational impairment. The course is usually characterised by gradual onset and chronic progressive decline. Other causes of dementia have to be excluded, these are other neurodegenerative disorders, severe systemic infections or including vitamin deficiencies, or substance abuse affecting the brain and consequently inducing dementia. The cognitive deficits must be chronic progressive and should not only appear during the course of delirium. The disturbance should not be better accounted by another psychiatric disorder such as major depressive disorder.

5.3. Vascular Dementia

Vascular dementia is characterised by the presence of cognitive deficits including memory impairment. These cognitive deficits should be severe enough to cause impairment in social and every day life. There should be a presence of neurological signs and symptoms, which indicate the presence of an underlying vascular disorder. Usually the clinical distinction between Alzheimer's disease and vascular dementia was based on the presence of neurological signs as well as different course of the symptoms. Subjects with vascular dementia are more likely to show signs of cardio-vascular problems or a history of stroke or myocardial infarctions (Hachinski et al. 1975). Vascular dementia is caused by insufficient cerebral blood flow to the brain cells. It can be caused by multiple cerebral infarcts, by single strategic infarcts damaging functional critical areas of the brain such as the hippocampus, thalamus, or forebrain, by various types of small vessel disease including Binswanger disease, by diffuse ischemic-hypoxic lesions, and by severe intracerebral haemorrhage (Roman 2002). There is considerable comorbidity between Alzheimer's disease and vascular dementia (Kalaria 2003).

5.4. Classification of the Depressions

Depressive disorders are predominantly classified by the number of symptoms and by the course; consent has been reached by recent classification systems such as DSM-IV and ICD 10:

Major depressive episode is defined by the presence of at least five depressive symptoms and the presence of these symptoms over at least two weeks. If major depressive episodes appear twice or more frequently, it is called a recurrent depressive disorder. The repetitive recurrence of depressive episodes might be also called a unipolar depression. In contrast subjects who experience depressive episodes as well as manic episodes during their lifetime will be specified as bipolar. Bipolar I disorder refers to the fact that objects have manic episodes as well as depressive episodes. Bipolar II disorder refers to the fact that patients have hypomanic as well as depressive episodes. Dysthymic disorder is defined by the presence of depressed mood for most of the day on more days than not over at least two years. It is not required that five depressive symptoms appear, however, first low mood and two additional symptoms including poor appetite or over-eating, insomnia, or hypersomnia, low energy or fatigue, low self-esteem, poor concentration or difficulty making decisions or feeling of hopelessness, must be present.

Cyclothymic disorder is characterised by chronic changing mood involving numerous episodes of hypomanic states and numerous episodes and depressive symptoms. However, the hypomanic symptoms as well as the depressive symptoms are of insufficient number, severity, persuasiveness or duration to meet full criteria for mania or major depression. During a two-year period the subjects should not be without symptoms for more than two months at a time.

Mood disorders including depression due to a general medical condition are characterised by the fact that the disturbance in mood is the direct psychological effect of a general medical condition. A large number of general medical conditions can cause mood problems such as Parkinson's Disease, Huntingdon's Disease and other neurodegenerative disorders, cerebrovascular problems including stroke, metabolic conditions such as prolonged vitamin B12 deficiency, endocrine disorders including hyper and hypothyroidism, hyper- and hypoadrenocorticism, autoimmune conditions including systemic lupus erythematodes, viral infections including hepatitis, humane immune deficiency and carcinomas as well as severe cardio-vascular problems. It is said that up to 30% of patient suffering severe neurological disorders including Parkinson's disease, Huntington's disease, multiple sclerosis, stroke and Alzheimer's disease, are prone to develop severe depressive disorders (Ernst and Angst 1995, Stordal et al. 2003).

Depression might also be induced by the chronic abuse of alcohol and other drugs. If this is diagnosed there should be a strong relationship between the presence of intoxication and the development and course of depression.

For the classification according to DSM-IV, there are several episode specifiers including severity of the depression, presence of psychotic symptoms, cause, presence of catatonic features, presence of melancholic features and post-partum on-set (see ICD 10 and DSM IV).

There have been discussions about classifying depression according to the age of onset (Heun et al. 2000). It has been observed that there is a higher familial aggregation of depression in subjects having a lower age-of-onset in contrast to subjects having a later age-of-onset (Maier et al. 1991). It has also been discussed that the course of late and early onset depression is different, however, even thought there might be some differences in that depression is less severe but prolonged in the elderly, there is no categorical classification (Gottfries 1998).

5.5. Aetiology of Depression

The aetiology of most depressive episodes is not known, however, as mentioned depression can be secondary to many disorders affecting the brain such as severe head trauma (Babin 2003).

Previous classifications of depression focused on hypothetical aetiology. The term reactive depression has been used for depressions where the episode was the consequence of a traumatic experience including that of a relative. Neurotic depression was defined as depression that was the long-term consequence of developmental problems during early and late childhood. Endogenous depression has been used for describing the fact that no cause could be found for the depression and that there was speculation about the endogeneity of the depression. These classifications had some therapeutical implications such as reactive depression was said to profit most from counselling and social support. Neurotic depression was said to profit most from psychological therapies including psychoanalysis and psychodynamic therapies. Endogenous depression was said to profit most from pharmacotherapy. However, previous attempts to classify these disorders were less helpful and it has been found that counselling, psychotherapy as well as pharmacotherapy is helpful in all three types of depression (Montgomery 1992).

5.6. Similarities and Differences in Classification and Aetiology

Depression is predominantly defined by the presence of symptoms and course of the disorder. This mostly refers to primary depressive disorders (secondary depressions are those which are induced by other major physical disorders). In contrast, the classification of the dementias is focussed on their aetiology. Here the course of the disorder is used as an indicator of the aetiology, e.g. subjects with Alzheimer's disease usually have a chronic progressive development of cognitive deficits whereas in vascular dementias the onset is more stepwise and fluctuating (Hachinski et al. 1975).

One important similarity between dementia and depression is that they both can be secondary to many other medical conditions. Severe medical conditions such as chronic kidney or liver disease can lead to affection of the brain which either responds by leading to depression or in long-term cases, leading to cognitive deficits which reach severity sufficient to call them dementia. The same applies to chronic substance abuse, chronic alcoholism as well as other drug abuse, can lead to severe depression and disabling dementing disorders.

6. Epidemiology of Dementia and Depression

6.1. Epidemiology of Dementia

Dementia is a disorder of the elderly, it is rare in subjects below 60 years, the prevalence in subjects above 60 years is around 5 %, it increases to 20% in subjects older than 80 years depending of the stringency of the diagnostic criteria (Förstl 1998, Hendrie 1998, Kukull and Ganguli 2000). Women have a higher risk to develop dementia, which is at least partially explained by the fact that their life expectancy is several years higher than that of men in all societies (e.g. Fratiglioni et al. 1997).

Risk factors for dementia may vary depending on the aetiology of the disorders. A series of potential risk factors have been identified for Alzheimer's disease: i.e. the presence of a apolipoprotein E4 Genotype (Finckh 2003), a familial aggregation of Down syndrome (van Duijn et al. 1991) increased parental age (Amaducci et al. 1986, Rocca et al. 1991), previous brain trauma (Mortimer et al 1991), a history of depression (Devenand et al. 1996), minor cognitive deficits (Bickel and Cooper 1994) subjective memory impairment (Schofield et al. 1997), lack of activity (Kondo and Yamashita 1990), low educational level and low professional achievement (Evans et al. 1997), exposion to environmental aluminium (Forbes et al. 1998), lack of vitamins in diet (Clarke et al. 1998) and others.

First-degree relatives of index cases with AD show a two- to three-fold increase in the occurrence of primary progressive dementias, as contrasted with control relatives (Silverman et al. 2000, Heun et al. 2001) which corresponds well to the relevance of many susceptibility factors including the presence of the apolipoprotein E4 allele (Finckh 2003). Twin studies of dementia support the relevance of genetic factors but are hampered by the fact that few twins survive to the age at highest risk.

6.2. Epidemiology of Depression

Major depressive disorder is one quite frequent disorder and probably the most common psychiatric disorder. However, the prevalence rates vary quite considerably according to the definitions. The American NIMH Epidemiological Catchment Area study reported a one month-prevalence of 1.5% and a lifetime prevalence of 4.4% (Weissman et al. 1988). However, in most other studies the lifetime prevalence is higher and goes up to 20%. Mean age of onset is in the middle twenties. There is no major variation of age-at-onset by sex, however, the prevalence and incidence is higher in women than in men, even though this seems influenced by social factors (Lucht et al. 2003). There have been some observations that younger age groups have a have an increase prevalence, which is called cohort effect (Cross-National Collaborative Group 1992). However, the cohort effect might be the result of memory bias. Major prospective studies would be necessary to rule out this bias.

There is a wealth of risk factors, which lead to depression, including female gender (Kessler et al. 1994), psychiatric disorders of the individual like cognitive impairment (Berger et al. 1999), previous depressive symptoms and episodes (Judd et al. 1997), alcohol as well as nicotine abuse (Breslau et al. 1993) and insomnia (Ford et al. 2001), medical disorders, i.e., chronic diseases (Roberts et al. 1997), perceived poor health (Barkow et al. 2001) and increasing disability (Roberts et al. 1997), social factors like marital status (Kivelä et al. 1996; Roberts et al. 1997), negative live events, social isolation (Kivelä et al. 1996), low income or financial problems and low level of education (Roberts et al. 1997).

Family studies indicate that the risk in first-degree relatives is increased in patients with depression in comparison to healthy controls and patients with other psychiatric disorders (Maier et al. 1991, Lieb et al. 2002). This indicates that there is some familial, possibly genetic, background leading to the disorder. Similarly, increased risks have been seen for occurrence of depression in relatives of bipolar I and II as well as early-onset univocal depressive patients (Heun and Maier 1993). Studies of late-onset depression (onset between 50 and 60 years) are less consistent. Maier et al. (1991) showed an increased risk of depression in first-degree relatives of the patients with late-onset (>60 years) depression in comparison with relatives of controls. In contrast, other authors observed comparable risks of depression in first-degree relatives of subjects with late-onset depression and in relatives of control subjects. Twin studies have also found an increased prevalence of depression in mono-psychotic twins in comparison with dicygotic twins (Kendler at al. 1993). However, the difference is higher in patients with bipolar disorder and more severe types of depression.

6.3. Similarities and Differences of Epidemiology of Dementia and Depression

Dementia and depression are very common disorders in the general population and in the elderly. They are both multifactorial disorders and there is considerable overlap concerning possible risk factors indicating that dementia and depression are common reactions to severe long-term damages of the brain. Genetic epidemiological studies have shown a diagnosis-specific familial aggregation of both individual disorders without any overlap (Heun et al.

2001), genetic factors are relevant in different types of dementia; in contrast, genetic factors causing depression have yet not been identified so far.

6.4. Other Similarities and Differences of Dementia and Depression

Similarities and differences in neurobiology and therapeutic approaches in depression and dementia will be dealt with in other chapter of this book.

7. Comorbidity of Depression and Dementia

Depression is a prevalent and important problem in old age (Copeland 1999, Wittchen et al. 1994). Cognitive dysfunction, including severe memory deficit, is frequent in subjects with geriatric depression (O'Connor et al. 1990, Deijen et al. 1993, Lichtenberg et al. 1995, Yaffe et al. 1999). When mental slowing and cognitive deficits are the main features of clinical presentation than the term of pseudo-dementia has been used. Pseudo-dementia indicates that the dementia is not true but only the result of severe cognitive deficits due to major depression. However, this term has rarely been used in previous years due to the fact that that the prefix pseudo refers to the fact that there might be something unreal or untrue. However, having cognitive deficits in severe depression is a realistic and disabilitating symptom. Sometimes, the only possibility to identify a pseudo-dementia syndrome is if cognitive deficits disappear when depression is improving.

On the other hand patients with dementia very often suffer from depression, depressive symptoms are common in subjects with Alzheimer's disease (Burns et al. 1990, Newman 1999, Emery and Oxman 1992). Depression in dementia not easy to identify due to the fact that some of the main features of depression such as lack of driving interest, are core symptoms of the dementia syndrome. Consequently a depressive syndrome should only be identified in patients with dementia if there is an episodic additional symptomatology of depression.

The reasons for this sort of symptom overlap in depressed and demented subjects are not yet clear. There are several possibilities to explain for this increased comorbidity (i.e. comorbidity above the rate expected by chance) of dementia and depression in the elderly:

(1) The depression and dementia are distinct disorders. The observed excess comorbidity is the result of an awareness bias because comorbid patients may contact physicians' awareness more often than patients with either dementia or depression.

(2) In the elderly, dementia, depression and the comorbid condition represent one single disorder with variable clinical presentations.

(3) The comorbid condition represents a distinct and independent disorder.

(4) Both disorders are causally linked, i.e. the presence of one disorder might induce the expression of the other disorder; e.g. cognitive deficits might induce depression, and vice versa.

(5) Identical confounding factors influence the expression of both disorders.

(6) Both disorders share common clinical features, which lower the threshold for the second disorder to be diagnosed if the first is present.

(7) Both disorders share common vulnerability factors, e.g. genetic factors, which increase the likelihood that the second disorder is developed if the first is already present.

Long-term prospective studies as well as thorough clinical and neurobiological investigations are needed to investigate these possibilities. We hope that the following chapters will help to clarify some of these issues, and will support unravelling some of these mysteries.

Acknowledgements

During the preparation of this manuscript, Prof. Heun and Prof. Goswami were International NHS Fellows at County Durham and Darlington Priority Service NHS Trust.

References

Amaducci LA, Fratiglioni L, Rocca WA, Fieschi C, Livrea P, Pedone D, Bracco L, Lippi A, Gandolfo C, Bino G, Prencipe M, Bonatti ML, Girotti F, Carella F, Tavolato B, Ferla S, Lenzi GL, Carolei A, Gambi A, Grigoletto F, Schoenberg BS (1986) Risk factors for clinically diagnosed Alzheimer's disease: A case-control study of an Italian population. *Neurology* **36**: 922-931.

American Psychiatric Association (1994) Diagnostic and Statistical Manual of Mental Disorders, Fourth Edition, Washington DC, American Psychiatric Association.

Au A, Chan AS, Chiu H. (2003) Verbal learning in Alzheimer's dementia. *J Int Neuropsychol Soc.* **9**: 363-75.

Babin PR. (2003) Diagnosing depression in persons with brain injuries: a look at theories, the DSM-IV and depression measures. *Brain Inj.* **17**: 889-900.

Barkow K, Maier W, Ustun TB, Gansicke M, Wittchen HU, Heun R. (2003) Risk factors for depression at 12-month follow-up in adult primary health care patients with major depression: an international prospective study. *J Affect Disord.* **76**: 157-69.

Berger AK, Fratiglioni L, Forsell Y, Winblad B, Backman L (1999) The occurrence of depressive symptoms in the preclinical phase of AD: a population-based study. *Neurology* **53**: 1998-2002.

Bickel H, Cooper B (1994) Incidence and relative risk of dementia in an urban elderly population: findings of a prospective field study. *Psychological Medicine*, **24**: 179-192.

Breslau N, Kilbey MM, Andreski P (1993) Nicotine dependence and major depression. New evidence from a prospective investigation. *Arch Gen Psychiatry* **50**: 31-35.

Burkart M, Heun R, Benkert O. (1998) Serial position effects in dementia of the Alzheimer type. *Dement Geriatr Cogn Disord.* **9**: 130-6.

Burns A, Jacoby R, Levy R. (1990) Psychiatric Phenomena in Alzheimer's Disease. III: Disorders of Mood. *Brit J Psychiatry* **157**: 81-86.

Clarke R, Smith AD, Jobst KA, Refsum H, Sutton L, Ueland PM (1998) Folate, Vitamin B12, and Serum Total Homocysteine Levels in Confirmed Alzheimer Disease. *Arch Neurol* **55**: 1449-1455.

Copeland JRM. (1999) Depression of older age. Origins of the study. *Brit J Psychiatry* **174**: 304-306.

Cross-National Collaborative Group (1992) The Changing Rate of Major Depression. Cross National Comparisons. *Journal of the American Medical Association* **268**: 3098-3105.

Deijen JB, Orlebeke JF, Rijsdijk FV. (1993) Effect of depression on psychomotor skills, eye movements and recognition-memory. *J Affect Dis* **29**: 33-40.

Devanand DP, Sano M, Tang M-X, Taylor S, Gurland BJ, Wilder D, Stern Y, Mayeux R (1996) Depressed Mood and the Incidence of Alzheimer's Disease in the Elderly Living in the Community. *Arch Gen Psychiatry,* **53**: 175-182.

Dew MA, Reynolds CF 3rd, Houck PR, Hall M, Buysse DJ, Frank E, Kupfer DJ (1997) Temporal profiles of the course of depression during treatment. Predictors of pathways toward recovery in the elderly. *Arch Gen Psychiatry* **54**: 1016-24.

Dorrego MF, Sabe L, Garcia Cuerva A, Kuzis G, Tiberti C, Boller F, Starkstein SE. (9199) Remote memory in Alzheimer's disease. *J Neuropsychiatry Clin Neurosci* 11: 490-7.

Edwards N. (2003) Differentiating the three D's: delirium, dementia, and depression. *Medsurg Nurs* **12**: 347-57.

Emery VO, Oxman TE. (1992) Update on the Dementia Spectrum of Depression. *Am J Psychiatry* **149**: 305-317.

Ernst C, Angst J. (1995) Depression in old age. Is there a real decrease in prevalence? A review. *Eur Arch Psychiatry Clin Neurosci* **245**: 272-87.

Evans DA, Hebert LE, Beckett LA, Scherr PA, Albert MS, Chown MJ, Pilgrim DM, Taylor JO (1997) Education and Other Measures of Socioeconomic Status and Risk of Incident Alzheimer Disease in a Defined Population of Older Persons. *Arch Neurol* **54**: 1399-1405.

Finckh U. (2003) The future of genetic association studies in Alzheimer disease. *J Neural Transm* **110**: 253-66.

Forbes WF, Hill GB (1998) Is Exposure to Aluminum a Risk Factor for the Development of Alzheimer Disease? - Yes. *Arch Neurol* **55**: 740-741.

Ford DE, Cooper-Patrick L (2001) Sleep disturbances and mood disorders: an epidemiologic perspective. *Depression and Anxiety* **14**: 3-6

Förstl H. (1998) Alzheimer's disease: the size of the problem, clinical manifestation and heterogeneity. *J Neural Transm Suppl* **54**: 1-8.

Fromholt P, Mortensen DB, Torpdahl P, Bender L, Larsen P, Rubin DC. (2003) Life-narrative and word-cued autobiographical memories in centenarians: comparisons with 80-year-old control, depressed, and dementia groups. *Memory* **11**: 81-8.

Gottfries CG. (1998) Is there a difference between elderly and younger patients with regard to the symptomatology and aetiology of depression? *Int Clin Psychopharmacol* **Suppl 5**: S13-8.

Hachinski VC, Iliff LD, Zilhka E, Du Boulay GH, McAllister VL, Marshall J, Russell RW, Symon L. (1975) Cerebral blood flow in dementia. *Arch Neurol* **32**: 632-7

Henderson VW, Finch CE. (1989) The neurobiology of Alzheimer's disease. *J Neurosurg* **70**: 335-53.

Heun R (1997) Demenzen bei andernorts klassifizierten Krankheitsbildern. In: Förstl H. (ed.) Lehrbuch der Gerontopsychiatrie. Enke, Stuttgart. 331-344

Heun R, Burkart M, Benkert O. (1997) Effect of repetition and inspection times on picture recall in patients with dementia of Alzheimer type. *Dement Geriatr Cogn Disord* **8**: 152-6.

Heun R, Kockler M, Papassotiropoulos A. (2000) Distinction of early- and late-onset depression in the elderly by their lifetime symptomatology. *Int J Geriatr Psychiatry* **15**: 1138-42.

Heun R, Maier W. (1993) The distinction of bipolar II disorder from bipolar I and recurrent unipolar depression: results of a controlled family study. *Acta Psychiatr Scand* **87**: 279-84.

Heun R, Mazanek M, Atzor KR, Tintera J, Gawehn J, Burkart M, Gansicke M, Falkai P, Stoeter P (1997) Amygdala-hippocampal atrophy and memory performance in dementia of Alzheimer type. *Dement Geriatr Cogn Disord* **8**: 329-36.

Heun R, Papassotiropoulos A, Jessen F, Maier W, Breitner JC. (2001) A family study of Alzheimer disease and early- and late-onset depression in elderly patients. *Arch Gen Psychiatry* **58**: 190-6.

Hier DB, Hagenlocker K, Shindler AG. (1985) Language disintegration in dementia: effects of etiology and severity. *Brain Lang* 25: 117-33

Jellinger KA. (2002) Vascular-ischemic dementia: an update. *J Neural Transm* Suppl **(62)**: 1-23.

Judd LL, Akiskal HS, Paulus MP (1997) The role and clinical significance of subsyndromal depressive symptoms (SSD) in unipolar major depressive disorder. *J Affect Disord* **45**: 17-18.

Kalaria RN. (2003) Comparison between Alzheimer's disease and vascular dementia: implications for treatment. *Neurol Res* **25**: 661-4.

Kendler KS, Neale MC, Kessler RC, Heath AC, Eaves LJ. (1993) A longitudinal twin study of personality and major depression in women. *Arch Gen Psychiatry* **50**: 853-62.

Kessing LV. (2004) Severity of depressive episodes according to ICD-10: prediction of risk of relapse and suicide. *Br J Psychiatry* **184**: 153-6.

Kessler RC, McGonagle KA, Nelson CB, Hughes M, Swartz M, Blazer DG. (1994) Sex and depression in the National Comorbidity Survey. II: Cohort effects. *J Affect Disord* **30**: 15-26.

Kiosses DN, Klimstra S, Murphy C, Alexopoulos GS. (2001) Executive dysfunction and disability in elderly patients with major depression. *Am J Geriatr Psychiatry* **9**: 269-74.

Kivelä SL, Kongas-Saviaro P, Laippala P, Pahkala K, Kesti E (1996) Social and psychosocial factors predicting depression in old age: a longitudinal study. *Int Psychogeriatr* 8: 635-44.

Kondo K, Yamashita I (1990) A case-control study of Alzheimer's disease in Japan: Association with inactive psychosocial behaviors. In: Hasegawa K, Homma A (eds.), Psychogeriatrics: Biomedical and Social Advances. Excerpta Medica, Amsterdam: 49-53.

Kramer JH, Duffy JM. (1996) Aphasia, apraxia, and agnosia in the diagnosis of dementia. *Dementia* **7**: 23-6.

Kukull WA, Ganguli M. (2000) Epidemiology of dementia: concepts and overview. *Neurol Clin* **18**: 923-50.

Lichtenberg PA, Ross T, Millis SR, Manning CA. (1995) The Relationship Between Depression and Cognition in Older Adults: A Cross-validity Study. *J Gerontol: Psychol Sci* **50B**: P25-P32.

Lieb R, Isensee B, Hofler M, Pfister H, Wittchen HU (2002) Parental major depression and the risk of depression and other mental disorders in the offspring: a prospective-longitudinal community study. *Arch Gen Psychiatry* **59**: 365-374.

Lucht M, Schaub RT, Meyer C, Hapke U, Rumpf HJ, Bartels T, von Houwald J, Barnow S, Freyberger HJ, Dilling H, John U. (2003) Gender differences in unipolar depression: a general population survey of adults between age 18 to 64 of German nationality. *J Affect Disord* **77**: 203-11.

Maier W, Lichtermann D, Minges J, Heun R, Hallmayer J, Klingler T. (1991) Unipolar depression in the aged: determinants of familial aggregation. *J Affect Disord* **23**: 53-61.

McBride T, Moberg PJ, Arnold SE, Mozley LH, Mahr RN, Gibney M, Kumar A, Gur RE. (2002) Neuropsychological functioning in elderly patients with schizophrenia and Alzheimer's disease. *Schizophr Res* **55**: 217-27

Montgomery SA. (1992) The advantages of paroxetine in different subgroups of depression. *Int Clin Psychopharmacol* **6 Suppl 4**: 91-100.

Moreaud O, David D, Charnallet A, Pellat J. (2001) Are semantic errors actually semantic?: Evidence from Alzheimer's disease. *Brain Lang* **77**: 176-86.

Mortimer JA, Van Duijn CM, Chandra V, Fratiglioni L, Graves AB, Heyman A, Jorm AF, Kokmen E, Kondo K, Rocca WA, Shalat SL, Soininen H, a Hofman for the EURODEM risk factors research group. (1991) Head Trauma as a Risk Factor for Alzheimer's Disease: A Collaborative Re-Analysis of Case-Control Studies. *International Journal of Epidemiology* **20 (Suppl 2)**: S28-S35.

Nanko S, Demura S. (1993) Life events and depression in Japan. *Acta Psychiatr Scand* **87**: 184-7.

Newman SC (1999) The prevalence of depression in Alzheimer's disease and vascular dementia in a population sample. *J Affect Dis* **52**: 169-176.

O'Connor DW, Pollitt PA, Roth M, Brook CPB, Reiss BB. (1990) Memory Complaints and Impairment in Normal, Depressed, and Demented Elderly Persons Identified in a Community Survey. Arch Gen Psychiatry 47: 224-227.

Potkin SG. (2002) The ABC of Alzheimer's disease: ADL and improving day-to-day functioning of patients. *Int Psychogeriatr* **14 Suppl 1**: 7-26.

Rainville C, Amieva H, Lafont S, Dartigues JF, Orgogozo JM, Fabrigoule C (2002) Executive function deficits in patients with dementia of the Alzheimer's type: a study with a Tower of London task. *Arch Clin Neuropsychol* **17**: 513-30.

Roberts RE, Kaplan GA, Shema SJ, Strawbridge WJ (1997) Prevalence and correlates of depression in an aging cohort: The Almeda County Study. *Journal of Gerontology* **52b**: 252-258.

Rocca WA, Van Duijn CM, Clayton D, Chandra V, Fratiglioni L, Graves AB, Heyman A, Jorm AF, Kommen E, Kondo K, Mortimer JA, Shalat SL, Soininen H, Hofman A (1991) Maternal Age and Alzheimer's Disease: A Collaborative Re-analysis of Case-Control Studies. *International Journal of Epidemiology* **20**: 21-27.

Roman GC. (2002) Vascular dementia revisited: diagnosis, pathogenesis, treatment, and prevention. *Med Clin North Am* **86**: 477-99.

Schofield PW, Marder K, Dooneief G, Jacobs DM, Sano M, Stern Y (1997) Association of Subjective Memory Complaints with Subsequent Cognitive Decline in Community-Dwelling Elderly Individuals with Baseline Cognitive Impairment. *Am J Psychiatry* **154**: 609-615.

Selkoe DJ. (2000) The genetics and molecular pathology of Alzheimer's disease: roles of amyloid and the presenilins. *Neurol Clin* **18**: 903-22.

Serretti A, Mandelli L, Lattuada E, Cusin C, Smeraldi E (2002) Clinical and demographic features of mood disorder subtypes. *Psychiatry Res* **112**: 195-210.

Silverman JM, Smith CM, Marin DB, Schmeidler J, Birstein S, Lantz M, Davis KL, Mohs RC (2000) Has familial aggregation in Alzheimer's disease been overestimated? *Int J Geriatr Psychiatry* **15**: 631-7.

Smith MZ, Esiri MM, Barnetson L, King E, Nagy Z. (2001) Constructional apraxia in Alzheimer's disease: association with occipital lobe pathology and accelerated cognitive decline. *Dement Geriatr Cogn Disord* **12**: 281-8.

Stordal E, Bjelland I, Dahl AA, Mykletun A. (2003) Anxiety and depression in individuals with somatic health problems. The Nord-Trondelag Health Study (HUNT). *Scand J Prim Health Care* **21**: 136-41.

Storosum JG, Elferink AJ, van Zwieten BJ, van den Brink W, Huyser J. (2004) Natural course and placebo response in short-term, placebo-controlled studies in major depression: a meta-analysis of published and non-published studies. *Pharmacopsychiatry* **37**: 32-6.

Tabaddor K, Mattis S, Zazula T. (1984) Cognitive sequelae and recovery course after moderate and severe head injury. *Neurosurgery* **14**: 701-8.

Tractenberg RE, Weiner MF, Patterson MB, Teri L, Thal LJ. (2003) Comorbidity of psychopathological domains in community-dwelling persons with Alzheimer's disease. *J Geriatr Psychiatry Neurol* **16**: 94-9.

Weissman MM, Leaf PJ, Tischler GL, Blazer DG, Karno M, Bruce ML, Florio LP (1988) Affective disorders in five United States communities. *Psychol Med* **18**: 141-53.

World Health Organization (1991) Tenth Revision of the International Classification of Diseases. Chapter V (F): Mental and Behavioural Disorders (including disorders of psychological development). Clinical Descriptions and Diagnostic Guidelines, WHO.

Wittchen H-U, Knäuper B, Kessler RC (1994) Lifetime Risk of Depression. *Brit J Psychiatry* **165 (suppl. 26)**: 16-22.

Yaffe K, Blackwell T, Gore R, Sands L, Reus V, Browner WS (1999) Depressive Symptoms and Cognitive decline in nondemented elderly women: a prospective study. *Arch Gen Psychiatry* **56**: 425-430.

In: Cognition and Mood Interactions
Editor: Miao-Kun Sun, pp. 19-32

ISBN 1-59454-229-5
2005 © Nova Science Publishers, Inc.

Chapter II

Monoamines in Mood and Cognition

---

*Chad E. Beyer and Lee E. Schechter**

Depression and Anxiety Research
Neuroscience Discovery Research, Wyeth Research, Princeton, New Jersey, USA

Over the past several decades, it has become convincingly clear that human psychiatric illnesses such as schizophrenia, depression and various anxiety-related disorders are comorbid with cognitive dysfunction. It should also be pointed out that patients diagnosed with Alzheimer's disease, where the primary diagnosis is cognitive impairment, and neurodegenerative motor disorders like Parkinson's disease and amyotrophic lateral sclerosis routinely exhibit clinical symptoms of both depression and cognitive dysfunction. While there is little doubt that a strong relationship between mood and cognition exists in many disease states, the challenge still remains to explain both the anatomical and neurochemical substrates underlying the manifestation of these comorbidities. In this regard, a role for the hippocampus and prefrontal cortical areas is associated with both disorders of mood and cognition. The fact that these brain regions may be interwoven in function (and presumably dysfunction) is not surprising based upon known preclinical and clinical work defining discrete yet specific afferent and efferent projections connecting these areas with subcortical regions. The precise neurochemical pathways, in particular the monoamines, and their balance in maintaining normal mood and cognition is more complex and various hypotheses have been put forth to explain the disturbances of these systems and how they regulate such functions. This review will highlight the clinical and preclinical notions integrating the pathology of depression and cognition and how these may be related to central monoaminergic systems.

1. Introduction

The finding that depressed patients frequently exhibit cognitive deficits is well documented and dates back to work done in the 1960s where it was reported that the efficacy of electroconvulsive shock (ECS) therapy to treat depression had parallel effects on memory

(Cronholm and Ottosson 1961). In particular, improvements in learning rather than retention seemed to correlate with amelioration of depressive symptoms. Since that time numerous findings have supported these clinical results showing that depressed patients demonstrate cognitive deficits. Thus, it is well accepted that these are most often observed as impairments in memory, attention and speed of processing; although the findings may differ depending upon the severity of the depressive state (Roy-Byrne et al. 1986; Wolfe et al. 1987; Austin et al. 1992; Brand et al. 1992). In severely depressed patients there also appears to be a deficit in executive functioning as described by the recent work of Goodwin and colleagues (1997). However, it should also be noted that no direct evidence exists in some studies (Moreaud et al. 1996; Purcell et al. 1997) where correlations were attempted to be drawn between Hamilton depression scores and neurocognitive task scores. This may be explained, in part, by differences in cognitive paradigms employed and the lack of a homogenous patient population.

The framework in which one can base the comorbidity of depression and cognitive deficits can certainly be related to overlapping and reciprocal neural networks in the brain (reviewed in Soares and Mann 1997; Phillips et al. 2003). From a preclinical standpoint, experimental work employing lesions to disrupt behavioral function have proven extremely helpful in determining a structure-function relationship. This has been more difficult in the clinical setting; in fact the organization of the brain can differ dramatically in the rodent making correlations between species somewhat unreliable. Nonetheless, it is well accepted that the hippocampus plays a central role in both mood and cognition. In this regard, Sheline and colleagues (Sheline 1996; Sheline et al. 1996) reported that hippocampal gray matter volumes as measured by MRI scans in subjects with a history of major recurrent depressive episodes were significantly smaller than a group of pair-wise matched normal controls. In contrast cerebral volumes were not significantly different when comparing depressed patients and controls. Indeed, widespread changes to the hippocampus make it difficult to pinpoint specific pathways involved and ultimately it most likely disrupts multiple and not just single neuronal connections. Further studies will need to determine the exact nature of decreased hippocampal volumes and recurrent depression. In terms of etiology of this finding it has been hypothesized that stress induces an enhancement of glutamate neurotoxicity that is most likely mediated by elevated levels of glucocorticoids.

Recent studies utilizing neural imaging technology and regional blood flow have begun to shed more light on gross macroscopic changes to brain regions involved in depression and cognition. There is rather strong evidence demonstrating that impaired function in the limbic loop certainly plays a role in affect, autonomic and vegetative domains (Cummings 1993). Mayberg and colleagues (1997) studied hospitalized unipolar patients using cerebral glucose metabolism and positron emission tomography (PET) to determine if treatment response could be correlated with activity in specific brain regions. Notably, rostral anterior cingulate metabolism differentiated treatment responders from non-responders in those patients receiving various antidepressant medications. Importantly these findings indicate that this area of the cingulate cortex may function as a bridge linking dorsal and ventral pathways necessary for the normal integrative processing of mood, motor, autonomic and cognitive behaviors, all of which are disrupted in depression. Similarly, recent functional imaging studies performed in depressed patients revealed metabolic changes in cortical and limbic areas following treatment with effective antidepressants and cognitive behavioral therapy (Goldapple et al. 2004). These findings corroborate results from PET imaging and cerebral glucose metabolism studies which show a decline in prefrontal cortex activity in both bipolar and depressed patients as compared to controls (Drevets et al. 1997), an effect at least partly attributed to the corresponding 39% and 48% reduction in cortical grey matter in bipolar and depressed patients, respectively (Drevets et al. 1997). While in fact these changes in brain morphology likely represent both direct and indirect alterations in monoaminergic innervation of the prefrontal cortex, only variable changes to neuroreceptor markers have been observed in the rostral cingulate regions.

The biochemical pathways relating to the anatomical correlates of depression and cognition have pointed towards monoaminergic dysfunction as a major etiological factor. The longstanding monoamine hypothesis of depression proposes that depression results from reduced levels of serotonin (5-HT) and norepinephrine (NE) in critical brain regions as discussed above. The involvement of both neurotransmitters can date back to the seminal work of Brodie and colleagues who demonstrated that depletion of these neurotransmitters with reserpine produced profound consequences on behavior in animals. This was later confirmed in clinical studies where a side effect of the use of reserpine in hypertensive patients resulted in profound depressive episodes (Beers and Passman 1990). To a certain extent, depletion studies have been used to examine the monoaminergic hypothesis of depression by using acute tryptophan depletion (ATD) to lower 5-HT levels and acute phenylalanine/tyrosine depletion (APTD) or the administration of alpha-methyl-para-tyrosine (AMPT) to lower NE and dopamine concentrations (see (Booij, Van der Does et al. 2003). Although a low 5-HT and NE model of depression is a rather simplistic view of the disease etiology and is consistent with the efficacy of known antidepressant drugs designed to augment monoaminergic neurotransmission, ATD does not worsen the symptoms of depressed patients (Delgado et al. 1994) and only induces mild dysphoria or no symptoms in healthy volunteers (Young et al. 1985). However this may not be surprising based on the notion that low 5-HT levels may act as a triggering biological factor in depression and may engage other biochemical and neuroreceptor changes required to produce a profound depressive episode in healthy volunteers (Van Praag et al. 1990; Booij et al. 2003). A similar postulation may also be true for lowered noradrenergic and dopaminergic neurotransmission. In general ATD and AMPT administered to individuals recently remitted, medicated patients or recovered depressed patients induced lowered mood or produced partial relapse (Booij et al. 2003). Interestingly, cognitive parameters were studied in some of these clinical investigations and revealed that a memory consolidation deficit was induced by ATD but improved focused attention whereas working memory impairments were denoted by APTD administration. Indeed the cognitive deficits in depression may differ dramatically from the biochemical pathology observed other psychiatric disorders but quite possibly some specific neural pathways may be disrupted and overlap in terms of cognitive dysfunction.

2. Role of Monoamines in Mood and Cognition

The hypothesis that the debilitating and often chronic symptoms of depression result from a perturbation of NE and 5-HT neurotransmission largely spawned from work done in the late 1950s and early 1960s showing that the early monoamine oxidase inhibitor, iproniazid, and the tricyclic antidepressant, imipramine, which are characterized by their ability to elevate monoamine levels by the preventing their breakdown and blocking their reuptake, respectively, were effective antidepressant agents (Eriksson 2000). In the 1980s and 1990s, these classes of compounds were superceded by the selective serotonin reuptake inhibitors (SSRIs), which work mainly by elevating 5-HT levels, although some work suggests that certain SSRIs may actually increase NE levels as well (Hughes and Stanford 1996; Owens et al. 2000). The most recent and novel class of effective antidepressant agents are the dual serotonin / norepinephrine reuptake inhibitors (SNRIs). In comparison to the SSRIs and tricyclic antidepressants, SNRIs such as venlafaxine exhibit a faster clinical onset of action (Clerc et al. 1995; Guelfi et al. 1995; Benkert et al. 1997) while being more effective in treating depression refractory to other types of antidepressants (Nierenberg et al. 1994; de Montigny et al. 1995). While these latter points remain somewhat controversial, the therapeutic utility of antidepressant agents exemplifies the important role of monoamines in clinically managing mood disorders. Moreover, their mechanism of action (i.e., elevating monoamines) may help explain the therapeutic pertinence of such neurotransmitters in related and / or comorbid disorders such as memory and cognitive dysfunction. Therefore, the proceeding sections will highlight work implicating monoaminergic systems in the neurobiology of depressive and cognitive disorders.

3. Serotonergic Systems

Serotonergic cell bodies in the central nervous system (CNS) are primarily restricted to a collection of neurons residing along the midline in the dorsal and median raphe nuclei. Together these nuclei comprise a serotonergic network that includes projections to the prefrontal cortex, dorsal and ventral hippocampus, nucleus accumbens, hypothalamus and amygdala. This widespread topographical distribution within the CNS has led to the postulation that 5-HT modulates numerous processes relevant to neuropsychiatric function. Serotonin is reported to exert marked effects on anxiety, mood, impulsivity, sleep, appetite, immune function and libido. Moreover, serotonergic dysfunction is characterized in considerable detail with respect to the etiology of psychiatric conditions including depression and anxiety; however, now that at least 14 receptor subtypes have been identified this role can easily be extended to other disorders including cognition and memory.

Several lines of evidence support the hypothesis that serotonergic systems are intimately related to the pathology and ultimate treatment of depressive disorders (reviewed in Owens and Nemeroff 1994; Nemeroff 1998). First, drug-free, depressed patients exhibit marked reductions in concentrations of 5-HT and metabolites, 5-HT transporter binding sites and in the 5-HT precursor molecule, tryptophan. Secondly, depressed patients show increased 5-HT$_2$ receptor binding sites. Thirdly, neuroendocrine and glucose utilization responses to serotonergic releasers such as fenfluramine are reported to be blunted in depressed patient populations compared to controls. And finally, drugs that elevate levels of 5-HT by either blocking its reuptake (e.g., selective 5-HT reuptake inhibitors or SSRIs) or breakdown (e.g., monoamine oxidase inhibitors) have extraordinary therapeutic benefit and clinical efficacy in treating depression.

In contrast to the undisputed role for 5-HT in mood and depressive disorders, serotonergic systems by themselves seem to exhibit only a moderate role in cognitive and memory function. Various nonselective 5-HT agonists including LSD and quipazine decrease rat performance in a serial reaction time task (Carli and Samanin 1992). Interestingly, these deficits were reversed by ritanserin, 5-HT$_{2A/2C}$ a 5-HT$_{2A/2C}$ antagonist, thus promoting the role of serotonergic receptor systems in modulating preclinical models of attention (Carli and Samanin 1992). mCPP and fenfluramine, 5-HT$_{1B/2C}$ agonist and 5-HT releasing agents, respectively, induce deficits in attention by increasing the error omission rate in the serial reaction time model (Carli and Samanin 1992). Additionally, rodent studies employing methods to deplete 5-HT concentrations yielded a variable range of results including impairments, improvements and no effect on performance in models of learning and memory (reviewed in Steckler and Sahgal 1995). While these seemingly disparate results can be partly explained by the extent and brain regions affected by the 5-HT lesion, differences in tone of the serotonergic system studied and the behavioral model examined, they do highlight the promiscuous involvement of 5-HT in mediating performance on preclinical cognitive / memory tasks. Because of these studies, considerable attention has been spent in not just understanding the role of 5-HT itself but also the direct influence and interactions this monoamine has on other neurotransmitter systems within discrete brain structures. Thus, the remaining portion of this section will focus on the relationship between serotonergic systems and other known modulators of cognition and memory – namely the acetylcholine (ACh) system.

There is definitive evidence revealing reciprocal relationships between central serotonergic and cholinergic neurotransmission. Localized lesions of the raphe nuclei reduce 5-HT concentrations in terminal areas and result in marked increases in ACh levels in the frontal cortex, hippocampus and limbic structures (Robinson 1983). These neurochemical findings, as well as other in vitro and in vivo studies (reviewed in Steckler and Sahgal 1995), strongly hint at a predominant inhibitory influence of 5-HT on cholinergic signaling. This is further supported by studies showing that administration of 5-HT alone decreases ACh levels in slice preparations from the hippocampus (Bianchi et al. 1989). Similarly, nonspecific 5-HT agonists and 5-HT releasing agents have been demonstrated to inhibit ACh release in the rat hippocampus and striatum (Maura et al. 1989; Maura et al. 1992). Additional work extending these findings proposes that 5-HT may work through inhibitory serotonergic autoreceptors to decrease ACh levels. Thus, in cases where elevations in ACh are paralleled by transient increases in 5-HT, authors claim that this release in 5-HT is sufficient to engage serotonergic autoreceptors, which in turn will ultimately decrease 5-HT release and remove the overall inhibitory tone of 5-HT on subsequent ACh (Bianchi et al. 1986).

The relationship between serotonergic autoreceptors and ACh release has also been explored. Acute administration of 8-OH-DPAT and buspirone, full and partial 5-HT$_{1A}$ receptor agonists, respectively, impairs performance on the Morris water maze and passive avoidance behavior models (see Myhrer 2003). Neurochemical studies in vivo as well as with synaptosomal preparations suggest that somatodendritic 5-HT$_{1A}$ autoreceptors in the raphe nuclei and not postsynaptic receptors in terminal areas (i.e., intra-cortical / hippocampal) constitute the primary circuitry through which 5-HT$_{1A}$ autoreceptors modulate the neurotransmission of ACh. Taken together, these results suggest that activation of 5-HT$_{1A}$ receptors actually result in deficits in memory processes at least at the preclinical level and provide evidence for the argument that selective 5-HT$_{1A}$ antagonists may exhibit promising effects in alleviating cognitive deficits. The potential therapeutic activity of a 5-HT$_{1A}$ antagonist is reviewed extensively by Schechter and colleagues (Schechter et al. 2002) who suggest that 5-HT$_{1A}$ receptor antagonists reverse cognitive deficits by effecting several neurotransmitter systems (e.g., glutamate).

The involvement of other 5-HT receptors (e.g., 5-HT$_{2A/2C/3/4}$) on learning and memory performance and to a certain extent cholinergic systems has also been examined (Myhrer 2003). However, very recent experimental efforts focused on the significance of 5-HT$_6$ receptors, the most recently identified of the 5-HT receptors, in preclinical models of cognitive performance. Initial microdialysis work revealed a distinct relationship between 5-HT$_6$ receptors and cholinergic systems and showed that antagonism of this receptor elevates ACh concentrations in the rat prefrontal cortex (Lacroix et al. 2004). Early behavioral studies report that administration of various 5-HT$_6$ receptor antagonists produces a yawning and stretching syndrome reminiscent to what is observed following administration of cholinergic agonists (Bourson et al. 1995). Similar patterns of behaviors are reported following treatment with antisense raised against the 5-HT$_6$ receptor (Bourson et al. 1995). Since these behaviors, whether induced by antisense or 5-HT$_6$ antagonists, were effectively blocked by cholinergic (but not dopaminergic) antagonists a relationship between serotonergic and cholinergic interactions is highly likely. Given the purported role of the cholinergic system in cognitive function the effects of 5-HT$_6$ receptor antagonists have been extensively studied in the Morris water maze, a test of spatial learning and memory. These studies showed that antagonism of the 5-HT$_6$ receptor enhanced retention of the learnt platform position without affecting acquisition of this behavior (Rogers et al. 2001; Lindner et al. 2003). Similarly, administration of a 5-HT$_6$ antagonist attenuated scopolamine-induced deficits in object discrimination tasks (Sleight et al. 1996; Woolley et al. 2003). Subsequent microdialysis studies actually showed that systemic administration of a 5-HT$_6$ antagonist produced a 2- and 3-fold increase in basal glutamate levels in the rat hippocampus and frontal cortex, respectively (Dawson et al. 2001). To our knowledge 5-HT$_6$ antagonists have not been shown to exhibit antidepressant-like activity in preclinical models but taken together, the preclinical behavioral and neurochemical effects provide a strong rationale for the pro-cognitive effects of selective 5-HT$_6$ receptor antagonists.

From the body of work discussed so far and from work cited, there is clear evidence that serotonergic systems, whether directly or indirectly, via effects on cholinergic and glutamatergic pathways, participate in mood and cognitive disorders. It is also clear that because these psychiatric illnesses are comprised of a constellation of symptoms that, undoubtedly, overlap and span a variety of physiological and behavioral arenas, it is unlikely that a single neurotransmitter system is involved. While 5-HT and related serotonergic receptor systems represent key neurochemical substrates underlying these disorders, their influence and reciprocal connections with other biochemical systems in numerous brain regions should not be understated or simply viewed in just one dimension. Thus, other monoamines, namely the noradrenergic and dopaminergic systems have been hypothesized to play an important role in the pathogenesis of depression as well as cognitive dysfunction.

4. Noradrenergic Systems

The majority of noradrenergic cell bodies are located in the locus coeruleus (LC), a hindbrain region consisting of dense axonal pathways that project throughout various cortical layers and subcortical structures including the hippocampus, amygdala, thalamus, nucleus accumbens and amygdala (Foote et al. 1983). The role of NE in the treatment of depressive disorders fits well with the widespread noradrenergic innervation and the fact that agents such as desipramine and more recently reboxetine, which selectively and potently block the reuptake up NE, appear to be at least as effective as SSRIs in the treatment of depression ((Nystrom and Hallstrom 1987; Dubini et al. 1997). Furthermore, compounds that facilitate noradrenergic neurotransmission by antagonizing NE autoreceptors also seem to possess antidepressant-like activity. Thus while other neurotransmitter systems play a role in the regulation of depressive disorders a role for the noradrenergic systems should not be excluded.

In addition to depressive disorders, the widespread distribution of central NE may also help explain a number of preclinical studies demonstrating a prominent role for this monoamine in modulating facets of executive cognitive function such as memory storage and acquisition (Arnsten and Goldman-Rakic 1985; Cole and Robbins 1992). Abercrombie and colleagues (Finlay et al. 1995) propose that noradrenergic cell bodies in the LC are partly responsible for the arousal and attention state of an organism. This postulation is supported by studies showing that in rodents, increases and decreases in LC neuronal activity corresponds with vigilance and drowsiness, respectively (Foote et al. 1991) while pharmacological or electrical stimulation of the LC has been demonstrated to elicit alert responses in nonhuman primates (see Usher et al. 1999). Finally, the fact that disturbances in NE transmission are often associated with various psychiatric illnesses including attention deficit hyperactivity disorder (ADHD) and schizophrenia, where in many cases severe cognitive deficits are comorbid findings, the central noradrenergic system, particularly innervations to the prefrontal cortex, is at least one common neurochemical pathway underlying the comorbidity of depression and cognitive deficits.

Experimental studies in primates show that noradrenergic projections from the LC modulate prefrontal cortex function via activation of local postsynaptic alpha adrenergic receptors. Specifically, basal NE release enhances cognitive performance and contents of working memory in primate frontal cortex by preferentially activating alpha 2A adrenoceptors (Arnsten et al. 1998), while nonselective alpha-2 adrenoceptor agonists like clonidine and guanfacine improve cognitive memory function in the delayed response and visual object discrimination tasks, models linked to adrenergic receptors in the dorsolateral and orbital prefrontal cortex, respectively. In addition, the nonselective alpha 2 receptor antagonist, yohimbine, is reported to impair performance on these tasks (Arnsten et al. 1998) and reverses deficits in delayed response performance in aged monkeys with cortical NE depletions (Coull 1994). Postsynaptic alpha 1 receptors in cortical areas, albeit seemingly in opposition to alpha 2 receptors, also are described to play a key role in executive function. Thus, under conditions of uncontrollable stress, NE levels in the frontal cortex are elevated above baseline conditions to engage local alpha 1 receptors resulting in deficits in spatial working memory tasks (Arnsten et al. 1998); Birnbaum et al. 1999; Mao et al. 1999). While these studies remain somewhat controversial, they highlight the important role of the noradrenergic system, via cortical alpha 1 and 2 adrenoceptors, in mediating executive functions such as arousal and memory in preclinical models. At this time the exact involvement of adrenergic receptor subtypes is not completely clear; however, the experimental work mentioned above suggests a common link between noradrenergic systems and anatomical brain regions in both mood and cognitive disorders.

The increases in NE observed after acute administration of 5-HT_6 receptor antagonists is also consistent with the purported role of the noradrenergic system in cognition. Lacroix and colleagues (2004) recently showed that systemic administration SB-271046, a selective $5\text{-}HT_6$ antagonist, elevates extracellular NE levels in the rat medial prefrontal cortex. Although these studies have yet to be confirmed by other research groups using this and other structurally unrelated 5-HT_6 antagonists, these results provide additional evidence supporting the role of 5-HT_6 receptor antagonists in the potential amelioration of cortical-related cognitive dysfunction. It is also interesting to mention that effective atypical antipsychotic agents, which also increase cortical NE levels in the cortex (Li et al. 1998), may relieve the negative symptoms and cognitive deficits in schizophrenics, in part, by possessing marked antagonist properties at 5-HT_6 receptors. Taken together, the neurochemical results collected to date indicate that noradrenergic systems can, by themselves and/or by indirect influences on other neurotransmitter systems, play a promiscuous role in human neuropsychiatric illness.

5. Dopaminergic Systems

Three prominent dopamine (DA) pathways exist in the brain. The nigrostriatal and tuberoinfudibular pathways mediate aspects of extrapyramidal motor movements and neuroendocrine function, respectively, while the mesocorticolimbic DA pathway, originating in the ventral tegmental area (VTA) with DA cell bodies innervating both cortical and limbic structures (Oades and Halliday 1987), plays a likely role in cognition, affect and motivation (Haracz 1982; Nieoullon 2002). The notion that DA and DA receptor systems modulate aspects of motor coordination, especially the motor deficits observed in patients suffering from Parkinson's disease, has been recognized since the 1960s (Bernheimer and Hornykiewicz 1965). The control of integrative aspects of behavior mediating facets of reward and the salient properties of reinforcing stimuli are likely controlled by central dopaminergic systems (Wise 1996; Nieoullon 2002). Alterations / dysfunctions in forebrain DA also correlate with several CNS disorders including Alzheimer's disease, Tourette's disease and ADHD. Finally, a role for DA in the pathology of depressive disorders is suggested by studies reporting bilateral increases in D2 receptor binding in the basal ganglia (D'Haenen H and Bossuyt 1994) and decreased levels of DA metabolites in the cerebrospinal fluid (CSF) of depressed patients (Reddy et al. 1992). Because all of these disorders are often comorbid with cognitive dysfunction, a critical role for DA in regulating a broad range of behavioral and cognitive processes has been emphasized (Nieoullon 2002).

With respective to the mesocorticolimbic DA pathways, DA innervation of the prefrontal cortex has been implicated both in the modulation of "normal" cognitive processes, in particular working memory, and in numerous neuropsychiatric disorder-induced and age-related memory deficits (Davis et al. 1991; Mattay et al. 2002; Volkow et al. 2002). Patients with other diseases, that undoubtedly result from dopaminergic alterations, such as schizophrenia or ADHD also exhibit alterations in cognitive functions. Preclinical studies support this notion and show that selective lesions of dopaminergic neurons in rats produce severe cognitive deficits, particularly when the mesocorticolimbic component of the dopaminergic systems is altered (Nieoullon 2002). More specifically, lesions of DA cell bodies in the rat VTA produce deficits in the retention of delayed-alternation behavior suggesting an inability of lesioned animals to "focus" on switching behaviors (Taghzouti et al. 1986). Poor performance on memory tasks have also been reported following discrete dopaminergic lesions of the hippocampus, amygdala and habenula (Le Moal and Simon 1991) leading to the conclusion that DA plays an integral role in normal function of memory and cognition.

Focal DA lesion studies of the prefrontal cortex were used to evaluate memory and cognitive performances in nonhuman primates. Thus, administration of the dopaminergic neurotoxin 6-OHDA into the prefrontal cortex, which destroys DA neurons in this area, results in marked impairments in monkey performance on delayed-alternation spatial tasks (Brozoski et al. 1979) suggesting cognitive deficits in lesioned monkeys. Conversely, similar cortical lesions of the DA system improve errors on a version of the Wisconsin card-sorting test (Roberts et al. 1994). These seemingly disparate results likely reflect differences in the activity of other DA systems in the brain, namely the nigrostriatal DA pathway. Taking all of these data together these experiments raise the question that extensive dopaminergic dysfunction in both cortical and subcortical areas may lead to cognitive deficits in neuropsychiatric disorders. While this argument may remain somewhat controversial, it is strengthened by the recent report demonstrating that extracellular cortical DA levels are increased following administration of selective $5\text{-}HT_6$ receptor antagonists. Moreover, these data indicate that pharmacotherapeutic agents designed to elevate DA transmission in the brain may help to enhance cognitive deficits related to neurologic or psychiatric diseases.

6. Conclusions

Mood and cognitive disorders involve several interconnecting brain regions and their disease pathology, while often overlapping, is complex and often cannot be simply defined by a single symptomology. Since these diseases are comprised of a constellation of symptoms and behavioral abnormalities such as disruptions in circadian rhythms, sleep, appetite, neuroendocrine and immune function, it is clear that not just one neurotransmitter system is responsible for the pathology. The preclinical and clinical data mentioned herein suggest that monoamines represent at least one common pathway mediating facets of depression and cognitive dysfunction. It is interesting to speculate that future development of novel pharmacotherapies will be able to treat these comorbid disorders.

References

Arnsten, A. F. and P. S. Goldman-Rakic (1985). "Catecholamines and cognitive decline in aged nonhuman primates." *Ann N Y Acad Sci* 444: 218-34.

Arnsten, A. F., J. C. Steere, D. J. Jentsch and B. M. Li (1998). "Noradrenergic influences on prefrontal cortical cognitive function: opposing actions at postjunctional alpha 1 versus alpha 2-adrenergic receptors." *Adv Pharmacol* 42: 764-7.

Austin, M. P., M. Ross, C. Murray, R. E. O'Carroll, K. P. Ebmeier and G. M. Goodwin (1992). "Cognitive function in major depression." *Journal of Affective Disorders.* 25(1): 21-9.

Beers, M. H. and L. J. Passman (1990). "Antihypertensive medications and depression." *Drugs* 40: 792-799.

Benkert, O., G. Grunder and H. Wetzel (1997). "Is there an advantage to venlafaxine in comparison with other antidepressants?" *Human Psychopharmacology* 12: 53-64.

Bernheimer, H. and O. Hornykiewicz (1965). "[Decreased homovanillic acid concentration in the brain in parkinsonian subjects as an expression of a disorder of central dopamine metabolism]." *Klin Wochenschr* 43(13): 711-5.

Bianchi, C., A. Siniscalchi and L. Beani (1986). "The influence of 5-hydroxytryptamine on the release of acetylcholine from guinea-pig brain ex vivo and in vitro." *Neuropharmacology* 25(9): 1043-9.

Bianchi, C., A. Siniscalchi and L. Beani (1989). "Effect of 5-hydroxytryptamine on [3H]-acetylcholine release from guinea-pig striatal slices." *Br J Pharmacol* 97(1): 213-21.

Birnbaum, S., K. T. Gobeske, J. Auerbach, J. R. Taylor and A. F. Arnsten (1999). "A role for norepinephrine in stress-induced cognitive deficits: alpha-1-adrenoceptor mediation in the prefrontal cortex." *Biol Psychiatry* 46(9): 1266-74.

Booij, L., A. J. W. Van der Does and W. J. Riedel (2003). "Monoamine depletion in psychiatric and healthy populations: review." *Mol Psychiatry* 8: 951-973.

Bourson, A., E. Borroni, R. Austin, F. Monsma Jr and A. Sleight (1995). "Determination of the role of the 5-HT6 receptor in the rat brain: A study using antisense oligonucleotides." *Journal of Pharmacology & Experimental Therapeutics.* 274: 173-180.

Brand, A. N., J. Jolles and C. Gispen-de Wied (1992). "Recall and recognition memory deficits in depression." *Journal of Affective Disorders.* 25(1): 77-86.

Brozoski, T. J., R. M. Brown, H. E. Rosvold and P. S. Goldman (1979). "Cognitive deficit caused by regional depletion of dopamine in prefrontal cortex of rhesus monkey." *Science* 205(4409): 929-32.

Carli, M. and R. Samanin (1992). "Serotonin2 receptor agonists and serotonergic anorectic drugs affect rats' performance differently in a five-choice serial reaction time task." *Psychopharmacology (Berl)* 106: 228-34.

Clerc, G. E., P. Ruimy and J. Verdeay-Pailles (1995). "A double blind comparison of venlafaxine and fluoxetine in patients hospitalized for major depression and melancholia." *International Clinical Psychopharmacology* 9: 138-143.

Cole, B. J. and T. W. Robbins (1992). "Forebrain norepinephrine: role in controlled information processing in the rat." *Neuropsychopharmacology* 7(2): 129-42.

Coull, J. T. (1994). "Pharmacological manipulations of the alpha 2-noradrenergic system. Effects on cognition." Drugs Aging 5(2): 116-26.

Cronholm, B. and J. O. Ottosson (1961). "Memory functions in endogenous depression before and after electroconvulsive therapy." Arch Gen Psychiatry 5: 193-9.

Cummings, J. L. (1993). "The neuroanatomy of depression." *J Clin Psychiatry* 54 Suppl: 14-20.

Davis, K. L., R. S. Kahn, G. Ko and M. Davidson (1991). "Dopamine in schizophrenia: a review and reconceptualization." *Am J Psychiatry* 148(11): 1474-86.

Dawson, L. A., H. Q. Nguyen and P. Li (2001). "The 5-HT(6) receptor antagonist SB-271046 selectively enhances excitatory neurotransmission in the rat frontal cortex and hippocampus." *Neuropsychopharmacology* 25(5): 662-8.

de Montigny, C., G. Debonnel, R. Bergeron, E. St Andre and P. Blier (1995). "Venlafaxine in treatment resistant depression: open label multicentre study." *Am Coll Neuropharmacol* 34: 158.

Delgado, P. L., L. H. Price, H. L. Miller, R. M. Salomon, G. K. Aghajanian, G. R. Heninger and D. S. Charney (1994). "Serotonin and the neurobiology of depression. Effects of tryptophan depletion in drug-free depressed patients." *Arch Gen Psychiatry* 51(11): 865-74.

D'Haenen H, A. and A. Bossuyt (1994). "Dopamine D2 receptors in depression measured with single photon emission computed tomography." *Biol Psychiatry* 35(2): 128-32.

Drevets, W. C., J. L. Price, J. R. Simpson Jr, R. D. Todd, T. Reich, M. Vannier and M. E. Raichle (1997). "Subgenual prefrontal cortex abnormalities in mood disorders." *Nature* 386: 824-827.

Dubini, A., M. Bosc and V. Polin (1997). "Noradrenaline-selective versus serotonin-selective antidepressant therapy: differential effects on social functioning." *J Psychopharmacol* 11(4 Suppl): S17-23.

Eriksson, E. (2000). "Antidepressant drugs: does it matter if they inhibit the reuptake of noradrenaline or serotonin." *Acta Psychiatr Scand* 101 (Suppl. 402): 12-17.

Finlay, J. M., M. J. Zigmond and E. D. Abercrombie (1995). "Increased dopamine and norepinephrine release in medial prefrontal cortex induced by acute and chronic stress: effects of diazepam." *Neuroscience* 64(3): 619-28.

Foote, S. L., C. W. Berridge, L. M. Adams and J. A. Pineda (1991). "Electrophysiological evidence for the involvement of the locus coeruleus in alerting, orienting, and attending." *Prog Brain Res* 88: 521-32.

Foote, S. L., F. E. Bloom and G. Aston-Jones (1983). "Nucleus locus ceruleus: new evidence of anatomical and physiological specificity." *Physiol Rev* 63(3): 844-914.

Goldapple, K., Z. Segal, C. Garson, M. Lau, P. Bieling, S. Kennedy and H. Mayberg (2004). "Modulation of cortical-limbic pathways in major depression: treatment-specific effects of cognitive behavior therapy." *Arch Gen Psychiatry* 61: 34-41.

Goodwin, G. M. (1997). "Neuropsychological and neuroimaging evidence for the involvement of the frontal lobes in depression." *J Psychopharmacol* 11(2): 115-22.

Guelfi, J. D., C. White, D. Hackett, J. Y. Guichoux and G. Magni (1995). "Effectiveness of venlafaxine in patients hospitalized for major depression and melancholia." *J Clin Psychiatry* 56: 450-458.

Haracz, J. L. (1982). "The dopamine hypothesis: an overview of studies with schizophrenic patients." *Schizophr Bull* 8(3): 438-69.

Hughes, Z. A. and S. C. Stanford (1996). "Increased noradrenaline efflux induced by local infusion of fluoxetine in the rat frontal cortex." *European Journal of Pharmacology.* 317: 83-90.

Lacroix, L. P., L. A. Dawson, J. J. Hagan and C. A. Heidbreder (2004). "5-HT6 receptor antagonist SB-271046 enhances extracellular levels of monoamines in the rat medial prefrontal cortex." *Synapse* 51(2): 158-64.

Le Moal, M. and H. Simon (1991). "Mesocorticolimbic dopaminergic network: functional and regulatory roles." *Physiol Rev* 71(1): 155-234.

Li, X. M., K. W. Perry, D. T. Wong and F. P. Bymaster (1998). "Olanzapine increases in vivo dopamine and norepinephrine release in rat prefrontal cortex, nucleus accumbens and striatum." *Psychopharmacology (Berl)* 136(2): 153-61.

Lindner, M. D., D. B. Hodges, Jr., J. B. Hogan, A. F. Orie, J. A. Corsa, D. M. Barten, C. Polson, B. J. Robertson, V. L. Guss, K. W. Gillman, J. E. Starrett, Jr., V. K. Gribkoff, M. L. Woolley, J. C. Bentley, A. J. Sleight, C. A. Marsden and K. C. Fone (2003). "An assessment of the effects of serotonin 6 (5-HT6) receptor antagonists in rodent models of learning." *J Pharmacol Exp Ther* 307(2): 682-91.

Mao, Z. M., B. M. Li and A. F. Arnsten (1999). "[Roles of alpha-2 adrenoceptor in prefrontal cortical cognitive functions]." *Sheng Li Ke Xue Jin Zhan* 30(1): 17-22.

Mattay, V. S., F. Fera, A. Tessitore, A. R. Hariri, S. Das, J. H. Callicott and D. R. Weinberger (2002). "Neurophysiological correlates of age-related changes in human motor function." *Neurology* 58(4): 630-5.

Maura, G., G. Andrioli, P. Cavazzani and M. Raiteri (1992). "5-Hydroxytryptamine3 receptors sited on cholinergic axon terminals of human cerebral cortex mediate inhibition of acetylcholine release." *J Neurochem* 58: 2334-7.

Maura, G., E. Fedele and M. Raiteri (1989). "Acetylcholine release from rat hippocampal slices is modulated by 5-hydroxytryptamine." *Eur J Pharmacol* 165: 173-9.

Mayberg, H. S., S. K. Brannan, R. K. Mahurin, P. A. Jerabek, J. S. Brickman, J. L. Tekell, J. A. Silva, S. McGinnis, T. G. Glass, C. C. Martin and P. T. Fox (1997). "Cingulate function in depression: a potential predictor of treatment response." *Neuroreport* 8(4): 1057-61.

Moreaud, O., B. Naegele, J. P. Chabannes, J. L. Roulin, B. Garbolino and J. Pellat (1996). "[Frontal lobe dysfunction and depressive state: relation to endogenous character of depression]." *Encephale* 22(1): 47-51.

Myhrer, T. (2003). "Neurotransmitter systems involved in learning and memory in the rat: a meta-analysis based on studies of four behavioral tasks." *Brain Res Rev* 41: 268-287.

Nemeroff, C. B. (1998). "Psychopharmacology of affective disorders in the 21st century." *Biological Psychiatry.* 44: 517-525.

Nieoullon, A. (2002). "Dopamine and the regulation of cognition and attention." *Prog Neurobiol* 67(1): 53-83.

Nierenberg, A. A., J. P. Feigner, R. Rudolph, J. O. Cole and J. Sullivan (1994). "Venlafaxine for treatment resistant unipolar depression." *J Clin Psychopharmacol* 4: 419-423.

Nystrom, C. and T. Hallstrom (1987). "Comparison between a serotonin and a noradrenaline reuptake blocker in the treatment of depressed outpatients. A cross-over study." *Acta Psychiatr Scand* 75(4): 377-82.

Oades, R. D. and G. M. Halliday (1987). "Ventral tegmental (A10) system: neurobiology. 1. Anatomy and connectivity." *Brain Res* 434(2): 117-65.

Owens, M. J., D. L. Knight and C. B. Nemeroff (2000). "Paroxetine Binding to the rat norepinephrine transporter in vivo." *Biological Psychiatry.* 47: 842-845.

Owens, M. J. and C. B. Nemeroff (1994). "The role of serotonin in the pathophysiology of depression: focus on the serotonin transporter." *Clin Chem* 40: 288-295.

Phillips, M. L., W. C. Drevets, S. L. Rauch and R. Lane (2003). "Neurobiology of emotion perception II: Implications for major psychiatric disorders." *Biological Psychiatry.* 54(5): 515-28.

Purcell, R., P. Maruff, M. Kyrios and C. Pantelis (1997). "Neuropsychological function in young patients with unipolar major depression." *Psychol Med* 27(6): 1277-85.

Reddy, P. L., S. Khanna, M. N. Subhash, S. M. Channabasavanna and B. S. Rao (1992). "CSF amine metabolites in depression." *Biol Psychiatry* 31(2): 112-8.

Roberts, A. C., M. A. De Salvia, L. S. Wilkinson, P. Collins, J. L. Muir, B. J. Everitt and T. W. Robbins (1994). "6-Hydroxydopamine lesions of the prefrontal cortex in monkeys enhance performance on an analog of the Wisconsin Card Sort Test: possible interactions with subcortical dopamine." *J Neurosci* 14(5 Pt 1): 2531-44.

Robinson, S. (1983). "Effect of specific serotonergic lesions on cholinergic neurons in the hippocampus, cortex and striatum." *Life Sciences* 32: 345-53.

Rogers, D.C. and Hagan, JJ (2001) "5-HT6 receptor antagonists enhance retention of a water maze task in the rat." *Psychopharmacology* 158:114-9.

Roy-Byrne, P. P., H. Weingartner, L. M. Bierer, K. Thompson and R. M. Post (1986). "Effortful and automatic cognitive processes in depression." *Archives of General Psychiatry.* 43(3): 265-7.

Schechter, L. E., L. A. Dawson and J. A. Harder (2002). "The potential utility of 5-HT1A receptor antagonists in the treatment of cognitive dysfunction associated with Alzheimer s disease." *Curr Pharm Des* 8(2): 139-45.

Sheline, Y. I. (1996). "Hippocampal atrophy in major depression: a result of depression-induced neurotoxicity?" *Mol Psychiatry* 1(4): 298-9.

Sheline, Y. I., P. W. Wang, M. H. Gado, J. G. Csernansky and M. W. Vannier (1996). "Hippocampal atrophy in recurrent major depression." *Proc Natl Acad Sci U S A* 93(9): 3908-13.

Sleight, A. J., F. J. Monsma, Jr., E. Borroni, R. H. Austin and A. Bourson (1996). "Effects of altered 5-ht6 expression in the rat: functional studies using antisense oligonucleotides." *Behav Brain Res* 73(1-2): 245-8.

Soares, J. C. and J. J. Mann (1997). "The anatomy of mood disorders--review of structural neuroimaging studies.[comment]." *Biological Psychiatry.* 41(1): 86-106.

Steckler, T. and A. Sahgal (1995). "The role of serotonergic-cholinergic interactions in the mediation of cognitive behaviour." *Behavioral Brain Research* 67: 165-199.

Taghzouti, K., H. Simon and M. Le Moal (1986). "Disturbances in exploratory behavior and functional recovery in the Y and radial mazes following dopamine depletion of the lateral septum." *Behav Neural Biol* 45(1): 48-56.

Usher, M., J. D. Cohen, D. Servan-Schreiber, J. Rajkowski and G. Aston-Jones (1999). "The role of locus coeruleus in the regulation of cognitive performance." *Science* 283(5401): 549-54.

Van Praag, H. M., G. M. Asnis, R. S. Kahn, S. L. Brown, M. Korn, J. M. Friedman and S. Wetzler (1990). "Nosological tunnel vision in biological psychiatry. A plea for a functional psychopathology." *Ann N Y Acad Sci* 600: 501-10.

Volkow, N. D., J. S. Fowler, G. J. Wang and R. Z. Goldstein (2002). "Role of dopamine, the frontal cortex and memory circuits in drug addiction: insight from imaging studies." *Neurobiol Learn Mem* 78(3): 610-24.

Wise, R. A. (1996). "Neurobiology of addiction." *Curr Opin Neurobiol* 6(2): 243-51.

Wolfe, J., E. Granholm, N. Butters, E. Saunders and D. Janowsky (1987). "Verbal memory deficits associated with major affective disorders: a comparison of unipolar and bipolar patients." *Journal of Affective Disorders.* 13(1): 83-92.

Woolley, M. L., C. A. Marsden, A. J. Sleight, K. C. Fone and A. Meneses (2003). "Reversal of a cholinergic-induced deficit in a rodent model of recognition memory by the selective 5-HT6 receptor antagonist, Ro 04-6790." *Psychopharmacology (Berl)* 170(4): 358-67.

Young, S. N., S. E. Smith, R. O. Pihl and F. R. Ervin (1985). "Tryptophan depletion causes a rapid lowering of mood in normal males." *Psychopharmacology (Berl)* 87(2): 173-7.

In: Cognition and Mood Interactions
Editor: Miao-Kun Sun, pp. 33-69

ISBN 1-59454-229-5
2005 © Nova Science Publishers, Inc.

Chapter III

Excitatory Amino Acids in Mood and Cognition

Miao-Kun Sun* and Daniel L. Alkon

Blânchette Rockefeller Neurosciences Institute, Rockville, MD, USA

Mood disorder and Alzheimer's disease research has been dominated by the monoamine hypothesis of depression and by the amyloid hypothesis, respectively. The glutamate system is now emerging as a crucial player in the pathophysiology of depression and dementia and as a target for development of medications for depression and Alzheimer's dementia. Activation of the glutamate receptors evokes a rapid Ca^{2+} influx into neurons, resulting in an activation of a variety of intracellular signal cascades, Ca^{2+} mobilization, and alterations in membrane channel activity and gene expression. The signal transduction mechanisms play a fundamental role in how the brain functions physiologically but are also at the core of neural injury and dysfunction. It has become gradually recognized that abnormal glutamate receptor activation lacks specified physiological functions and underlies the development of depressive symptoms and of many forms of dementia. The evidence that glutamate receptor antagonists can reduce memory and mood deficits provides further support for the notion that the glutamate system is involved in the pathogenesis of dementia and depression. Some of them show a promising profile as therapeutic agents, not just as symptom-relievers, with a more rapid onset. In most cases, a functional inhibition of the glutamate system may represent an effective approach to antidepressive and antidementic therapies. Agents that have antagonistic activity at different sites show differential structure-activity relationships, possess distinct pharmacological profiles, and therefore have different therapeutic potentials. This chapter summarizes current knowledge and developments concerning a variety of agents that affect the glutamate system and discusses their potential as pharmacological drugs in the treatments of depression and dementia.

1. Introduction

Depression and dementia, two major entities of brain dysfunction, are devastating diseases that affect the quality of life in a large segment of the population and represent a tremendous challenge to modern medicine and science. Despite decades of intensive research, we are still far from a complete understanding of the detailed cellular/molecular mechanisms and cascades responsible for the mood and memory collapse. There are, however, promising leads in the fight against depression and dementia. These two disorders appear to share some common molecular mechanisms and cascades and attack a similar brain circuit (Nestler et al., 2002; Sun and Alkon 2002a). Among the variety of neurotransmitter systems, a normal operation of the glutamate neurotransmission is gradually recognized as essential to the status of mood and levels of cognition. Developing agents that act on this system may yield effective therapeutic drugs for antidepressive and antidementic medications.

As discussed in Chapter I of this book, mood disorders are among the most prevalent forms of mental illness. They are recurrent, life threatening (due to the risk of suicide), and a major cause of morbidity worldwide. Stressful life events, such as threat, loss, humiliation, or defeat, play a central role in the onset and course of depression, resulting in a lasting mood status: feelings of worthlessness, hopelessness, guilt, doom, and suicidality among other symptoms. Whether such stressful experiences lead to depression, however, may partly depend on the subjects' genetic makeup (Caspi et al., 2003). Nevertheless, several forms of depression affect 2%-5% of the U.S. population, and up to 20% of the population suffer from milder forms of the illness. In fact, most adults will suffer one or more depressive episodes during their lifetime. Depression, one of the five leading causes of disease burden worldwide (Murray and Lopez, 1997), is almost twice as common in females than males. Another roughly 1-2% are afflicted by bipolar disorder (also known as manic-depressive illness), which affects females and males equally. Depression has been described by humankind for several millennia. Yet, it wasn't until the middle part of the 19th century that the brain became the focus of efforts to understand its pathophysiology. The effectiveness of antidepressants that affect the monoaminergic systems is the real drive for the scientific research focusing on the behavioral aspects and pharmacology of monoamine agents. These agents have revolutionized antidepressive treatment, yet, may have slowed down the efforts to attain a broad understanding of mood dys-regulation. However, an important role of glutamate systems in the pathophysiology of mood regulation is becoming recognized and deserves intensive investigation.

Dementia, on the other hand, is a progressive decline of memory and cognitive abilities, including a loss of memory, decreased attention, reduced ability in learning, judgment, and decision-making. The most common form of dementia is Alzheimer's dementia (AD), which affects 4 million Americans and about 20-30 million worldwide (Selkoe and Schenk, 2003), especially the elders. As the population ages, the number of AD patients is expected to triple in the next three decades. Investigation into the etiology for AD reveals that the vast majority of AD cases are probably caused by multiple undefined factors. Only less than 10% of the AD cases, those with early onset familial AD, can be traced to autosomal dominant mutations in the genes. The AD research has been dominated by the amyloid hypothesis, i.e., all the AD pathophysiological changes/impairments are either leading to or as a consequence of neurotoxic amyloid accumulation. Focusing on reducing the amyloid production and removing amyloid plaques has yielded promising leads. However, it is becoming clear that AD is a synaptic disorder. Abnormal operation of the glutamate system plays a more important role in AD pathogenesis than has been realized. In addition, a cure cannot be achieved without restoring the normal glutamate transmission, which is at the core of signal processing that defines many types of learning and memory.

2. The Glutamate Receptors

L-Glutamate, the major excitatory amino acid in the brain, serves as the endogenous agonist for both the ligand-gated ionotropic glutamate receptor (iGluR) and the G-protein-linked metabotropic glutamate receptors (mGluR) (Collingridge and Lester, 1989; Sun, 1996; Michaelis, 1998; de Blasi et al., 2001; Riedel et al., 2003). Defining receptor/subunit specificity is important in glutamate pharmacology since it determines the particular pharmacodynamic profile and adverse effects.

Based on their preferential interaction with particular ligands, iGluRs in the mammalian forebrain are further subclassed into three major receptors: NMDA receptors (NR), α-amino-3-hydroxy-5-methyl-4-isoxazoleproprionate (AMPA) receptors, and kainate receptors. The AMPA receptors and the kainate receptors are often referred to as the non-NMDA receptors. The NMDA and non-NMDA receptors are co-localized in individual synapses, especially in adults (Bekkers and Stevens, 1989). The basic structures of iGluRs include a large extracellular N-terminal region, 3 transmembrane segments (TM1, TM3, and TM4), a P loop region (initially named as TM2) that forms the pore selectivity filter, and a cytoplasmic C-terminal region (Dingledine et al., 1999). The N-terminal domain is responsible for Mg^{2+} metal ion binding and channel activity, whereas the transmembrane domains are important for ion channel formation. The TM3 segment may function as a transduction element, whose conformational change couples ligand binding with channel opening (Jones et al., 2002), while the TM2-3 loop of NR2 may modulate Ca^{2+}-dependent inactivation by interacting with the NR1 C terminus (Vissel et al., 2002). The intracellular domain is involved in regulating receptor activity, subcellular localization, and even gene expression (Holmes et al., 2002) after a process termed regulated intramembrane proteolysis (Brown et al., 2000).

The NRs are heteromeric channels, consisting of mostly the NR1 and NR2A-D subunits, while three families of the NR subunits have been identified: NR1, NR2, and NR3. The NRs are thought to be either tetramers (Laube et al., 1998) or pentamers that are composed of at least two NR1, at least two NR2 subunits (Laube et al., 1998), and less commonly an NR3 subunit (Das et al., 1998; Chatterton et al., 2002). The NRs are unique in their glycine co-agonist-binding sites. The activation of the NRs requires occupation of two independent glutamate binding sites and two glycine-binding sites (Benveniste and Mayer, 1991; Clements and Westbrook, 1991). In frog oocytes, NR1 expression itself forms homomeric ion channels that can be activated by NMDA and L-glutamate, requiring glycine for full activation. NR2 expression alone does not form functional NRs. Coexpression of NR1 with NR2 subunits, on the other hand, forms ion channels that exhibit very similar ion conductance to those NRs in neurons (Zeron et al., 2002). The NRs are mobile, moving laterally between synaptic and extrasynaptic pools (Tovar and Westbrook, 2002). They form complexes in the postsynaptic density (PSD) with other proteins, such as α-actinin, tyrosine-kinases, Ca^{2+}-calmodulin, PSD95 (alternative nomenclature SAP90), SAP97 (or hdlg), and SAP102 (Yu et al., 1997; Kennedy, 1998; Tezuka et al., 1999; Soderling and Derkach, 2000). Targeting the intracellular signal cascades of the NRs may provide a more specific therapeutic action.

The NR1 subunit is widely distributed throughout the brain and is a product of a single gene expressed as eight alternatively spliced mRNAs. The NR2 subunits, however, show distinct regional and developmental patterns of expression, providing most of the structural basis for heterogeneity in the NRs. In the adult rat hippocampus and cerebral cortex, the predominant NR2 subunits are NR2A and NR2B. The NR2C, on the other hand, is expressed almost exclusively in the cerebellum and several nuclei, while the NR2D is expressed mainly in the diencephalon and midbrain. From a pharmacological point of view, blocking the particular NR2 subunits would thus have better side-effect profiles than would an antagonism of the NR1 subunits.

The AMPA receptors, whose activation with 2 molecules of glutamate per receptor characteristically produces a fast excitatory synaptic signaling, are composed of the glutamate receptor (GluR)1, GluR2, GluR3, and GluR4 subunits. Their affinity for glutamate is lower than the NRs' and they show a more rapid dissociation from ligand binding. The kainate receptors, existing presynaptically and postsynaptically with physiological roles remaining to be defined, are composed of the GluR5, GluR6, GluR7, kainite receptor 1, and kainite receptor 2 subunits.

The mGluRs are G protein-coupled receptors and are assumed to have seven transmembrane regions, similar to other G protein-coupled receptors. The mGluRs can be either a homo- or heteromer. Eight types of mGluR have been cloned, dividing into three subgroups according to their signal transduction pathway. The group I mGluR is located both presynaptically and postsynaptically and consists of the mGluR1 (a,b,c,d) and mGluR5 (a,b). They interact with the Gp/11 subunit of G-protein, activating the enzyme phospholipase C as well as activating the inositide triphosphate/calcium and diacylglycerol/protein kinase C cascades through phosphoinositide hydrolysis. In the rat brain, mGluR5 is widely expressed in the whole hippocampus. The dentate gyrus expresses the highest level of mGluR5, located at the distal dendritic compartments of the dentate gyrus molecular layer and on the interneurons. The group II and III mGluRs are located presynaptically. The group II mGluRs include the mGluR2 and the mGluR3. Their activation leads to an inhibition of the adenyl cyclase enzyme. The group III mGluR consists of mGluR4 (a,b), mGluR6, mGluR7 (a,b), and mGluR8 (a,b), whose activation leads to an inhibition of the adenyl cyclase and an interaction with the enzyme phosphodiesterase, changing cGMP concentrations.

3. Physiology and Pathophysiology

Glutamate receptors play an important role in neural communication, serving functions in neural development and plasticity (Reidel et al., 2003). The GluRs are involved in almost all types of brain functions, ranging from consciousness, thoughts, mood, cognition, to cardiorespiratory control and nociceptive sensation. The GluRs are also regulated by other transmitter receptors (Lee et al., 2002) and are involved in many neurological disorders, including stroke, epileptiform seizures, Huntington's disease, Parkinson's disease, AD, amyotrophic lateral sclerosis, and nociception (Dingledine et al., 1986; Rothman and Olney, 1995; Liu et al., 1997; Doble, 1999; Sun, 1999; Covasa et al., 2000; Woolf and Salter, 2000; Chizh et al., 2001; Le and Lipton, 2001; Gill et al., 2002; Peeters et al., 2002; Planells-Cases et al., 2002; Zeron et al., 2002).

The main function of the AMPA receptor activation is to provide a fast synaptic signal and of the NR to provide ligand-gated brief Ca^{2+} influx. The physiological role of kainite receptor activation, on the other hand, has not been defined. Activation through the mGluRs either provides a pathway to regulate intracellular signal cascades through G proteins or modulate operation of the glutamate system. In the hippocampus, activation of the AMPA receptors leads to relieving the voltage-dependent blockade of the NR by Mg^{2+}. The Ca^{2+} oscillation or infrequent mobilization, affects not only dramatically and dynamically the synaptic plasticity but also efficiency and specificity of gene expression (Dolmetsch et al., 1998). The transcription of the glutamate system itself, however, appears to be tightly controlled in the mammals. Out of 19 glutamatergic gene promoters (13 glutamate receptor subunits, 4 transporters, and 2 metabolizing enzymes), none was found to have a polymorphism that changes the ability of the sequence to initiate transcription by a factor of more than 1.35-fold (Smith et al., 2003), too weak a change to result in corresponding effects after compensation. Expression of glutamate receptors and transporters is thus unusually tightly controlled, suggesting that non-coding polymorphisms are unlikely to make a significant contribution to cognitive-psychiatric phenotypes.

3.1. Synaptic Transmission

Synaptic transmission is the best-studied function involving glutamate neurotransmission. The AMPA receptors activate fast, show rapid desensitization, and are responsible for the fast, immediate postsynaptic response to glutamate release. The NRs are coupled with an ion channel, which is voltage-dependent, owing to a voltage-dependent blockade by Mg^{2+}, and permeable to Ca^{2+} and Na^+ when open. Depolarization by AMPA receptor activation removes this block. Thus, the NR is use-dependent: NMDA is more effective at opening the ion channels when the cell is depolarized to overcome the Mg^{2+} block, acting as a coincidence detector linking neurotransmitter activation with the electric state of the neuron. Ca^{2+} transients in dendritic spines evoked by single synaptic stimuli through NR activation can then trigger Ca^{2+} release from internal stores in individual spines of the CA1 neurons (Emptage et al., 1999; Kovalchuk et al., 2000). The voltage-dependent Mg^{2+} blockade of the NRs is essential to normal operation of the glutamate system. What would happen if the glutamate action is not brief and the cell membrane cannot return to its hyperpolarization phase? The NRs lose their sensitivity to Mg^{2+} blockade! Loss of this Mg^{2+} blockade of the NRs because of overexcitation due to excessive glutamate release or insufficient reuptake underlies pathogenesis of many neurodegenerative disorders, mood deregulation, and dementia.

Although activation of the NRs requires the presence of both glutamate and glycine, L-glutamate has the neurotransmitter role since it is released from presynaptic terminals in an activity-dependent manner, while glycine acts as a modulator, which is present in the extracellular fluid at more constant levels. Aspartate binds and activates the NRs and competes with L-glutamate for transport across the plasma membrane. Its role as a neurotransmitter remains to be established since it is not taken into synaptic vesicles (Osen et al., 1995; Fykse and Fonnum, 1996).

The mGluR transmission is much slower and more modulatory in nature. Activation of the mGluR1 results in an increase in intracellular Ca^{2+} concentrations, a direct depolarization of the CA1 pyramidal cells, an increased frequency of spontaneous inhibitory postsynaptic potentials, and an inhibition of synaptic transmission in the CA1 region (Mannaioni et al., 2001). A mGluR5 activation, on the other hand, leads to suppression of the Ca^{2+}-activated K current (I_{AHP}) and a potentiation of NMDA receptor-mediated currents (Jia et al., 1998; Attucci et al., 2001; Mannaioni et al., 2001). The impact of mGluR activation through second messenger systems on neuronal functions and plasticity represents an important research area in signal transduction.

3.2. Synaptic Plasticity

Functional relevance of the glutamate receptors cannot be discussed without mentioning their essentiality for induction of long-term potentiation (LTP) of the synaptic inputs. In 1973, Bliss and Lømo (1973) discovered that a burst of high-frequency electric stimulation of the glutamatergic inputs, including the Schaeffer collateral pathway, induced a lasting enhanced postsynaptic response (about double) to the inputs in the hippocampus. Since the hippocampus is a key region for declarative memory and is involved in memory formation of objects and space (Milner et al., 1998), the results were viewed as cellular equivalence to learning and memory, literally opening the doors to decades of memory research. Glutamatergic synaptic plasticity involves a cooperation of the NR and the AMPA receptors. The depolarization initiated by AMPA receptor activation removes the voltage-dependent Mg^{2+} blockade of the NR and thus activates the NR, whereas expression of the LTP is mediated largely by the AMPA receptors (Benke et al., 1998; Winblad and Poritis, 1999; Soderling and Derkach, 2000). The consistent finding of LTP at these glutamatergic synapses is that LTP cannot be induced if the NRs are blocked (O'Connor et al., 1995). The NMDA receptor proteins are relatively fixed, whereas the AMPA receptor trafficking is controlled by neuronal activity (Bredt and Nicoll, 2003), signaling the synaptic membranes on and off. In the hippocampal CA1 pyramidal cells, from which most of the current understanding of LTP is derived, the NRs are located in the dendritic spine. The central role of NR activation in the initiation of LTP is to provide the Ca^{2+} influx that is needed for evoking the cascade leading to synaptic plasticity.

The role of mGluR in synaptic plasticity is less well studied. AMPA is reported to increase the glucocorticoid-inducible kinase mRNA levels in the rat hippocampus (Lee et al., 2003). In mice lacking mGluR5, hippocampal LTP has been found normal but spatial learning and fear conditioning are both impaired (Lu et al., 1997; Jia et al., 1998).

While correlation between LTP and memory remains controversial, there are reports that enhancing LTP, such as through over-expression NR2B, enhances declarative memory (Han and Stevens, 1999; Tang et al., 1999) and that interruption of LTP through NMDA gene knockout or receptor antagonism impairs spatial memory (Tsien et al., 1996; Mayford and Kandel, 1999; Shimizu et al., 2000; Ekstrom et al., 2001). Ablating the NR gene in CA3 in mice only has also been reported to have normal learning and memory in a full-cue environment but a reduction in memory upon partial cue removal, suggesting an involvement of the recurrent NRs in CA3 in the response (Nakazawa et al., 2002). Others, however, cannot find such correlation (Nosten-Bertrand et al., 1996; Cain, 1998; Zamanillo et al., 1999). An effective blockade of the NRs eliminated LTP but had no effect on spatial learning/memory in rats (Saucier and Cain, 1995). In mice lacking the AMPA receptor subunit GluR-A, CA3-CA1 LTP is absent but water maze spatial memory is not impaired (Zamanillo et al., 1999). In a recent study, rats with an isolated CA1 area, isolated from CA3, show a normal acquisition of a spatial recognition task (Brun et al., 2002), suggesting that the direct entorhinal-CA1 system is sufficient for recollection-based recognition memory and that the CA3-CA1 connection may be required in recall.

LTP is not the only form of synaptic plasticity that depends on functional integrity of the glutamate receptors. Low frequency stimulation (1-3 Hz; 900 stimuli) in the CA1 region of the hippocampus of neonatal rodents (e.g., 12-20 days-old rats) induces a lasting period of depressed postsynaptic response (LTD; Lee et al., 1998; Hendricson et al., 2002). The induction also depends on NR activation (Dudek and Bear, 1992; Mulkey and Malenka, 1992; Hendricson et al., 2002; Mockett et al., 2002; van Dam et al., 2002; but see Bolshakov and Siegelbaum, 1994). Direct brief bath application of NMDA (3 min of 20 μM) in a hippocampal slice has also been reported to produce a postsynaptic, reversible, saturable, and postnatal age-dependent LTD, through dephosphorylation of the GluR1 subunit of the AMPA receptors (Tovar and Westbrook, 2002), or decreased postsynaptic protein kinase C substrate phosphorylation (van Dam et al., 2002). One study shows that the NR-dependent LTD in the hippocampus relies mainly on activation of the receptor population containing the NR2C/D subunits (Hrabetova et al., 2000). The fact that the NR2D subunit expression decreases abruptly during the transition to adulthood in rats (Monyer et al., 1994) may account for the drastic developmental changes in the age-dependent efficacy in LTD induction. At the cerebellar synapses between parallel fibers and Purkinje cells, LTD has been shown to depend on activation of the presynaptic NRs and to require no spatial integration of multiple inputs, since the effect is observed when the input is restricted to a single fiber (Casado et al., 2002).

3.3. Excitotoxic Damage

One of the central mechanisms that relate to a variety of neurodegenerative disorders is the release of an excessive amount of excitatory amino acids into the extracellular space. Excitotoxicity, first described by Olney (Olney, 1969), is characterized by an excessive release of glutamate, which results in neuronal injury, neurodegeneration, and neuronal death and exhibits no specified signal transduction roles. Glutamate excitotoxicity has been implicated as an underlying pathogenic mechanism in cerebral ischemia/hypoxia, amyotrophic lateral sclerosis, Huntington's disease, AD, mood disorders, and Parkinson's disease (Lipton and Rosenberg, 1994; Block and Schwarz 1996; Heintz and Zoghbi, 2000; Ikonomidou et al., 2000; Carpenedo et al., 2002; Hirbec et al., 2002). Over-activation of NR, AMPA receptors, kainate receptors, or mGluR is neurotoxic. The NRs of a depolarized neuron are no longer sensitive to Mg^{2+} blockade. Overexcitation and a lasting increase in intracellular Ca^{2+} concentrations activate a variety of enzymes and triggers apopotosis. The neuronal damage/death in AD appears to mainly depend on NR activation (Greenamyre and Young, 1989). Depression is associated with atrophy and a significantly decreased brain volume centered in the hippocampus. Rat hippocampal neurons exposed to 0.5 mM NMDA for 10 min produced more cytoplasmic vacuolization (a two-fold increase) than in control neurons, a change observed 90 min later (Bown et al., 2003). Neuroprotection from this neurotoxic damage may underlie antidementic and antidepressive pharmacology.

The brains of depressed and AD patients are well known to exhibit reduced cerebral vascular perfusion/metabolism, especially in those neural structures involved in mood regulation and memory. NR activation plays an essential role in neurodegenerative disorders, such as ischemic and traumatic brain injury, because of its high permeability to Ca^{2+}, high affinity for glutamate, and its relative lack of desensitization during prolonged activation (Lipton and Rosenberg, 1994). Acute and chronic insults result in a marked accumulation of glutamate in the extracellular space. Global ischemia, for instance, leads to selective neural damage in the CA1 sector of the hippocampus (Block, 1999), largely through a hypoxic/ischemic switch in favor of the NR-mediated synaptic transmission/Ca^{2+} influx and consequent internal Ca^{2+} release (Belousov et al., 1995). Anoxia/hypoxia is known to induce LTP in the hippocampus (Hammond et al., 1994). The anoxic LTP is mediated exclusively by the NRs (Przegalinski et al., 1997). NR activation also mediates reactive oxygen species-induced pathophysiology in rat hippocampal slices, including epileptiform activity (Avshalumov and Rice, 2002). Lasting stimulation of the NRs (100-500 μM NMDA) has been shown to activate calpain in hippocampal neurons (del Cerro et al., 1994), leading to changed activity of the neural transcription factor NF-κB (see below). The effects of NR agonists on neurological injury would be consistent with evidence that oxidative damage and mitochondrial abnormalities occur early in AD (Hirai et al., 2001).

One important factor mediating oxidative damage and apoptosis is the apoptosis-inducing factor (AIF), whose structure is similar to glutathione peroxidase, a potent scavenger of peroxides in mammalian cells (Mate et al., 2002). AIF is expressed in the hippocampus, dentate gyrus, olfactory bulb, cerebral cortex and various brainstem nuclei. The functions of AIF have been proposed (Klein et al., 2002) as that under normal physiological conditions, it resides in the mitochondrial membrane to act as a free radical scavenger, since mutant cerebellar granule cells are susceptible to exogenous and endogenous peroxide-mediated apoptosis (Klein et al., 2002). Under conditions leading to apoptosis, AIF translocates from the mitochondria, resulting in large-scale DNA fragmentation.

3.4. Gene Transcription

Some of the glutamate-induced effects depend on gene expression, through regulation of nuclear gene transcription factors. Several signaling cascades may be involved, such as the cAMP/Ca^{2+}-responsive element binding protein and NF-κB (Denny et al., 1990; Freudenthal and Romano, 2000; Touyarot et al., 2002; Schölzke et al., 2003; Lamprecht and LeDoux, 2004).

Glutamate activates NF-κB (Guerrini et al., 1995,1997; Kaltschmidt et al., 1995), with a neuronal effect of either pro- or antiapoptosis (Chan and Mattson, 1999; Mattson et al., 2000; Pizzi et al., 2002; Syntichaki et al., 2002; de Erausquin et al., 2003). All three subtypes of iGluR activate NF-κB, while mGluR activation appears to inhibit NF-κB activation in striatal neurons (Wang et al., 1999). NF-κB activation by calpain may mediate long-term effects of glutamate on neuronal survival, memory formation, or death. In primary murine cerebellar granule cells, glutamate (0.3 mM for 20-90 min) induced a rapid reduction of IκBα levels, an endogenous NF-κB inhibitor and a key step in NF-κB activation, and nuclear translocation of the NF-κB subunit p65 (Schölzke et al., 2003). Degradation of IκBα is triggered by phosphorylation of serine-32 and serine-36 by the IκB kinase, with the resulting phosphorylated IκBα being degraded by the proteasome. The glutamate-induced IκBα reduction is blocked by MK-801 (10 μM; Figure 3.1), but not by specific inhibitors of the proteasome, caspase 3, and the phosphoinositide 3-kinase. This is consistent with the evidence that most neurons contain the calpains μ-calpain and m-calpain, which are activated by an increase in the cytosolic Ca^{2+} concentrations and glutamate (Wang, 2000). Calpeptin (10 μM, 30 pretreatment), an inhibitor of the glutamate-activated Ca^{2+}-dependent protease calpain, blocked the IκBα reduction and reduced the nuclear translocation of p65 and glutamate-induced cell death (Schölzke et al., 2003). If glutamate indeed mediates neuronal damage in dementia and depression through activation of the transcription factors as new evidence indicates, removal of the overexcitation through NR antagonism would be an effective strategy to prevent or cure the disorders.

3.5. Aging

Interest has been raised by the gradual replacement of the NR2B subunits in the NRs in the hippocampus by the NR2A subunits with aging, possibly a use-dependent phenomenon (Barria and Malinow, 2002; Loftis et al., 2003). The NR2B subunit is expressed prenatally. Thus, neonatal NRs are more sensitive to ifenprodil (Figure 3.1), an NR2B-selective antagonist, and may be less susceptible to a voltage-dependent Mg^{2+} blockade. A progressively increased expression of NR2A subunits in the NRs alters kinetic properties of the NRs and has been proposed to be responsible for the decreased plasticity in older age.

4. Glutamate Receptor Antagonists

From a therapeutic point of view, blocking glutamate receptors, the NRs and the mGluRs, is suggested for antidepressive and antidementic pharmacology. One exception is the AMPA receptors, whose positive modulators are reported to have antidepressant and antidementic activity, although a direct and potent activation of the AMPA receptors is neurotoxic. Strategies for inhibiting the glutamate receptor-mediated function involve the use of antagonists that block the iGluRs and mGluRs.

4.1. The NRs

Blockade of the NR/complex can be achieved at different sites: the NR glutamate-binding site; the ion channel binding site; the glycine co-agonist site; polyamine binding site; and the redox modulatory site(s).

NR antagonists that block the glutamate-binding site of the NRs include D-2-amino-5-phosphopentanoic acid (AP-5), D-2-amino-7-phosphoheptanoic acid (AP-7), [3-[(±)-carboxypiperazin-4-yl]prop-1-yl]-phosphonic acid (CPP), [3-[(±)-2-carboxypeprazin-4-yl]-propen-1-yl]-phosphonic acid (CPP-ene), LY235959, selfotel ([[(±)-2-carboxypiperidin-4-yl]methyl-4-yl]phosphonic acid, CGS19755), (±)-(E)-2-amino-4-propyl-5-phosphono-pentenoic acid (CGP39653), and CGP-40116. Their activity depends on the length of the molecular chains, which are longer than those of the agonists. Ligands that act at the glutamate or at the glycine-binding site show low selectivity between different subtypes of the receptors (Priestley et al., 1995; Grimwood et al., 1996). These antagonists are potent but will cause significant and unacceptable psychiatric adverse effects, such as paranoia and delirium (Muir and Lees, 1995; Lees, 1997). They are important pharmacological tools. None of them, however, has found clinical usage. Selfotel, a competitive NR antagonist, was terminated during phase III trials because of a trend toward increased mortality (Davis et al., 2000).

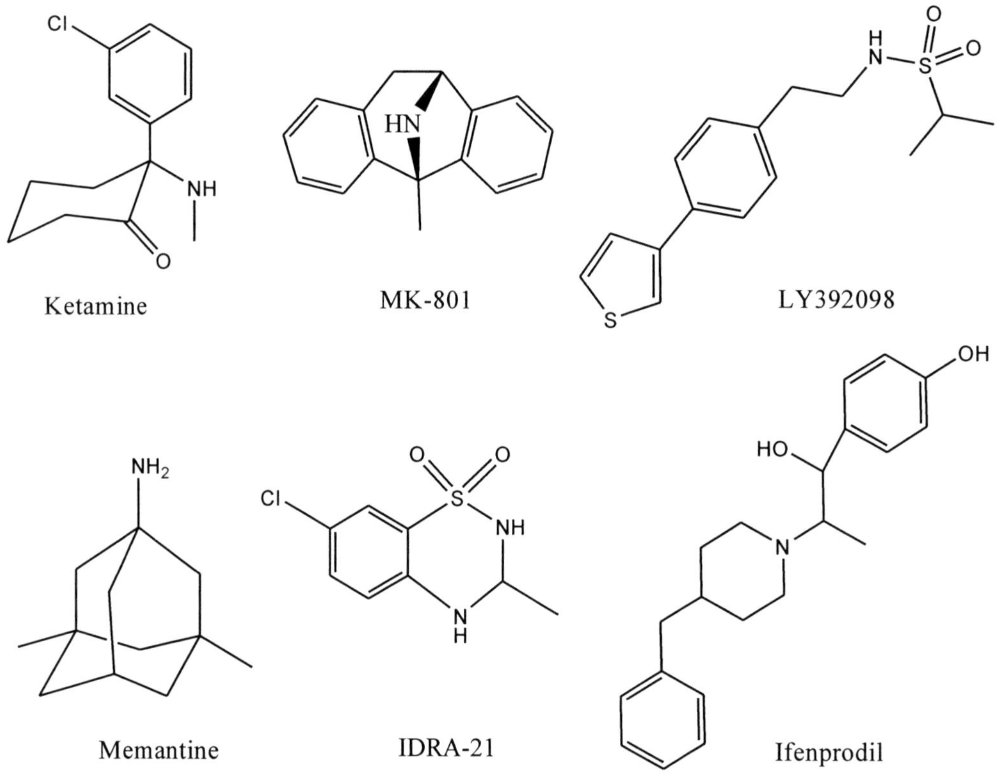

Figure 3.1. Chemical structures of some agents that act on the glutamatergic system and exhibit an antidepressive and/or antidementic action.

A number of structurally diverse compounds, including analogues of phencyclidine (PCP), ketamine (Figure 3.1), dizocilpine (MK-801), dextromethorphan, aptiganel, 3,3-diphenylpropyl-N-glycinamide, memantine (Figure 3.1), remacemide, and N-(2-chloro-5-(methylmercapto) phenyl)-N'-(3-(methylmercapto) phenyl-N'-methylguanidine monohydrochloride (CNS 5161; Walters et al., 2002), are known to act on the ionic channel site (or PCP binding site). NR antagonists that block the channel with high affinity and potency cause significant and unacceptable psychiatric adverse effects (Muir and Lees, 1995; Lees, 1997), while the agents with moderate affinity are better tolerated clinically. N-alkylglycines (such as 3,3-diphenylpropyl-N-glycinamide, inhibition with micromolar affinity, fast on-off kinetics, and strong voltage-dependence) have been found to saturate the blocker-binding site of MK-801 and efficiently prevent excitotoxic neurodegeneration of cerebellar and hippocampal neurons (Planells-Cases et al., 2002). Memantine, a close congener of the antiviral and antiparkinsonian drug amantadine, is a low affinity ion channel blocker of the NR complex, with IC_{50} of about 2 μM (Danysz et al., 1997), as compared with MK-801's 25 nM. It is relatively clinically safe. Analysis of structure-affinity relationships of 1,3,5-alkylsubstituted cyclohexylamines at the NR PCP site shows that they are moderate affinity NR antagonists (Jirgensons et al., 2000).

The NR is unique in that it has an absolute requirement for the presence of glycine for receptor activation. Many different classes of antagonists at the glycine site of the NR have been identified, including 7-cholorokynurenic acid, 5,7-diCl-kynurenic acid, HA-966, gavestinel (GV-150526), licostinel (ACEA-1021), HA966, ACPC, L-701252, and felbamate. For instance, derivatives of 4,6-dichloroindole-2-carboxylic acid are well known as antagonists of the glycine site. A recent study reveals that its hydantoin-substituted compounds at position 3 exhibit higher affinity for the site (Jansen et al., 2003). Thus, secondary amine (NHCH$_2$Ph; substitution at position 3) possesses the lowest affinity, while NHCOPh substitution exhibits 10-times higher affinity than the sulfonamide NHSO$_2$Ph (Jansen et al., 2003). Urea or hydantoin substitution results in compounds with further improved affinity, indicating the importance of a hydrogen bond acceptor function. The advantage of antagonists at the glycine site of the NR is that, unlike the competitive NR antagonists, these antagonists show little psychomimetic side effects and no vacuolization. Gavestinel, an antagonist at the glycine site of the NR, however, has been reported to show no benefits in stroke patients, though without significant adverse effects (Lees et al., 2000).

The polyamines spermine and spermidine are potent positive modulators of the NRs and produce excitotoxic effects in neurons. Antagonists at the site are therefore neuroprotective. Ifenprodil, a phenylethanolamine originally developed as a vasodilating agent based on its activity as a α_1-adrenergic antagonist, is NR2B-selective, binding to the N-terminal LIVBP-like domain of NR2B (Perin-Dureau et al., 2002), but whether its interaction with the polyamine binding site defines its pharmacological action as an NR antagonist remains to be studied (Williams, 2001). Several phenylethanolamines are neuroprotective in both *in vivo* and *in vitro* models of a variety of neurological disorders and lack many of the side effects associated with non-subunit-selective NR antagonists (Kew and Kemp, 1998).

NR2B selective antagonists exhibit a distinct structural requirement in comparison to other NR antagonists. The initial compounds, ifenprodil, haloperidol, and eliprodil, all have a common motif (Nikam and Meltzer, 2002): a tertiary basic amine attached via 2 linkers to 2 aryl rings, respectively; a non-polar ring; and a polar ring. Both the aryl rings seem important with one of the rings being non-polar and the other polar with a hydrogen bond donor. Haloperidol and eliprodil, however, do not have the B-ring hydrogen bond donor. The distance between the two rings is important and could be 9-11 or 17-18 angstroms, with the linkers holding the rings in preferred orientation. Consistent with this finding is the evidence that conformationally constrained linkers in CP-283,097, retain good activity at the NR2B receptor. The second-generation NR2B antagonists (Monyer et al., 1994; Pinard, et al., 2001), such as CP101,606, CP-283,097, and Ro25,6981, are significantly more selective at the receptors.

The redox site is affected by chemical reducing and oxidizing agents. Oxidation may favor disulphide bond formation (S-S) over free thiol (-SH) groups and thus downregulate the channel activity. At least one of the NRs' redox modulatory sites can also be downregulated by nitric oxide (NO) group transfer (defined as S-nitrosylation), which may facilitate disulphide bond formation. This reaction leads to a less NMDA-evoked Ca^{2+} influx and thus neuroprotection. It is blocked by agents that specifically interact with sulfhydryl groups, including N-ethyl-maleimide and methanethiosulfonates such as 2-(trimethylammonium) ethyl methanethiosulfonate and nitroglycerin (Lipton et al., 1998; Le and Lipton, 2001).

There is also a high affinity (nM range) voltage-independent Zn^{2+} site and lower affinity (μM range) voltage-dependent Zn^{2+} site for inhibition (Choi and Lipton, 1999). Zn^{2+} is considered as NR2A-selective, binding on the leucine/isoleucine/valine-binding protein (LIVBP)-like domain of NR2A with high affinity (Paoletti et al., 2000). The NR2A and NR2B subunits are also subject to tyrosine-residue phosphorylation. Phosphorylation of the intracellular, C-terminal tyrosine residues relieves a basal zinc inhibition of NRs (Zheng et al., 1998). Infusion of tyrosine kinases potentiates the current through NR1-NR2A or NR1-NR2B recombinant channels.

Ethanol has a potent and selective effect on NRs (Lovinger et al., 1989), although the exact sites(s) and molecular mechanism(s) by which ethanol inhibits the NRs in the brain have not been identified. Candidates include several NR modulatory sites recognized by glycine, Mg^{2+}, Zn^{2+}, polyamines, and redox agents. Alternatively, it may involve an interaction between ethanol and a hydrophobic region of the NR-channel protein, a region that is exposed to and is only accessible from the extracellular environment (Peoples and Stewart, 2000). There is a report that ethanol has a biphasic action on NMDA-activated currents in hippocampal pyramidal cells. At 2-9 mM, ethanol enhances the NMDA response (Lima-Landman and Albuquerque, 1989). At 10-25 mM, it produces inhibition of NMDA-stimulated Ca^{2+} influx (Hoffman et al., 1989). The NR antagonism is the most consistently reported. Many other behavioral actions of ethanol are produced at such high concentrations, probably via a nonspecific perturbation of neuronal membrane lipids (Hunt, 1985).

4.2. The AMPA Receptors

The AMPA receptors have 3 separate binding sites: the glutamate/AMPA-binding site, a desensitization-binding site, and an intra-ion channel-binding site. Activation of the AMPA-binding site of the AMPA receptors is neurotoxic even when the agonists are applied at low concentrations, limiting their use in behavioral pharmacology. The desensitization-binding site is more interesting, since effects are more of potentiation devoid of neurotoxic side effects (such as aniracetam, cyclothiazide, IDRA-21 (Figure 3.1), or benzylpiperidines). The ion channel can be blocked by compounds such as Joro spider toxin.

4.3. The mGluRs

The importance and contribution of the mGluR activation to mood regulation and cognition have not been well studied. A selective mGluR5 antagonist 2-methyl-6-(phenylethynyl)pyridine has been reported to produce impairments of rat LTP, reference memory, and working memory in an eight-arm radial maze when the agent is i.c.v. administered (Naie and Manahan-Vaughan, 2004). Activation of the group II mGluRs with an mGluR 2/3 agonist, aminopyrrolidine dicarboxylate has also been shown to decrease performance on a working memory task, an effect blocked by the mGluR 2/3 antagonist LY341494 (Aultman and Moghaddam 2001; Gregory et al., 2003).

5. Pharmacological Actions of Glutamate Receptor Antagonists

Glutamate is involved in a variety of brain functions and neural disorders. Thus, the potential therapeutic application of agents acting on the GluRs is enormous. Preclinical studies have in fact provided evidence that NR antagonists have therapeutic potential to treat stroke, AD, epilepsy, traumatic brain injury, Parkinson's disease, Huntington's disease, tardive dyskinesias (Richter and Löscher, 1998; but see Richter, 2003), nociception, anxiety and depression (Sanacora et al., 2003). The limitation to their clinical application is their severe side effects, including impact on respiratory and cardiovascular control, perceptual disturbances, hallucinations, possible cognitive and motor deficits, and neuronal cell death. However, the tremendous therapeutic promise of agents that act on the glutamate system is still a major impetus to develop effective compounds that lack these side effects.

5.1. Enhancing Monoaminergic Transmission

Blocking the NR results in an enhanced monoaminergic transmission (Yan et al., 1997), an action fundamental to the antidepressant effects of various NR antagonists. For example, in the raphe nucleus, activation of the NRs induces inhibitory postsynaptic currents (Jolas and Aghajanian, 1997). Blocking the NRs increases raphe neural activity (Lejeune et al., 1994) and 5-HT release, as measured with microdialysis in the medial prefrontal cortex and dorsal hippocampus (Martin et al., 1998). In mice, blocking NR function has also been reported to increase monoamine activity (Miyamoto et al., 2001).

5.2. Blocking Excitotoxicity

It is generally believed that the NRs play a major role in neurotoxicity, due to their high Ca^{2+} permeability. Blocking the GluRs generally, and blocking the NRs specially, makes a fundamental difference with regard to neuronal survival and functions when facing insult. The NRs have been therefore considered prime therapeutic targets for the development of useful neuroprotective strategies. The protective action has been shown in a variety of preparations *in vitro* and *in vivo*. Several NR antagonists have been reported to show antidepressive and/or antidementic activity (see below). Dextromethorphan, an antagonist at the NR, administered 20 min before global ischemia (4VO for 20 min in rats) and on day 1, 3, and 5 after, significantly reduces functional deficits in Morris water maze performance and CA1 neuronal damage (Block and Schwarz, 1996). Consistent with these findings is the evidence that facilitating kynurenine metabolism toward formation of kynurenic acid, an endogenous iGluR antagonist, reduces ischemic cell death in organotypic hippocampal slices (Carpenedo et al., 2002). The success of pharmacology based on NR antagonism depends on whether the agents are able to target overactivated receptors without arresting synaptic transmission. Drugs such as MK-801 and PCP are nanomolar affinity open channel blockers that efficiently protect neurons but possess significant side effects. Submicromolar affinity blockers such as memantine have a better therapeutic profile (see below).

5.3. Blocking Neuronal Amyloid Uptake

NR antagonists are found to be able to protect neurons from neurodegenerative damage. One underlying mechanism is the involvement of NR activation in neuronal uptake of neurotoxic amyloid β peptide (Aβ). Evidence has been provided that NR activation stimulates APP processing to produce Aβ (Gordon-Krajcer et al., 2002). Aβ formation and aggregation characterize one of the major pathophysiological features of the AD brain and its uptake into neurons is known to be an essential step in triggering intracellular neurofibrillary tangles. Blocking the NRs thus reduces $Aβ_{1-42}$ uptake and the pathogenic changes of hippocampal neurons (Bi et al., 2002). In rat nucleus basalis, blocking the NRs with MK-801 has been reported to antagonize Aβ neurotoxicity: delayed cell death and loss of cholinergic fiber projections to the neocortex (Harkany et al., 2000). These observations are consistent with the evidence that senile plaques are known to increase the neurotoxic effects of glutamate *in vivo* and *in vitro* (Koh et al., 1990; Kowall et al., 1991).

6. Antidepressive and Antidementic Effects of Glutamate Receptor Modulators/Antagonists

Glutamatergic transmission is involved in signal processing in mood regulation and memory consolidation (Day et al., 2003) and is damaged in depression and AD. Excitotoxicity, due to excessive release of glutamate leading to over-excitation of neurons and neuronal injury and death, is the basis for pharmacology of glutamate receptor antagonists. Excitotoxicity is involved in the development of mood disorders and memory impairments. Blocking the NRs produces antidepressive and antidementia effects in various experimental studies and clinical trials. This strategy would suggest that a common excitotoxicity, though at a different network, is mostly responsible for the abnormal neural control of mood and memory functions and is supported by clinical and experimental observations. One benefit of these compounds is their unique profile of rapid onset of antidepressive effects (Krystal et al., 2002).

In a majority of the cases, antagonists for the iGluRs and the mGluRs have antidepressive and antidemetic action. However, evidence suggests that positive allosteric modulators of the AMPA receptors are effective in antidepressant action in animal models (Li et al., 2001; Skolnick et al., 2001; Quirk and Nisenbaum, 2002). Similar agents have also been shown to enhance some aspects of memory in humans (Ingvar et al., 1997; Lynch et al., 1997).

6.1. Antidepressant Therapy

Glutamate neurotransmission plays an important role in depression and antidepressant activity of monoamine antidepressants (Paul and Skolnick, 2003). Exposure to inescapable stress is known to increase glutamate release (Gilad et al., 1990; Moghaddam, 1993). NR abnormalities are observed in human major depressives (Law and Deakin 2001) and suicide victims (Nowak et al., 1995).

The involvement of NRs in mood regulation and abnormality is suggested by the observations that successful chronic antidepressant treatments alter NR binding (Skolnick, 1999; Petrie et al., 2000). Evidence has been provided that some antidepressant drugs either inhibit NR binding (Reynolds and Miller, 1988), change NR binding properties, or modulate the release or reuptake of glutamate (Paul and Skolnick, 2003). Fluoxetine, an effective SSRI, decreases glutamate exocytosis (Wang et al., 2003). It remains to be determined, however, whether this is part of the action underlying its antidepressive effect.

Agents that are related to glutamate neurotransmission and that have been shown to exhibit antidepressant activity include NR antagonists, group I mGluR antagonists, and positive modulators of AMPA receptors. In early observations, D-cycloserine, an antibiotic developed to treat tuberculosis with NR glycine-binding site partial antagonist profile, although not known at the time, was reported to exhibit antidepressant effects in a high proportion of the depressed tuberculoiss patients (Crane, 1959, 1961). MK-801 has been found effective in animal tests used to detect antidepressant properties (Trullas and Skolnick, 1990; Maj et al., 1992). Chronic MK-801 treatment reverses deficit in rewarded behavior (anhedonia), a decrease in sucrose consumption, in mildly stressed rats (Papp and Moryl, 1993). Amantadine, initially developed as an antiviral agent but with a low-affinity uncompetitive NR antagonist, has antidepressant effects (Parkes et al., 1970; Vale et al., 1971; Huber et a., 1999). Since then, NR antagonists for various NR subtypes have been found to have antidepressant effects (Skolnick, 1999; Berman et al., 2000; Petrie et al., 2000; Stewart and Reid, 2002; Sun and Alkon, 2002a; Zomkowski et al., 2002), including competitive and non-competitive NR antagonists (Trullas and Skolnick, 1990; Maj et al., 1992; Przegalinski et al., 1997; Berman et al., 2000). For instance, significant improvement in depressive symptoms is observed in depressive patients, within 72 hours after i.v.

administration of ketamine hydrochloride (0.5 mg/kg Berman et al., 2000). The use of ketamine anesthesia in depressed patients undergoing orthopedic surgery was reported to produce a prolonged antidepressant effect (Koduh et al., 2002), consistent with the observation in an animal model of depression (Yilmaz et al., 2002). These agents are generally found to exhibit no effects on locomotor activity while producing antidepressant effects. This specificity of action is important because it is generally accepted that general behavioral stimulants, such as various dopamine stimulants at doses that increase locomotor or exploratory activity, can induce false positive effects in the forced swimming test, the leading animal model of depression. However, the apparent antidepressant action of NMDA receptor antagonists is reported to be a false-positive effect caused by dopamine-related motor-stimulant activity (Panconi et al., 1993). Activation of the NRs in the ventral, but not in the dorsal, hippocampus has been shown to increase locomotor activity (Zhang et al., 2002a). I.c.v. administration of agmatine, has also been found to reduce the immobility in the forced swimming test and to significantly enhance the antidepressant effect of imipramine, while its mechanisms may involve an interaction with NRs, NO, and α_2-adrenoceptors (Zomkowski et al., 2002). Similarly, there is also evidence that co-administration of NR antagonists (such as memantine, 2.5 and 5 mg/kg) with traditional antidepressants produces a greater antidepressant effect in the rat forced swimming test, without increasing locomotor activity significantly (Rogóż et al., 2002). Riluzole, an agent with antiglutamatergic properties (MacIver et al., 1996), has been reported to exhibit antidepressant activity (Zarate et al., 2002, 2004; Coric et al., 2003).

Severe mood disorders are associated with impairments of structural plasticity (Zarate et al., 2002). The plasticity enhancing strategies include NR antagonists and glutamate release-reducing agents. Thus, AMPA receptor potentiator LY392098 (Figure 3.1) has been reported to produce an antidepressant-like effect in rats and mice (Li et al., 2001).

Chronic antidepressant treatment also alters the mGluR groups I, II, and III (Pilc and Legutko, 1995; Pilc et al., 1998). mGluR2/3 (and group III) receptor agonists are able to modulate 5-HT$_{2A}$ receptors (Marek and Aghajanian, 1998; Aghajanian and Marek, 2000), a potential target in mood pharmacology. The mGluR II/III agonists have preclinical antianxiety, antipsychotic, and neuroprotectant properties (Schoepp, 2001) and both agonists and antagonists indirectly affect serotonin neurotransmission (Marek et al., 2000).

6.2. Antidementia Therapy

Although AD has been the major focus of dementia, the dementia discussed here includes other memory disorders as well as those in aging. This makes sense, since few cases diagnosed using clinical criteria do not have some evidence of mixed pathology (Holmes et al., 1999).

The AD brain is characterized by a gradual deposit of amyloid plaques and neurofibrillary tangles. It takes 3.4 years on average for an intact neuron affected by neurofibrillary pathology to become a ghost tangle (Bobinski et al., 1998). What is important is that neural damage occurs before the amyloid deposit and tangle formation. Synaptic function, especially those in the hippocampus, is sensitive to neurotoxic amyloid (Sun and Alkon, 2002b). The underlying mechanisms, evoked by soluble amyloid and/or related pathological factors, are mediated by excitotoxic agents and oxidative species. The current AD drug developments are focused on 4 fronts: eliminating amyloid deposition; blocking abnormal phosphorylation of τ protein; reducing the amyloid-induced oxidative stress and inflammatory response; and restoring the impaired neurotransmission and network. Neuronal uptake of neurotoxic amyloid represents an important pathogenic step in AD neurodegenerative disorders and is mediated by NR activation. Blocking the NRs, thus, may offer a neuroprotective mechanism, since the blockade reduces amyloid uptake. A combined therapy including NR antagonists and agents that reduce the amyloid production and/or remove amyloid (DeMattos et al., 2002; Matsuoka et al., 2003) may form a better therapeutic strategy. In cultured hippocampal slices, NR antagonism completely blocks internalization of $A\beta_{1-42}$ and pathogenic effects (Bi et al., 2002). In animal AD models of dementia, treatment with MK-801 analogs has been found to dramatically improve learning ability and memory in the active avoidance test and Morris water maze test (Bachurin et al., 2001). In addition to the effects of NR antagonism on amyloid pathology, NR antagonism has been shown to increase production of new granule neurons in the aged rat hippocampus (Nacher et al., 2003). However, it has not been established how important neurogenesis is in learning and memory. Nevertheless, the therapeutic value of NR antagonism on AD dementia would suggest an involvement of some common pathophysiologcal cascades in a variety of neurodegenerative disorders. It is not surprising that other types of dementia share many pathological features of AD dementia. For instance, it is well established that $A\beta$ and amyloid angiopathy result in vascular hypoperfusion and release of excitatory amino acids (Cacabelos et al., 1999; Sun and Alkon, 2001).

Another major type of dementia is stroke and stroke-related dementia, including ischemic or vascular dementia (Sun et al., 2002a). Stroke is the third most common cause of death from human diseases and accounts for the loss of 175,000 lives in US each year (Brott and Bogousslavsky, 2000). The ischemic damage is mainly mediated by excitotoxic injury, caused by the excitatory amino acids. Because of the extreme sensitivity of the memory-related neural structures, such as the hippocampus, to ischemia and hypoxia, dementia is the major consequent symptom in those who survived stroke episodes and in ischemic patients. Blocking the NRs, especially when the antagonists are applied before the ischemia, effectively ameliorates the deficits in spatial learning and memory induced by global ischemia (Block, 1999). Thus, pretreatment with ketamine dramatically reduces the cytochrome c release from the mitochondria and increased expression of procaspase-3 in rat hippocampal cells induced by 15 min global ischemia (Zhang et al., 2002b). SM-31900, an NR glycine-binding site antagonist, has been found to reduce infarct volume induced by permanent middle cerebral artery occlusion in rats, when administered even 60 min after the onset of ischemia (Ohtani et al., 2003). Postischemic MK-801, a potent non-competitive NR antagonist, has also been shown to improve the spatial performance of ischemic rats (Rod et al., 1990).

Nonselective NR antagonists with high affinity are the most consistently neuroprotective agents in animal models of stroke, but clinical trials in stroke and traumatic brain injury with these NR antagonists have so far mostly failed. The problem is not that the NR antagonists do not work in humans but that the levels of drugs achieved in humans have been consistently below those needed for maximal neuroprotection in animal models. The limitation for achieving higher levels of the drugs in humans is a number of adverse effects, including hallucinations, a central nervous system-mediated increase in blood pressure, and at high doses, catatonia and anesthesia. Some clinical trials using NR antagonists have been aborted due to their severe psychomimetic adverse effects. However, use-dependent antagonists with moderate/low affinity appear clinically safer: such as memantine and nitroglycerine (Lipton et al., 1994; Lipton et al., 1998; Winblad and Poritis, 1999; Le and Lipton, 2001; Danysz and Parsons, 2003). Nitroglycerine acts through NO release to down-regulate NR activation through S-nitrosylation but occasionally causes syncope due to hypotension and bradycardia (Melenovsky et al., 2002). Clinically, 10 weeks of D-cycloserine have been found to provide mild benefits in improving the implicit memory of AD patients (Schwartz et al., 1996). Memantine, a low-affinity voltage-dependent NR antagonist at the open channel site (with K_i of 0.54 µM for replacing [^{3}H]MK-801 binding from postmorten human brain; Kornhuber and Weller, 1997), has been tried in all forms of dementia and shown to improve memory in moderate-to-severe and severe dementia (Winblad and Poritis, 1999; Le and Lipton, 2001; Helmuth, 2002; Orgogozo et al., 2002; Reisberg et al., 2003; Rogawski and Wenk, 2003). Unlike MK-801, which causes a progressive use-dependent accumulation of block leading to a complete inhibition, memantine does not accumulate in the pore. With a daily maintenance dose of 20 mg in humans, the serum levels of memantine are within the range of 0.5 to 1.0 µM, only minimally inhibiting the NR channel conductance and leaving some NR-mediated synaptic transmission. Unlike cholinesterase inhibitors, memantine is likely to show neuroprotective effects and to slow down disease progression. Some of the mechanisms underlying memantine effects may include an induction of brain-derived neurotrophic factor and trkB receptor expression (Marvanová et al., 2001). The moderate/low affinity antagonists may allow neurons to maintain critical Ca^{2+} homeostasis, thus a safer side effect profile.

Positive modulators of the AMPA receptor are reported to enhance memory performance. For instance, oral IDRA-21 (0.15 – 10 mg/kg), an agent that inhibits the rate of desensitization of the AMPA receptor during prolonged exposure to competitive agonists, improves the performance of a delayed matching-to-sample task by young adult rhesus monkeys and task accuracy in aged monkeys (Buccafusco et al., 2004).

7. Adverse and Toxic Effects

The glutamate receptor pharmacology is characterized by a balance of the receptor antagonists and side effects. Many of the antagonists can easily achieve a complete blockade of the receptors but have no clinical usefulness because of severe side effects associated with such an effective blockade. Because glutamatergic transmission represents the most predominant excitatory neurotransmitter in the brain, a general blockade of its receptors may induce a variety of adverse effects or side effects, depending on the doses applied and the agents used. For instance, although most of the NR antagonists effectively reduce glutamate neurotoxicity *in vitro*, their *in vivo* utility has been heavily questioned due to serious side effects at clinically effective doses. In humans, antagonists at glutamate or glycine site are less selective to the receptors and produce more profound side effects, including light-headedness, dizziness, paresthesia, and agitation at low doses, nystagmus, hallucinations, somnolence, and blood pressure increases at moderate doses, and catatonia and "dissociative anesthesia" at high doses. Some of the adverse side effects of NR antagonists may result from their pharmacological profile such as impact on arousal or release of other neurotransmitters. Ketamine and MK-801 are known to decrease acetylcholine release in the pontine reticular formation, resulting in alterations in breath and disruption of sleep (Lydic et al., 2002). PCP intoxication, for example, induces psychomimetic responses and repetitive motor movements including rocking and head shaking from side to side (Breese et al., 2002). The general assumption is that to maximize therapeutic effects and minimize adverse effects of the NR antagonists in antidepressive and antidementic therapies, the antagonists should target over-excitation, but avoid the normal synaptic transmission, although the mechanisms involved in the pathophysiology of depression and dementia and in pharmacological therapy are undefined.

Competitive or potent non-competitive antagonists at the NR or glycine co-agonist binding sites have the most severe adverse effects because of a powerful blockade of the normal synaptic transmission, occurring at low agonist concentrations. To block the pathophysiological excitotoxicity that occurs at high concentrations of the agonists, these potent antagonists would eliminate the normal synaptic transmission. They may therefore have no clinical value as therapeutic agents in depression and dementia. But they are the most potent in the receptor blockade and their short-term acute value in stroke therapy may deserve further evaluation. In addition, their impact on basal and chemoreflex control of cardiovascular and respiratory systems needs careful monitoring (Sun, 1995; Sun and Reis, 1995; Sun, 1996; Sun and Reis, 1996). For instance, CNS 5161 has an effective NR antagonism with ED_{80} against necrotic effects of NMDA of 4 mg/kg in neonatal rats (Hu et al., 1997). Small doses are well tolerated in healthy volunteers, while an arterial blood pressure increase becomes obviously too severe when the dose reaches 2 mg/kg (i.v.) (Walters et al., 2002).

Because of differentiation in the NR subunit expression in different brain areas and developmental stages, antagonists that are selective for a particular subunit represents attractive compounds to dramatically reduce potential side effects. For instance, many of the severe side effects that limit effective therapeutic application of the potent and competitive and non-competitive NR antagonists can be traced to their blockade of the NR1/NR2A, which is widely expressed in the adult mammal. The NR2B, on the other hand, is expressed in the forebrain, including the cortex, striatum, and hippocampus, areas that are most severely affected by neurotoxicity in neurodegenerative disorders. Thus, targeting the NR2B appears to provide optimal therapeutic benefit without inducing side effects that are associated with blocking other NR subunits. There are indeed reports that selective blockade of the NR subunits may have distinct pharmacological properties. For instance, conantokin-G and ifenprodil, NR2B subunit-selective NR antagonists, are reported to significantly increase the survival rate in primary rat forebrain cultures against staurosporin-induced apoptosis, while the non-selective NR antagonist dizocilpine does not (Williams et al., 2002).

In a similar vein, weak and/or partial antagonists, especially those antagonists acting on the open channels, would have fewer adverse effects. The relative blockade of the physiological and pathophysiological response would depend on their relative extent, favoring an antagonism of the overwhelming NR over-activation. A weak blockade of the physiological response would also leave the door open for an easier compensation by the neural mechanisms to minimize impact due to interruption of vital functions by the agents. In view of the suggestion that affinity for the NR2A subunit is responsible for the severe side effects, another possibility that might be related to a better safety profile of the low-affinity antagonists is to develop antagonists that display less inhibition of the NR1/NR2A receptor subtypes and more preferential affinities for the NR1/NR2C,D subtypes (Gregory et al., 2000; Palmer, 2001), as discussed above.

Chronic NR antagonist administration (14 days) is likely to result in an up-regulated expression in the hippocampus of genes for mitogen-activated protein kinase (MAP kinase 1), proteosome subunit β precursor, protein kinase C B-I and B-II types, mGluR2, and acetylcholinesterase; and a down-regulated expression of genes for NR1, adenosine A1 receptor, preprolactin (O'Donneli et al., 2003). The impact of such alterations needs further evaluation.

8. Concluding Remarks

Targeting glutamatergic neurotransmission is a highly sophisticated matter due to the ambiguous functions of glutamate in physiological and pathophysiological conditions. The balance between blocking excitotoxicity and allowing some glutamatergic neurotransmission is a critical one. Such a balance needs to be worked out in several additional fronts. AMPA receptor agonists or positive modulators are reported to have beneficial effects. But, more research is needed to evaluate the potential neurotoxic influence of enhancing glutamate transmission. Indeed, AMPA receptor antagonists have been reported to be neuroprotective (Weiser, 2002). Similarly, NR antagonists have been proposed and tested to improve cognition, while NR2B subunit overexpression has been shown to exhibit better learning and memory (Tang et al., 1999). Transfection of the wild-type serum and glucocorticoid-inducible kinase gene has been reported to enhance spatial learning (Tsai et al., 2002), while glucorticoid is believed to underlie stress-mediated hippocampal atrophy and impairments of mood and cognition, including spatial learning deficits. In addition, although the slower onset of clinical antidepressant effects and antidepressive action of Brain-derived neurotrophic factor (BDNF) would suggest a crucial role of neuroprotection/neurogenesis in antidepressive pharmacology, the evidence that patients successively treated with SSRIs show a rapid depressive relapse following tryptophan depletion diets (Aberg-Wistedt et al., 1998; Delgado et al., 1991,1999) suggests that the involvement of monoamine transmission in mood regulation, pathogenesis, and pharmacology cannot be ruled out.

Cholinesterase inhibitors are the antidementic drugs clinically available for AD, have limited success in relieving symptoms temporally, but do not slow the decline of the disorder. Targeting the underlying pathogenic mechanisms would lead to better medications. Nevertheless, the search for better agents has led to a rich pharmacology and a number of promising candidates for the treatment of behavioral and cognitive disorders. Several lines of evidence suggest that antidementic and antidepressive treatments can be achieved through NR antagonism, by using effective NR antagonists with fewer and less severe side effects. Ifenprodil (NR2B subtype-selective NR antagonist) and memantine, for instance, show promise to adequately separate antidementia and antidepressant effects from unacceptable side effects. Memantine has been reported to produce behavioral improvement across a number of dimensions in patients with AD (Ambrozi and Danielczyk, 1988; Gortelmeyer and Erbler, 1992). Ifenprodil has also high affinities for α_1-adrenoceptors and serotonin receptors (Nikam and Meltzer, 2002). Newer NR2B-selective compounds (CP-10606, Ro256981, and CI1041) seem better tolerated than ifenprodil and eliprodil in initial studies. Ro-256981, though, still causes cardiovascular side effects and has an antagonistic action at the α_1-adrenoceptors with K_i of 0.18 μM (Pinard et al., 2001). More selective compounds might yield effective agents with fewer side effects in the near future. Another question is whether targeting the NR2B subunit would selectively impair memory, since mice that overexpress the NR2B subunit have been reported to exhibit superior ability in performing learning and memory tasks (Doyle et al., 1998; Tang et al., 1999).

One possibility to achieve effective NR blockade without severe side effects is to target intracellular signal cascades of NR activation, such as PSD-95, although such agents would not be viewed as NR antagonists. Interruption of the NR-PSD-95 interaction may represent an effective therapeutic strategy in ischemic therapy without blocking synaptic activity and Ca^{2+} influx (Aarts et al., 2002). PSD-95 appears to play an important role in maturation of excitatory synapses (El-Husseini et al., 2000), synaptic plasticity (Migaud et al., 1998) probably through an activity-dependent palmitate cycling on PSD-95 (El-Husseini et al., 2002), and ischemic brain damage (Aarts et al., 2002). Through its second PDZ domain (PDZ2), PSD-95 binds the COOH-terminus tSXV motif of NR2 subunits as well as neuronal NOS. PSD-95 causes a reduction in the NR/channel gating (Rutter et al., 2002). Mutant mice lacking PSD-95 have been reported to exhibit enhanced CA1 LTP and impaired water maze spatial learning and memory (Migaud et al., 1998), while PSD-95 over-expression has been found to enhance the probability of observing long-term depression (Beique and Andrade, 2003). In general, however, NR activity is unaffected by genetically disrupting PSD-95 in vivo (Migaud et al., 1998) or by suppressing its expression in vitro (Sattler et al., 1999). PSD-95 deletion or interruption of the NR-PSD-95 interaction dissociates NR activity from NO production and suppresses excitotoxicity (Sattler et al., 1999; Aarts et al., 2002). The neuroprotection against ischemic damage in rats is effective *in vitro* and *in vivo* 1 hour after the insult (Aarts et al., 2002). However, others have reported that PSD-deficiency induces significant neuronal cell death within 24 hours, both in primary hippocampal neurons and in organotypic hippocampal slices (Gardoni et al., 2002).

Current antidepressants are sub-optimal, since many patients do not respond to the antidepressants available, some drugs cause side effects that are intolerable in some patients, and the antidepressant medications are better viewed as ways to relieving symptoms rather than curing the disease. Evidence supporting an antidepressant effect of NR antagonists is enormous. Development of NR antagonists may also lead to new antidepressants, especially those having a faster onset of action and effective in cases un-responsive to current antidepressants. Several agents that affect glutamate neurotransmission appear to possess such profiles. The main problem limiting the use of NR antagonists as clinical antidepressants and antidementia drugs is their adverse effects that cannot be tolerated clinically. However, as detailed molecular and physiological properties of the NR-channel complex and pharmacological properties of the antagonists become evident (Patankar and Jurs, 2002), perhaps, the next generation of compounds will finally realize their full clinical potential.

References

Aarts M, Liu Y, Liu L, Besshoh S, Arundine M, Gurd JW, Wang Y-T, Salter MW, Tymianski M. Treatment of ischemic brain damage by perturbing NMDA receptor-PSD-95 protein interactions. *Science* **298**: 846-850, 2002.

Aberg-Wistedt A, Hasselmark L, Stain-Malmgren R, Aperia B, Kjellman BF, Mathe AA. Serotonergic 'vulnerability' in affective disorder: A study of the tryptophan depletion test and relationships between peripheral and central serotonin indexes in citalopram-responders. *Acta Psychistr Scand* **97**: 374-380, 1998.

Aghajanian GK, Marek GJ. Serotonin model of schizophrenia: emerging role of glutamate mechanisms. *Brain Res Brain Res Rev* **31**: 302-312, 2000.

Ambrozi, L., Danielczyk, W. Treatment of impaired cerebral function in psychogeriatric patients with memantine – results of a phase II double-blind study. *Pharmacopsychiatry* **21**: 144-146, 1988.

Attucci S, Carla V, Mannaioni G, Moroni F. Activation of type 5 metabotropic glutamate receptors enhances NMDA responses in mice cortical wedges. *Br J Pharmacol* **132**: 799-806, 2001.

Aultman JM, Moghaddam B. Distinct contribution of glutamate and dopamine receptors to temporal aspects of rodent working memory using a clinically relevant task. *Psychopharmacology* **153**: 353-364, 2001.

Avshalumov MV, Rice ME. NMDA receptor activation mediates hydrogen peroxide-induced pathophysiology in rat hippocampal slices. *J Neurophysiol* **87**: 2896-2903, 2002.

Bachurin S, Tkachenko S, Baskin I, Lermontova N, Mukhina T, Petrova L, Ustinov A, Proshin A, Grigoriev V, Lukoyanov N, Palyulin V, Zefirov N. Neuroprotective and cognition-enhancing properties of MK-801 flexible analog. Structure-activity relationships. *Ann New York Acad Sci* **939**: 219-236, 2001.

Barria A, Malinow R. Subunit-specific NMDA receptor trafficking to synapses. *Neuron* **35**: 345-353, 2002.

Beique JC, Andrade R. PSD-95 regulates synaptic transmission and plasticity in rat cerebral cortex. *J Physiol (Lond)* **546**: 859-867, 2003.

Bekkers JM, Stevens CF. NMDA and non-NMDA receptors are co-localized at individual excitatory synapses in cultured rat hippocampus. *Nature* **341**: 230-233, 1989.

Belousov AB, Godfraind J-M, Krnjević K. Internal Ca^{2+} stores involved in anoxic responses of rat hippocampal neurons. *J Physiol* **486**: 547-556, 1995.

Benke TA, Lüthi A, Isaac JTR, Collingridge GL. Modulation of AMMPA receptor unitary conductance by synaptic activity. *Nature* **393**: 793-797, 1998.

Benveniste M, Mayer ML. Structure-activity analysis of binding kinetics for NMDA receptor competitive antagonists: the influence of conformational restriction. *Biophysical J* **59**: 560-573, 1991.

Berman RM, Cappiello A, Anand A, Oren DA, Heninger GR, Charney DS, Krystal JH. Antidepressant effects of ketamine in depressed patients. *Biol Psychiatry* **47**: 351-354, 2000.

Bi X, Gall CM, Zhou J, Lynch G. Uptake and pathogenic effects of amyloid beta 1-42 are enhanced by integrin antagonists and blocked by NMDA receptor antagonists. *Neuroscience* **112**: 827-840, 2002.

Bliss TV, Lømo T. Long-lasting potentiation of synaptic transmission in the dentate area of the anaesthetized rabbit following stimulation of the perforant path. *J Physiol* **232**: 331-356, 1973.

Block F. Global ischemia and behavioral deficits. *Prog Neurobiol* **58**: 279-295, 1999.

Block F, Schwarz M. Dextromethorphan reduces functional deficits and neuronal damage after global ischemia in rats. *Brain Res* **741**: 153-159, 1996.

Bobinski M, Wegiel J, Tarnawski M, Bobinski M, de Leon M, Reisberg B, Miller DC, Wisniewski HM. Duration of neurofibrillary changes in the hippocampal pyramidal neurons. *Brain Res* **799**: 156-158, 1998.

Bolshakov VY, Siegelbaum SA. Postsynaptic induction and presynaptic expression of hippocampal long-term depression. *Science* **264**: 1148-, 1994.

Bown CD, Wang JF, Young LT. Attenuation of *N*-methyl-D-aspartate-mediated cytoplasmic vacuolization in primary rat hippocampal neurons by mood stabilizers. *Neuroscience* **117**: 949-955, 2003.

Bredt DS, Nicoll RA. AMPA receptor trafficking at excitatory synapses. *Neuron* **40**: 361-379, 2003.

Breese GR, Knapp DJ, Moy SS. Integrative role for serotonergic and glutamatergic receptor mechanisms in the action of NMDA antagonists: potential relationships to antipsychotic drug actions on NMDA antagonist responsiveness. *Neurosci Biobehav Rev* **26**: 441-455, 2002.

Brott T, Bogousslavsky J. Treatment of acute ischemic stroke. *N Eng J Med* **343**: 710-722, 2000.

Brown MS, Ye J, Rawson RB, Goldstein JL. Regulated intramembrane proteolysis: a control mechanism conserved from bacteria to humans. *Cell* **100**: 391-398, 2000.

Brun VH, Otnæss MK, Molden S, Steffenach H-A, Witter MP, Moser M-B, Moser EI. Place cells and place recognition maintained by direct entorhinal-hippocampal circuitry. *Science* **296**: 2243-2246, 2002.

Buccafusco JJ, Weiser T, Winter K, Klinder K, Terry AV Jr. The Effects of IDRA 21, a positive modulator of the AMPA receptor, on delayed matching performance by young and aged rhesus monkeys. *Neuropharmacology* **46**: 10-22, 2004.

Cacabelos R, Takeda M, Winblad B. The glutamatergic system and neurodegeneration in dementia: preventive strategies in Alzheimer's disease. *Int J Geriatr Psychiatry* **14**: 3-47, 1999.

Cain DP. Testing the NMDA, long –term potentiation, and cholinergic hypothesis of spatial learning. *Neurosci Biobehav Rev* **22**: 181-193, 1998.

Carpenedo R, Meli E, Peruginelli F, Pellegrini-Giampietro DE, Moroni F. Kynurenine 3-mono-oxygenase inhibitors attenuate post-ischemic neuronal death in organotypic hippocampal slice cultures. *J Neurochem* **82**: 1465-1471, 2002.

Casado M, Isope P, Ascher P. Involvement of presynaptic N-methyl-D-aspartate receptors in cerebellar long-term depression. *Neuron* **33**: 123-130, 2002.

Caspi A, Sugden K, Moffitt TE, Tyalor A, Craig IW, Harrington H, McClay J, Mill J, Martin J, Braithwaite A, Poulton R. Influence of life stress on depression: moderation by a polymorphism in the 5-HTT gene. *Science* **301**: 386-389, 2003.

Chatterton JE, Awobuluyi M, Premkumar LS, Takahashi H, Talantova M, Shin Y, Cui J, Tu S, Sevarino KA, Nakanishi N, Tong G, Lipton SA, Zhang D. Excitatory glycine receptors containing the NR3 family of NMDA receptor subunits. *Nature* **415**: 793-798, 2002.

Chan SL, Mattson MP. Caspase and calpain substrates: roles in synaptic plasticity and cell death. *J Neurosci Res* **58**: 167-190, 1999.

Chizh BA, Headley PM, Tzschentke TM. NMDA receptor antagonists as analgesics: focus on the NR2B subtype. *Trends Pharmacol Sci* **22**: 636-642, 2001.

Choi Y-B, Lipton SA. Identification and mechanism of action of two histidine residues underlying high-affinity Zn^{2+} inhibition of the NMDA receptor. *Neuron* **23**: 171-180, 1999.

Clements JD, Westbrook GL. Activation kinetics reveal the number of glutamate and glycine bonding sites on the *N*-methyl-D-aspartate receptor. *Neuron* **7**: 605-613, 1991.

Collingridge GL, Lester RA. Excitatory amino acids receptors in the vertebrate central nervous system. *Pharmacol Rev* **41**: 143-210, 1989.

Coric V, Milanovic S, Wasylink S, Patel P, Malison R, Krystal JH. Beneficial effects of the antiglutamatergic agent riluzole in a patient diagnosed with obsessive-compulsive disorder and major depressive disorder. *Psychopharmacology* **167**: 219-220, 2003.

Covasa M, Ritter RC, Burns GA. NMDA receptor participation in control of food intake by the stomach. *Am J Physiol* **278**: R1362-R1368, 2000.

Crane, G.E. Cycloserine as an antidepressant agent. *Am J Psychiatry* **115**: 1025-1026, 1959.

Crane, G.E. The psychotropic effect of cycloserine: a new use of an antibiotic. *Comp Psychiatry* **2**: 51-59, 1961.

Danysz W, Parsons CG, Kornhuber J, Schmidt WJ, Quack G. Aminoadamantanes as NMDA receptor antagonists and antiparkinsonian agents – preclinical studies. *Neurosci Biobehav Rev* **21**: 455-468, 1997.

Danysz W, Parsons CG. The NMDA receptor antagonist memantine as a symptomatological and neuroprotective treatment for Alzheimer's disease: preclinical evidence. *Int J Geriatr Psychiatry* **18**: S23-S32, 2003.

Das S, Sasaki YF, Rothe T, Premkumar LS, Takasu M, Crandall JE, Dikkes P, Conner DA, Rayudu PV, Cheung W, Chen HS, Lipton SA, Nakanishi N. Increased NMDA current and spine density in mice lacking the NMDA receptor NR3A. *Nature* **393**: 377-381, 1998.

Davis SM, Lees KR, Albers GW, Diener HC, Markabi S, Karlsson G, Norris J. Selfotel in acute ischemic stroke: possible neurotoxic effects of an NMDA antagonist. *Stroke* **31**: 347-354, 2000.

Day M, Langston R, Morris RGM. Glutamate-receptor-mediated encoding and retrieval of paired-associate learning. *Nature* **424**: 205-209, 2003.

de Blasi A, Conn PJ, Pin J-P, Nicoletti F. Molecular determinants of metabotropic glutamate receptor signaling. *Trends Pharmacol Sci* **22**: 114-120, 2001.

de Erausquin GA, Hyrc K, Dorsey DA, Mamah D, Dokucu M, Masco DH, Walton T, Dikranain K, Soriano M, Garcia Verdugo JM, Goldberg MP, Dugan LL. Nuclear translocation of nuclear transcription factor-κ B by alpha-amino-3-hydroxy-5-methyl-4-isoxazolepropionic acid receptors leads to transcription of p53 and cell death in dopaminergic neurons. *Mol Pharmacol* **63**: 784-790, 2003.

del Cerro S, Arai A, Kessler M, Bahr BA, Vanderklish P, Rivera S, Lynch G. Stimulation of NMDA receptors activates calpain in cultured hippocampal slices. *Neurosci Lett* **167**: 149-152, 1994.

Delgado, PL, Price LH, Miller HL, Salomon RM, Licinio J, Krystal JH, Heninger GR, Charney DS. Rapid serotonin depletion as a provocative challenge test for patients with major depression: Relevance to antidepressant action and the neurobiology of depression. *Psychpharmacol Bull* **27**: 321-330, 1991.

Delgado PL, Miller HL, Salomon RM, Licinio J, Krystal JH, Moreno FA, Heninger GR, Charney DS. Tryptophan-depletion challenge in depressed patients treated with desipramine or fluoxetine: implications for the role of serotonin in the mechanism of antidepressant action. *Biol Psychiatry* **46**: 212-220, 1999.

DeMattos RB, Bales KR, Cummings DJ, Paul SM, Holtzman DM. Brain to plasma amyloid-beta efflux: a measure of brain amyloid burden in a mouse model of Alzheimer's disease. *Science* **295**: 2264-2267, 2002.

Denny JB, Polan-Curtain J, Ghuman A, Wayner MJ, Armstrong DL. Calpain inhibitors block long-term potentiation. *Brain Res* **534**: 317-320, 1990.

Dingledine R, Hynes MA, King GL. Involvement of N-methyl D-aspartate receptors in epileptiform bursting in the rat hippocampal slice. *J Physiol* **380**: 175-189, 1986.

Dingledine R, Borges K, Bowie D, Traynelis SF. The glutamate receptor ion channels. *Pharmacol Rev* **51**: 7-61, 1999.

Doble A. The role of excitotoxicity in neurodegenerative disease: implications for therapy. *Pharmacol Ther* **81**: 163-221, 1999.

Dolmetsch RE, Xu K, Lewis RS. Calcium oscillations increase the efficacy and specificity of gene expression. *Nature* **392**: 933-936, 1998.

Doyle KM, Feerick S, Kirkby DL, Eddleston A, Higgins GA. Comparison of various N-methyl-D-aspartate receptor antagonists in a model of short-term memory and on overt behaviour. *Behav Pharmacol* **9**: 671-681, 1998.

Dudek SM, Bear MF. Homosynaptic long-term depression in area CA1 of hippocampus and effects of N-methyl-D-aspartate receptor blockade. *Proc Natl Acad Sci USA* **89**: 4363-4367, 1992.

Ekstrom AD, Meltzer J, McNaughton BL, Barnes CA. NMDA receptor antagonism blocks experience-dependent expansion of hippocampal "place fields". *Neuron* **31**: 631-638, 2001.

El-Husseini AE, Schnell E, Chetkovich DM, Nicoll RA, Bredt DS. PSD-95 involvement in maturation of excitatory synapses. *Science* **290**: 1364-1368, 2000.

El-Husseini AE, Schnell E, Dakoji S, Sweeney N, Zhou Q, Prange O, Gauthier-Campbell C, Aguilera A, Nicoll RA, Bredt DA. Synaptic strength regulated by palmitate cycling on PSD-95. *Cell* **108**: 849-863, 2002.

Emptage N, Bliss TVP, Fine A. Single synaptic events evoke NMDA receptor-mediated release of calcium from internal stores in hippocampal dendritic spines. *Neuron* **22**: 115-124, 1999.

Freudenthal R, Romano A. Participation of Rel/NF-κB transcription factors in long-term memory in the crab Chasmagnathus. *Brain Res* **855**: 274-281, 2000.

Fykse EM, Fonnum F. Amino acid neurotransmission: dynamics of vesicular uptake. *Neurochem Res* **21**: 1053-1060, 1996.

Gardoni F, Bellone C, Viviani B, Marinovich M, Meli E, Pellegrini-Giampietro DE, Cattabeni F, Di Luca M. Lack of PSD-95 drives hippocampal neuronal cell death through activation of an alpha CaMKII transduction pathway. *Eur J Neurosci* **16**: 777-786, 2002.

Gilad GM, Gilad VH, Wyatt RJ, Tizabi Y. Region-selective stress-induced increase of glutamate uptake and release in rat forebrain. *Brain Res* **525**: 335-338, 1990.

Gill R, Alanine A, Bourson A, Buttelmann B, Fischer G, Heitz M-P, Kew JNC, Levet-Trafit B, Lorez H-P, Malherbe P, Miss M-T, Muttel V, Pinaro E, Roever S, Schimitt M, Trube G, Wybrecht R, Wyler R, Kemp JA. Pharmacological characterization of Ro 63-1908(1-l2-(4-hydroxy-phenoxy)-ethyl]-4-(4-methyl-benzyl)-piperidin-4-ol), a novel subtype-selective N-methyl-D-aspartate antagonists. *J Pharmacol Exp Ther* **302**: 940-948, 2002.

Gordon-Krajcer W, Salinska E, Lazarewicz JW. *N*-methyl-D-aspartate receptor-mediated processing of beta- amyloid precursor protein in rat hippocampal slices: in vitro-superfusion study. *Folia Neuropathol* **40**: 13-17, 2002.

Gortelmeyer, R., Erbler, H. Memantine in the treatment of mild to moderate dementia syndrome. A double-blind placebo-controlled study. *Arzneimittel-Forschung* **42**: 904-913, 1992.

Greenamyre JT, Young AB. Excitatory amino acids and Alzheimer's disease. *Neurobiol Aging* **10**: 593-602, 1989.

Gregory TF, Wright JL, Wise LD, Meltzer LT, Serpa KA, Konkoy CS, Whittemore ER, Woodward RM. Parallel synthesis of a series of subtype-selective NMDA receptor antagonists. *Bioorg Med Chem Lett* **10**: 527-529, 2000.

Gregory ML, Stech NE, Owens RW, Kalivas, PW. Prefrontal group II metabotropic glutamate receptor activation decreases performance on a working memory task. *Ann NY Acad Sci* **1003**: 405-409, 2003.

Grimwood S, Le Bourdelles B, Atack JR, Barton C, Cockett W, Cook SM, Gilbert E, Hutson PH, McKernan RM, Myers J, Ragan CI, Wingrove PB, Whiting PJ. Generation and characterization of stable cell lines recombinant human N-methyl-D-aspartate receptor subtypes. *J Neurochem* **66**: 2239-2247, 1996.

Guerrini L, Blass F, Denis-Dinini S. Synaptic activation of NF-κB by glutamate in cerebellar granule neurons in vitro. *Proc Natl Acad Sci USA* **92**: 9077-9081, 1995.

Guerrini L, Molteni A, Wirth T, Kistler B, Blasi F. Glutamate-dependent activation of NF-κB during mouse cerebellum development. *J Neurosci* **17**: 6057-6063, 1997.

Hammond C, Crépel V, Gozlan H, Ben-Ari Y. Anoxic LTP sheds light on the multiple facets of NMDA receptors. *Trends Neurosci* **17**: 497-503, 1994.

Han EB, Stevens CF. Of mice and memory. *Learn Mem* **6**: 539-541, 1999.

Harkany T, Abraham I, Timmerman W, Laskay G, Toth B, Sasvari M, Konya C, Sebens JB, Korf J, Nyakas C, Zarandi M, Soos K, Penke B, Luiten PG. Beta-amyloid neurotoxicity is mediated by a glutamate-triggered excitotoxic cascade in rat nucleus basalis. *Eur J Neurosci* **12**: 2735-2745, 2000.

Heintz N, Zoghbi HY. Insights from mouse models into the molecular basis of neurodegeneration. *Annu Rev Physiol* **62**: 779-802, 2000.

Helmuth L. New therapies. New Alzheimer's treatments that may ease the mind. *Science* **297**: 1260-1262, 2002.

Hendricson AW, Miao CLK, Lippmann MJ, Morrisett RA. Ifenprodil and ethanol enhance NMDA receptor-dependent long-term depression. *J Pharmacol Exp Ther* **301**: 938-944, 2002.

Hirai K, Aliev G, Nunomura A, Fujioka H, Russell RL, Atwood CS, Johnson AB, Kress Y, Vinters HV, Tabaton M, Shimohama S, Cash AD, Siedlak SL, Harris PLR, Jones PK, Petersen RB, Perry G, Smith MA. Mitochondrial abnormalities in Alzheimer's disease. *J Neurosci* **21**: 3017-3023, 2001.

Hirbec H, Hausset AL, Kamenka JM, Privat A, Vignon J. Re-evaluation of phencyclidine low-affinity or "non-NMDA" binding sites. *J Neurosci Res* **68**: 305-314, 2002.

Hoffman PL, Rabe CS, Moses F, Tabakoff B. *N*-methyl-D-aspartate receptors and ethanol: inhibition of calcium flux and cyclic GMP production. *J Neurochem* **52**: 1937-1940, 1989.

Holmes C, Cairns N, Lantos P, Mann A. Validity of current clinical criteria for Alzheimer's disease, vascular dementia and dementia with Levy bodies. *Br J Psychiatry* **174**: 45-50, 1999.

Holmes KD, Mattar P, Marsh DR, Jordan V, Weaver LC, Dekaban GA. The C-terminal C1 cassette of the *N*-methyl-D-aspartate receptor 1 subunit contains a bi-partite nuclear localization sequence. *J Neurochem* **81**: 1152-1165, 2002.

Hrabetova S, Serrano P, Blace N, Tse HW, Skifter DA, Jane DE, Monaghan DT, Sacktor TC. Direct NMDA receptor subpopulations contribute to long-term potentiation and long-term depression induction. *J Neurosci* **20**: RC81, 2000.

Hu L-Y, Guo J, Magar SS, Fischer JB, Burke-Howie KJ, Durant GJ. Synthesis and pharmacological evaluation of N-(2,5-disubstituted phenyl)-N'-(3-substituted phenyl)-N'-methylguanidines as N-methyl-D-aspartate receptor ion-channel blockers. *J Med Chem* **40**: 4281-4289, 1997.

Huber, T.J., Dietrich, D.E., Emrich, H.M. Possible use of amantadine in depression. *Pharmacopsychiatry* **32**: 47-55, 1999.

Hunt WA. *Alcohol and Biological Membranes*, The Guilford Press: New York, 1985.

Ikonomidou C, Stefovka V, Turski L. Neuronal death enhanced by N-methyl-D-aspartate antagonists. *Proc Natl Acad Sci USA* **97**: 12885-12890, 2000.

Ingvar M, Ambros-Ingerson J, Davis M, Granger R, Kesster M, Rogers GA, Schehr RS, Lynch G. Enhancement by an ampakine of memory encoding in humans. *Exp Neurol* **146**: 553-559, 1997.

Jansen M, Potschka H, Brandt C, Löscher W, Dannhardt G. Hydantoin-substituted 4,6-dichloroindole-2-carboxylic acids as ligands with high affinity for the glycine binding site of the NMDA receptor. *J Med Chem* **46**: 64-73, 2003.

Jia Z, Lu Y, Henderson J, Taverna F, Romano C, Abramow-Newerly W, Wojtowicz JM, Roder J. Selective abolition of the NMDA component of long-term potentiation in mice lacking mGluR5. *Lear Mem* **5**: 331-343, 1998.

Jirgensons A, Kauss V, Kalvinsh I, Gold MR, Danysz W, Parsons CG, Quack G. Synthesis and structure-affinity relationships of 1,3,5-alkylsubstituted cyclohexylamines binding at NMDA receptor PCP site. *Eur J Med Chem* **35**: 555-565, 2000.

Jolas T, Aghajanian GK. Opioids suppress spontaneous and NMDA-induced inhibitory postsynaptic currents in the dorsal raphe nucleus of the rat in vitro. *Brain Res* **755**: 229-245, 1997.

Jones KS, VanDongen HMA, VanDongen AM. The NMDA receptor M3 segment is a conserved transduction element coupling ligand binding to channel opening. *J Neurosci* **22**: 2044-2053, 2002.

Kaltschmidt C, Kaltschmidt B, Baeuerle PA. Stimulation of ionotropic glutamate receptors activates transcription factor NF-κB in primary neurons. *Proc Natl Acad Sci USA* **92**: 9618-9622, 1995.

Kennedy MB. Signal transduction molecules at the glutamatergic postsynaptic membrane. *Brain Res Brain Res Rev* **26**: 243-257, 1998.

Kew JN, Kemp JA. An allosteric interaction between the NMDA receptor polyamine and ifenprodil sites in rat cultured cortical neurons. *J Physiol Lond* **512**: 17-28, 1998.

Klein J, Longo-Guess CM, Rossmann MP, Seburn KL, Hurd RE, Frankel WN, Bronson RT, Ackerman SL. The harlequin mouse mutation downregulates apoptosis-inducing factor. *Nature* **419**: 367-374, 2002.

Koh J, Yang LL, Cotman CW. Beta-amyloid protein increases the vulnerability of cultured cortical neurons to excitotoxic damage. *Brain Res* **533**: 315-320, 1990.

Kornhuber J, Wellwe M. Psychotogenicity and *N*-methyl-D-aspartate receptor antagonism: implications for neuroprotective pharmacotherapy. *Biol Psychiatry* **41**: 135-144, 1997.

Kovalchuk Y, Eilers J, Lisman J, Konnerth A. NMDA receptor-mediated subthreshold Ca^{2+} signals in spines of hippocampal neurons. *J Neurosci* **20**: 1791-1799, 2000.

Kowall NW, Beal MF, Busciglio J, Duffy LK, Yankner BA. An in vivo model for the neurodegenerative effects of beta amyloid and protection by substance P. *Proc Natl Acad Sci. USA* **88**: 7247-7251, 1991.

Krystal JH, Sanacora G, Blumberg H, Anand A, Charney DS, Marek G, Epperson CN, Goddard A, Mason GF. Glutamate and GABA systems as targets for novel antidepressant and mood-stabilizing treatments. *Mol Psychiatry*

Kudoh A, Takahira Y, Katagai H, Takazawa T. Small-dose ketamine improves the postoperative state of depressed patients. *Anesth Analg* **95**: 114-118, 2002.

Lamprecht R, LeDoux J. Structural plasticity and memory. *Nature Rev Neurosci* **5**: 45-54, 2004.

Laube B, Kuhse J, Betz H. Evidence for a tetrameric structure of recombinant NMDA receptors. *J Neurosci* **18**: 2954-2961, 1998.

Law AJ, Deakin JF. Asymmetrical reductions of hippocampal NMDAR1 glutamate receptor mRNA in the psychoses. *NeuroReport* **12:** 2971-2974, 2001.

Le DA, Lipton SA. Potential and current use of *N*-methyl-D-aspartate (NMDA) receptor antagonists in disease of aging. *Drugs Aging* **18:** 717-724, 2001.

Lee H-K, Kameyama K, Huganir RL, Bear MF. NMDA induces long-term synaptic depression and phosphorylation of the GluR1 subunit of AMPA receptors in hippocampus. *Neuron* **21:** 1151-1162, 1998.

Lee FJ, Xue S, Pei L, Vukusic B, Chéry N, Wang Y, Wang YT, Niznik HB, Yu X-M, Liu F. Dual regulation of NMDA receptor functions by direct protein-protein interactions with the dopamine D1 receptor. *Cell* **111:** 219-230, 2002.

Lee EHY, Hsu WL, Ma YL, Lee PJ, Chao CC. Enrichment enhances the expression of *sgk*, a glucocorticoid-induced gene, and facilitates spatial learning through glutamate AMPA receptor mediation. *Eur J Neurosci* **18:** 2842-2852, 2003.

Lees KR. Cerestat and other NMDA antagonists in ischemic stroke. *Neurology* **49 Suppl. 4:** S66-S69, 1997.

Lees KR, Asplund K, Carolei AD, Davis SM, Diener HC, Kaste M, Orgogozo JM, Whitehead J. Glycine antagonist (gavestinel) in neuroprotection (GAIN International) in patients with acute stroke: a randomized controlled trial. *Lancet* **335:** 1949-1954, 2000.

Lejeune F, Gobert A, Rivet JM, Millan MJ. Blockade of transmission at NMDA receptors facilitates the electrical and synthetic activity of ascending serotonergic neurons. *Brain Res* **656:** 427-431, 1994.

Li X, Tizzano JP, Griffey K, Clay M, Lindstrom T, Skolnick P. Antidepressant-like actions of an AMPA receptor potentiator (LY392098). *Neuropharmacology* **40:** 1028-1033, 2001.

Lima-Landman MT, Albuquerque EX. Ethanol potentiates and blocks NMDA-activated single-channel currents in rat hippocampal pyramidal cells. *FEBS Lett* **247:** 61-67, 1989.

Lipton SA, Rosenberg PA. Excitatory amino acids as a final common pathway for neurologic disorders. *N Engl J Med* **330:** 613-622, 1994.

Lipton SA, Singel DJ, Stamler JS. Nitric oxide in the central nervous system. *Prog Brain Res* **103:** 359-364, 1994.

Lipton SA, Rayudu PV, Choi YB, Sucher NJ, Chen HS. Redox modulation of the NMDA receptor by NO-related species. *Prog Brain Res* **118:** 73-82, 1998.

Liu H, Mantyh P, Basbaum A. NMDA-receptor regulation of substance P release from primary afferent nociceptors. *Nature* **386:** 721-724, 1997.

Loftis JM, Janowsky A. The N-methyl-D-aspartate receptor subunit NR2B: localization, functional properties, regulation, and clinical implications. *Pharmacol Ther* **97:** 55-85, 2003.

Lovinger DM, White G, Weight FF. Ethanol inhibits NMDA-activated ion current in hippocampal neurons. *Science* **243:** 1721-1724, 1989.

Lu YM, Jia Z, Janus C, Henderson JT, Gerlai R, Wojtowicz JM, Roder JC. Mice lacking metabotropic glutamate receptor 5 show impaired learning and reduced CA1 long-term potentiation (LTP) but normal CA3 LTP. *J Neurosci* **17:** 5196-5205, 1997.

Lydic R, Baghdoyan HA. Ketamine and MK-801 decrease acetylcholine release in the pontine reticular formation, slow breathing, and disrupt sleep. *Sleep* **25:** 617-622, 2002.

Lynch G, Granger R, Ambros-Ingerson J, Davis CM, Kessler M, Schehr R. Evidence that a positive modulator of AMPA-type glutamate receptors improved recall in aged humans. *Exp Neurol* **145**: 89-92, 1997.

MacIver MB, Amagasu SM, Mikulec AA, Monroe FA. Riluzole anesthesia: use-dependent block of presynaptic glutamate fibers. *Anesthesiology* **85**: 626-634, 1996.

Maj J, Rogoz Z, Skuza G, Sowinska H. Effects of MK-801 and antidepressant drugs in the forced swimming test in rats. *Eur J Neuropsychopharmacol* **2**: 37-41, 1992.

Mannaioni G, Marino MJ, Valenti O, Traynelis SF, Conn PJ. Metabotropic glutamate receptors 1 and 5 differentially regulate CA1 pyramidal cell function. *J Neurosci* **21**: 5925-5934, 2001.

MarekGJ, Aghajanian GK. 5-Hydroxytryptamine-induced excitatory postsynaptic currents in neo-cortical layer V pyramidal cells: suppression by mu-opiate receptor activation. *Neuroscience* **86**: 485-497, 1998.

Marek GJ, Wright RA, Schoepp DD, Monn JA, Aghajanian GK. Physiological antagonism between 5-hydroxytryptamine(2A) and group II metabotropic glutamate receptors in prefrontal cortex. *J Pharmacol Exp Ther* **292**: 76-87, 2000.

Martin P, Carlsson ML, Hjorth S. Systemic PCP treatment elevates brain extracellular 5-HT: a microdialysis study in awake rats. *NeuroReport* **9**: 2985-2988, 1998.

Marvanová M, Lakso M, Pirhonen J, Nawa H, Wong G, Castrén E. The neuroprotective agent memantine induces brain-derived neurotrophic factor and trkB receptor expression in rat brain. *Mol Cell Neurosci* **18**: 247-258, 2001.

Mate MJ, Ortiz-Lombardia M, Boitel B, Haouz A, Tello D, Susin SA, Penninger J, Kroemer G, Alzari PM. The crystal structure of the mouse apoptosis-inducing factor AIF. *Nat Struct Biol* **9**: 442-446, 2002.

Matsuoka Y, Saito M, LaFrancois J, Saito M, Gaynor K, Olm V, Wang L, Casey E, Lu Y, Shiratori C, Lenere C, Duff K. Novel therapeutic approach for the treatment of Alzheimer's disease by peripheral administration of agents with an affinity to beta-amyloid. *J Neurosci* **23**: 29-33, 2003.

Mayford M, Kandel ER. Genetic approaches to memory storage. *Trends Genet* **15**: 463-470, 1999.

Melenovsky V, Wichterle D, Malik J, Simek J, Hradec J, Ceska R, Malik M. Nitroglycerine induced syncope occurs in subjects with delayed phase shift of baroreflex action. *Pacing Clin Eelctrophysiol* **25**: 828-832, 2002.

Michaelis EK. Molecular biology of glutamate receptors in the central nervous system and their role in excitotoxicity, oxidative stress and aging. *Prog Neurobiol* **54**: 369-415, 1998.

Migaud M, Charlesworth P, Dempster M, Webster LC, Watabe AM, Makhinson M, He Y, Ramsay MF, Morris RGM, Morrison JH, O'Dell TJ, Grant SGN. Enhanced long-term potentiation and impaired learning in mice with mutant postsynaptic density-95 protein. *Nature* **396**: 433-439, 1998.

Milner B, Squire LR, Kandel ER. Cognitive neuroscience and the study of memory. *Neuron* **20**: 445-468, 1998.

Miyamoto Y, Yamada K, Noda Y, Mori H, Mishina M, Nabeshima T. Hyperfunction of dopaminergic and serotonergic neuronal systems in mice lacking the NMDA receptor epsilon1 subunit. *J Neurosci* **21**: 750-757, 2001.

Mockett B, Coussens C, Abraham WC. NMDA receptor-mediated metaplasticity during the induction of long-term depression by low-frequency stimulation. *Eur J Neurosci* **15**: 1819-1826, 2002.

Moghaddam B. Stress preferentially increases extraneuronal levels of excitatory amino acids in the prefrontal cortex: comparison to hippocampus and basal ganglia. *J Neurochem* **60**: 1650-1657, 1993.

Monyer H, Burnashev N, Laurie DJ, Sakmann B, Seeburg PH. Developmental and regional expression in the rat brain and functional properties of four NMDA receptors. *Neuron* **12**: 529-540, 1994.

Muir KW, Lees KR. Clinical experience with excitatory amino acid antagonist drugs. *Stroke* **26**: 503-513, 1995.

Mulkey RM, Malenka RC. Mechanism underlying induction of homosynaptic long-term depression in area CA1 of the hippocampus. *Neuron* **9**: 967-975, 1992.

Murray CJ, Lopez AD Alternative projections of mortality and disability by cause 1990-2020: Global Burden of Disease Study. *Lancet* **349**: 1498-1504.

Nacher J, Alonso-Llosa G, Rosell DR, McEwen BS. NMDA receptor antagonist treatment increases the production of new neurons in the aged rat hippocampus. *Neurobiol Aging* **24**: 273-284, 2003.

Naie K, Manahan-Vaughan D. Regulation by metabotropic glutamate receptor 5 of LTP in the dentate gyrus of freely moving rats: relevance for learning and memory formation. *Cerebral Cortex* **14**: 189-198, 2004.

Nakazawa K, Quirk MC, Chitwood RA, Watanabe M, Yeckel MF, Sun LD, Kato A, Carr CA, Johnston DL, Wilson MA, Tonegawa S. Requirement for hippocampal CA3 NMDA receptors in associative memory recall. *Science* **297**: 211-218, 2002.

Nestler EJ, Barrot M, DiLeone RJ, Eisch AJ, Gold SJ, Monteggia LM. Neurobiology of depression. *Neuron* **34**: 13-25, 2002.

Nikam SS, Meltzer LT. NR2B selective NMDA receptor antagonists. *Current Pharmaceut Design* **8**: 845-855, 2002.

Nosten-Bertrand M, Errington ML, Murphy KPSJ, Tokugawa Y, Barboni E, Kozlova E, Michalovich D, Morris RGM, Silver J, Stewart CL, Bliss TV, Morris RJ. Normal spatial learning despite regional inhibition of LTP in mice lacking Thy-1. *Nature* **379**: 826-829, 1996.

Nowak G, Ordway GA, Paul LA. Alterations in the *N*-methyl-D-aspartate (NMDA) receptor complex in the frontal cortex of suicide victims. *Brain Res* **675**: 157-164, 1995.

O'Connor JJ, Rowan MJ, Anwyl R. Potentiation of *N*-methyl-D-aspartate-receptor-mediated currents detected using the excised patch technique in the hippocampal dentate gyrus. *J Neurosci* **15**: 2013-2020, 1995.

O'Donnell J, Stemmelin J, Nitta A, Brouillette J, Quirion R. Gene expression profiling following chronic NMDA receptor blockade-induced learning deficits in rats. *Synapse* **50**: 171-180, 2003.

Ohtani K-I, Tanaka H, Ohno Y. SM-31900, a novel NMDA receptor glycine-binding site antagonist, reduces infarct volume induced by permanent middle cerebral artery occlusion in spontaneously hypertensive rats. *Neurochem Int* **42**: 375-384, 2003.

Olney JW. Brain lesions, obesity, and other disturbances in mice treated with monosodium glutamate. *Science* **164**: 719-721, 1969.

Orgogozo J-M, Rigaud A-S, Stöffler A, Möbius H-J, Forette F. Efficacy and safety of memantine in patients with mild to moderate vascular dementia: a randomized, placebo-controlled trial (MMM 300). *Stroke* **33**: 1834-1839, 2002.

Osen KK, Storm-Mathisen J, Ottersen OP, Dihle B. Glutamate is concentrated in and released from parallel fiber terminals in the dorsal cochlear nucleus: a quantitative immunocytochemical analysis in guinea pig. *J Comp Neurol* **357**: 482-500, 1995.

Palmer GC. Neuroprotection by NMDA receptor antagonists in a variety of neuropathologies. *Curr Drug Targ* **2**: 241-271, 2001.

Panconi E, Roux J, Altenbaumer M, Hampe S, Porsolt RD. MK-801 and enantiomers: potential antidepressants or false positives in classical screening models? *Pharmacol. Biochem Behav* **46**: 15-20, 1993.

Paoletti P, Perin-Dureau F, Fayyazuddin A, Le Goff A, Callebaut I, Neyton J. Molecular organization of a zinc binding n-terminal modulatory domain in a NMDA receptor subunit. *Neuron* **28**: 911-925, 2000.

Papp M, Moryl E. New evidence for the antidepressant activity of MK-801, a non-competitive antagonist of NMDA receptors. *Pol J Pharmacol* **45**: 549-553, 1993.

Parkes, J.D., Zilkha, K.J., Marsden, P., Baxter, R.C., Knill-Jones, R.P. Amantadine doses in treatment of Parkinson's disease. *Lancet* **1**: 1130-1133, 1970.

Patankar SJ, Jurs PC. Prediction of glycine/NMDA receptor antagonists inhibition from molecular structure. *J Chem Inf Comput Sci* **42**: 1053-1068, 2002.

Paul IA, Skolnick P. Glutamate and depression. *Ann NY Acad Sci* **1003**: 250-272, 2003.

Peeters M, Page G, Maloteaux J-M, Hermans E. Hypersensitivity of dopamine transmission in the rat striatum after treatment with the NMDA receptor antagonist amantadine. *Brain Res* **949**: 32-41, 2002.

Peoples RW, Stewart RR. Alcohol inhibit N-methyl-D-aspartate receptors via a site exposed to the extracellular environment. *Neuropharmacology* **39**: 1681-1691, 2000.

Perin-Dureau F, Rachline J, Neyton J, Paoletti P. Mapping the binding site of the neuroprotectant ifenprodil on NMDA receptors. *J Neurosci* **22**: 5955-5965, 2002.

Petrie R, Reid IC, Stewart CA. The *N*-methyl-D-aspartate receptor, synaptic plasticity, and depressive disorder. A critical review. *Pharmacol Ther* **87**: 11-25, 2000.

Pilc A, Legutko B. The influence of prolonged antidepressant treatment on the changes in cyclic AMP accumulation induced by excitatory amino acids in rat cerebral cortical slices. *NeuroReport* **7**: 85-88, 1995.

Pilc A, Branski P, Palucha A, Tokarski K, Bijak M. Antidepressant treatment influences group I of glutamate metabotropic receptors in slices from hippocampal CA1 region. *Eur J Pharmacol* **349**: 83-87, 1998.

Pinard E, Alanine A, Bourson A, Büttelmann B, Gill R, Heitz M-P, Jaeschke G, Mutel V, Trube G, Wyler R. Discovery of (R)-1-[2-hydroxy-3-(4-hydroxy-phenyl)-propyl]-4-(4-

methyl-benzyl)-piperidin-4-ol: a novel NR1/2B subtype selective NMDA receptor antagonist. *Bioorgan Med Chem Lett* **11**: 2173-2176, 2001.

Pizzi M, Goffi F, Boroni F, Benarese M, Perkins SE, Liou HC, Spano P. Opposing roles for NF-κB/Rel factor p65 and c-Rel in the modulation of neuron survival elicited by glutamate and interleukin-1β. *J Biol Chem* **277**: 717-720, 2002.

Planells-Cases R, Montoliu C, Humet M, Fernández AM, Garcia-Martimez C, Valera E, Merino JM, Perez-Paya E, Messeguer A, Felipo V, Ferrer-Montiel A. A novel N-methyl-D-aspartate receptor open channel blocker with in vivo neuroprotectant activity. *J Pharmacol Exp Ther* **302**: 163-173, 2002.

Priestley T, Laughton P, Myers J, Le Bourdelles B, Kerby J, Whiting PJ. Pharmacological properties of recombinant human N-methyl-D-aspartate receptors comprising NR1A/NR2A and NR1A/NR2B subunit assemblies expressed in permanently transfected mouse fibroblast cells. *Mol Pharmacol* **48**: 841-848, 1995.

Przegalinski E, Tatarczynska E, Deren-Wesolek A, Chojnacka-Wojcik E. Antidepressant-like effects of a partial agonist at strychnine-insensitive glycine receptors and a competitive NMDA receptor antagonist. *Neuropharmacology* **36**: 31-37, 1997.

Quirk JC, Nisenbaum ES. LY404187: A novel positive allosteric modulator of AMPA receptors. *CNS Drug Rev* **8**: 255-282, 2002.

Reisberg B, Doody R, Stöffler A, Schmitt F, Ferris S, Möbius HJ. Memantine in moderate-to-severe Alzheimer's disease. *N Engl J Med* **348**: 1333-1341, 2003.

Reynolds IJ, Miller RJ. Tricyclic antidepressants block N-methyl-D-aspartate receptors: similarities to the action of zinc. *Br J Pharmacol* **95**: 95-102, 1988.

Richter A. The NMDA receptor NR2B subtype selective antagonist Ro 25-6981 aggravates paroxysmal dyskinesia in the dt(sz) mutant. *Eur J Pharmacol* **458**: 107-110, 2003.

Richter A, Löscher W. Pathology of idiopathic dystonia: findings from genetic animal models. *Prog Neurobiol* **54**: 633-677, 1998.

Riedel G, Platt B, Micheau J. Glutamate receptor function in learning and memory. *Behav Brain Res* **140**: 1-47, 2003.

Rod MR, Wishaw IQ, Auer RN. The relationship of structural ischemic brain damage to neurobehavioural deficit: the effect of postischemic MK-801. *Can J Psychol* **44**: 196-209, 1990.

Rogawski MA and Wenk GL. The neuropharmacological basis for the use of memantine in the treatment of Alzheimer's disease. *CNS Drug Rev* **9**: 275-308, 2003.

Rogóż Z, Skuza G, Maj J, Danysz W. Synergistic effect of uncompetitive NMDA receptor antagonists and antidepressant drugs in the forced swimming test in rats. *Neuropharmacology* **42**: 1024-1030, 2002.

Rothman SM, Olney JW. Excitotoxicity and the NMDA receptor – still lethal after eight years. *Trends Neurosci* **18**: 57-58, 1995.

Rutter AR, Freeman FM, Stephenson FA. Further characterization of the molecular interaction between PSD-95 and NMDA receptors: the effect of the NR1 splice variant and evidence for modulation of channel gating. *J Neurochem* **81**: 1298-1307, 2002.

Sanacora G, Rothman DL, Mason G, Krystal JH. Clinical studies implementing glutamate neurotransmission in mood disorders. *Ann NY Acad Sci* **1003**: 292-308, 2003.

Sattler R, Xiong Z, Lu WY, Hafner M, MacDonald JF, Tymianski M. Specific coupling of NMDA receptor activation to nitric oxide neurotoxicity by PSD-95 protein. *Science* **284:** 1845-1848, 1999.

Saucier D, Cain DP. Spatial learning without NMDA receptor-dependent long-term potentiation. *Nature* **378:** 186-189, 1995.

Schoepp DD. Unveiling the functions of presynaptic metabotropic glutamate receptors in the central nervous system. *J Pharmacol Exp Ther* **299:** 12-20, 2001.

Schölzke MN, Potrovita I, Subramaniam S, Prinz S, Schwaninger M. Glutamate activates NF-κB through calpain in neurons. *Eur J Neurosci* **18:** 3305-3310, 2003.

Schwartz BL, Hashtroudi S, Herting RL, Schwartz P, Deutsch SI. d-Cycloserine enhances implicit memory in Alzheimer's patients. *Neurology* **46:** 420-424, 1996.

Selkoe DJ, Schenk D. Alzheimer's disease: Molecular understanding predicts amyloid-based therapeutics. *Annu Rev Pharmacol Toxicol* **43:** 545-584, 2003.

Shimizu E, Tang Y-P, Rampon C, Tsien JZ. NMDA receptor-dependent synaptic reinforcement as a crucial process for memory consolidation. *Science* **290:** 1170-1174, 2000.

Skolnick P. Antidepressants for the new millennium. *Eur J Pharmacol* **375:** 31-40, 1999.

Skolnick P, Legutko B, Li X, Bymaster FP. Current perspective on the development of non-biogenic amine-based antidepressants. *Pharmacol Res* **43:** 411-423, 2001.

Smith SK, Hoogendoorn B, Guy CA, Coleman SL, O'Donovan MC, Buckland PR. Lack of functional promoter polymorphisms in genes involved in glutamate neurotransmission. *Psychiatric Genet* **13:** 193-199, 2003.

Soderling TR, Derkach VA. Postsynaptic protein phosphorylation and LTP. *Trends Neurosci* **23:** 75-80, 2000.

Stewart CA, Reid IC. Antidepressant mechanisms: functional and molecular correlates of excitatory amino acid neurotransmission. *Mol Psychiatry* **7:** S15-S22, 2002.

Sun M-K. Central neural organization and control of sympathetic nervous system in mammals. *Prog Neurobiol* **47:** 157-233, 1995.

Sun M-K. Pharmacology of reticulospinal vasomotor neurons in cardiovascular regulation. *Pharmacol Rev* **48:** 465-494, 1996.

Sun M-K. Hypoxia, ischemic stroke, and memory deficits: prospects for therapy. *IUBMB Life* **48:** 373-378, 1999.

Sun M-K, Alkon DL. Perspectives on the cell biology underlying Alzheimer's disease and the potential for therapy. *LifeXY* **1:** 1075-1086, 2001.

Sun M-K, Alkon DL. Depressed or demented: common CNS drug targets? ! *Curr Drug Targets – CNS Neurol Disord* **1:** 575-592, 2002a.

Sun M-K, Alkon DL. Impairment of hippocampal CA1 heterosynaptic transformation and spatial memory by β-amyloid$_{25-35}$. *J Neurophysiol* **87:** 2441-2449, 2002b.

Sun M-K, Reis DJ. NMDA receptor-mediated sympathetic chemoreflex excitation of RVL-spinal vasomotor neurones in rats. *J Physiol (Lond)* **482:** 53-68, 1995.

Sun M-K, Reis DJ. Excitatory amino acid-mediated chemoreflex excitation of respiratory neurones in rostral ventrolateral medulla in rats. *J Physiol (Lond)* **492:** 559-571, 1996.

Sun M-K, Xu H, Alkon DL. Protection of synaptic function, spatial learning, and memory from transient hypoxia in rats. *J Pharmacol Exp Ther* **300:** 408-416, 2002a.

Syntichaki P, Xu K, Driscoll M, Tavernarakis N. Specific aspartyl and calpain proteases are required for neurodegeneration in C. elegans. *Nature* **419**: 939-944, 2002.

Tamiz AP, Whittemore ER, Zhou Z-L, Huang J-C, Drewe JA, Chen J-C, Cai S-X, Weber E, Woodward RM, Keana JFW. Structure-activity relationships for a series of bis(phenylalkyl)amines: potent subtype-selective inhibitors of *N*-methyl-D-aspartate receptors. *J Med Chem* **41**: 3499-3506, 1998.

Tamiz AP, Whittemore ER, Woodward RM, Upasani RB, Keana FW. Structure-activity relationship for a series of 2-substituted 1,2,3,4-tetrahydro-9*H*-pyrido[3,4-*b*]indoles: potent subtype-selective inhibitors of *N*-methyl-D-aspartate (NMDA) receptors. *Bioorg Med Chem Lett* **9**: 1619-1624, 1999a.

Tamiz AP, Cai SX, Zhou Z-L, Yuen P-W, Schelkun RM, Whittemore ER, Weber E, Woodward RM, Keana JFW. Structure-activity relationship of *N*-(phenylalkyl)cinnamides as novel NR2B subtype-selective NMDA receptor antagonists. *J Med Chem* **42**: 3412-3420, 1999b.

Tang YP, Shimizu E, Duber R, Rampon C, Kechner GA, Zhuo M, Lie G, Tsien JZ. Genetic enhancement of learning and memory in mice. *Nature* **401**: 63-69, 1999.

Tezuka T, Umemori H, Akiyama T, Nakanishi S, Yamamoto T. PSD-95 promotes Fyn-mediated tyrosine phosphorylation of the *N*-methyl-D-aspartate receptor subunit NR2A. *Proc Natl Acad Sci USA* **96**: 435-440, 1999.

Touyarot K, Poussard S, Cortes-Torrea C, Cottin P, Micheau J. Effect of chronic inhibition of calpain in the hippocampus on spatial discrimination learning and protein kinase C. *Behav Brain Res* **136**: 439-48, 2002.

Tovar KR, Westbrook GL. Mobile NMDA receptor at hippocampal synapses. *Neuron* **34**: 255-264, 2002.

Trullas R, Skolnick P. Functional antagonists at the NMDA receptor complex exhibit antidepressant actions. *Eur J Pharmacol* **185**: 1-10, 1990.

Tsai KJ, Chen SK, Ma YL, Hsu WL, Lee EHY. *sgk*, a primary glucorticoid-induced gene, facilitates memory consolidation of spatial learning in rats. *Proc Natl Acad Sci USA* **99**: 3990-3995, 2002.

Tsien JZ, Heurta PT, Tonegawa S. The essential role of hippocampal CA1 NMDA receptor-dependent synaptic plasticity in spatial memory. *Cell* **87**: 1327-1338, 1996.

Vale, S., Espejel, M.A., Dominguez, J.C. Amantadine in depression. *Lancet* **2**: 437, 1971.

van Dam EJ, Ruiter B, Kamal A, Ramakers GM, Gispen WH, de Graan PN. *N*-methyl-D-aspartate-induced long-term depression is associated with a decrease in postsynaptic protein kinase C substrate phosphorylation in rat hippocampal slices. *Neurosci Lett* **320**: 129-132, 2002.

Vissel B, Krupp JJ, Heinemann SF, Westbrook GL. Intracellular domains of NR2 alter calcium-dependent inactivation of N-methyl-D-aspartate receptors. *Mol Pharmacol* **61**: 595-605, 2002.

Walters MR, Bradford APJ, Fischer J, Lees KR. Early clinical experience with an novel NMDA receptor antagonist CNS 5161. *Br J Clin Pharmacol* **53**: 305-311, 2002.

Wang KK. Calpain and caspase: can you tell the difference? *Trends Neurosci* **23**: 20-26, 2000.

Wang Y, Qin ZH, Nakai M, Chen RW, Chuang DM, Chase TN. Co-stimulation of cyclic-AMP-linked metabotropic glutamate receptors in rat striatum attenuates excitotoxin-induced nuclear factor-κB activation and apoptosis. *Neuroscience* **94**: 1153-1162, 1999.

Wang SJ, Su CF, Kuo YH. Fluoxetine depresses glutamate exocytosis in the rat cerebrocortical nerve terminals (synaptosomes) via inhibition of P/Q-type Ca^{2+} channels. *Synapse* **48**: 170-177, 2003.

Weiser T. AMPA receptor antagonists with additional mechanisms of action: new opportunities for neuroprotective drugs? *Curr Pharmaceut Design* **8**: 941-951, 2002.

Williams K. Ifenprodil, a novel NMDA receptor antagonist: site and mechanism of action. *Current Drug Targets* **2**: 285-298, 2001.

Williams A, Dave J, Lu X, Ling G, Tortella F. Selective NR2B NMDA receptor antagonists are protective against staurosporine-induced apoptosis. *Eur J Pharmacol* **452**: 135-136, 2002.

Winblad B, Poritis N. Memantine in severe dementia: results of the 9M-best study (benefit and efficacy in severely demented patients during treatment with memantine. *Int J Geristr Psychiatry* **14**: 135-146, 1999.

Woolf CJ, Salter MW. Neuronal plasticity: increasing the gain in pain. *Science* **288**: 1765-1769, 2000.

Yan QS, Reith ME, Jobe PC, Dailey JW. Dizocilpine (MK-801) increases not only dopamine but also serotonin and norepinephrine transmissions in the nucleus accumbens as measured by microdialysis in freely moving rats. *Brain Res* **765**: 149-158, 1997.

Yilmaz A, Schulz D, Aksoy A, Canbeyli R. Prolonged effect of an anesthetic dose of ketamine on behavioral despair. *Pharmacol Biochem Behav* **71**: 341-344, 2002.

Yu XM, Askalan R, Keil GJ2[nd], Salter MW. NMDA channel regulation by channel-associated protein tyrosine kinase Src. *Science* **275**: 674-678, 1997.

Zamanillo D, Sprengel R, Hvalby O, Jense V, Burnashev N, Rozov A, Kaiser KM, Koster HJ, Borchardt T, Worley P, Lubke J, Frotscher M, Kelly PH, Sommer B, Andersen P, Seeburg PH, Sakmann B. Importance of AMPA receptors for hippocampal synaptic plasticity but not for spatial learning. *Science* **284**: 1805-1811, 1999.

Zarate CA, Quiroz J, Payne J, Manji HK. Modulators of the glutamatergic system: implications for the development of improved therapeutics in mood disorders. *Psychpharmacol Bull* **36**: 35-83, 2002.

Zarate CA, Payne JL, Quiroz J, Sporn J, Denicoff KK, Luckenbaugh D, Charney DS, Manji HK. An open-label trial of riluzole in patients with treatment-resistant major depression. *Am J Psychiatry* **161**: 171-174, 2004.

Zeron MM, Hansson O, Chen N, Wellington CL, Leavitt BR, Brundin P, Hayden MR, Raymond LA. Increased sensitivity to N-methyl-D-aspartate receptor-mediated excitotoxicity in a mouse model of Huntington's disease. *Neuron* **33**: 849-860, 2002.

Zhang WN, Bast T, Feldon J. Effects of hippocampal *N*-methyl-D-aspartate infusion on locomotor activity and prepulse inhibition: differences between the dorsal and ventral hippocampus. *Behav Neurosci* **116**: 72-84, 2002a.

Zhang C, Shen W, Zhang G. *N*-methyl-D-aspartate receptor and L-type voltage-gated Ca^{2+} channel antagonists suppress the release of cytochrome c and the expression of procaspase-3 in rat hippocampus after global brain ischemia. *Neurosci Lett* **328:** 265-268, 2002b.

Zheng F, Gingrich MB, Traynelis SF, Conn PJ. Tyrosine kinase potentiates NMDA receptor currents by reducing tonic zinc inhibition. *Nature Neurosci* **1:** 185-191, 1998.

Zomkowski AD, Hammes L, Lin J, Calixto JB, Santos AR, Rodrigues AL. Agmatine produces antidepressant-like effects in two models of depression in mice. *NeuroReport* **13:** 387-391, 2002.

In: Cognition and Mood Interactions
Editor: Miao-Kun Sun, pp. 71-88

ISBN 1-59454-229-5
2005 © Nova Science Publishers, Inc.

Chapter IV

Angiotensin in Mood and Cognition

*Paul R. Gard**

School of Pharmacy & Biomolecular Sciences, University of Brighton, UK

The brain Renin-Angiotensin System, which is comprised of a variety of peptides including angiotensin II, angiotensin III and angiotensin IV acting on AT_1, AT_2 and AT_4 receptors, is best known for its effects on the cardiovascular system and its role in hypertension but it is also important in cognition and behaviour. Although confusing and contradictory, animal studies suggest that angiotensin II reduces learning and memory, increases anxiety and possibly has some role in depressive-like behaviour. Studies with transgenic animals generally support these findings, although the particular receptor subtypes involved remain unresolved. Related to these experimental findings in animals, drugs which decrease brain angiotensin II function appear to have cognitive enhancing, anxiolytic and antidepressant effects.

Data from humans studies are less clear, evidence of anxiolytic and antidepressant actions remain anecdotal or subsumed within claims of improved 'Quality of Life' but there is now good evidence that angiotensin II antagonists may not only prevent age-related cognitive decline, but may improve cognition. The involvement of the brain renin-angiotensin system in the aetiology of common human psychological disorders remains to be fully appreciated, as does the potential for its manipulation in their treatment.

1. Introduction

In 1897 Tiegerstedt and Bergman discovered a pressor substance contained in saline extracts of the kidney, which they named "renin". It was not until 1940, however, that Braun-Menendez and his colleagues in Argentina and Page and Helmer in the United States independently reported that renin was, in fact, an enzyme that acted on a plasma protein to produce another peptide with pressor activity. This newly discovered peptide was given the name hypertensin by Braun-Menendez and his colleagues and angiotonin by Page and Helmer; they later agreed to rename the substance using the hybrid term angiotensin and to call the plasma protein substrate angiotensinogen. It is now recognised that, in humans, angiotensinogen is a 14 amino acid peptide which is converted to a decapeptide, now called angiotensin I, by the actions of renin. angiotensin I is then converted to the octapeptide angiotensin II by Angiotensin Converting Enzyme (ACE) which is present within the endothelium of most blood vessels but has highest concentrations within the pulmonary vasculature. This synthetic cascade is represented in figure 4.1. Angiotensin II is the bioactive peptide originally identified by Braun-Menendez and his colleagues and by Page and Helmer.

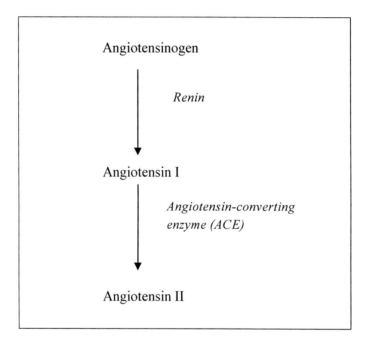

Figure. 4.1 Synthetic pathway for angiotensin II.

The recognition that renin, the angiotensins and ACE are of paramount importance in the control of blood pressure and fluid balance, and the discovery of a naturally occurring inhibitor of ACE in the venom of the Arrowheaded Viper (*Bothrops Jararaca*), meant that the 'Renin-Angiotensin System' became the focus of intense research in the latter half of the twentieth century. This research, because of the history of the discovery of renin and angiotensin II, was concentrated on the development of agents for the treatment of cardiovascular disorders. The cardiovascular system, however, is not the only system in which renin and angiotensin system play a role.

2. The Renin- Angiotensin System

The true complexity of the renin- angiotensin system has only emerged over the last few years. Synthesis of the angiotensins begins with the conversion of angiotensinogen, a circulating peptide produced predominantly by the liver but also produced in the brain, to angiotensin I by renin. ACE then converts angiotensin I to angiotensin II, the most active of the angiotensins. ACE (also named EC 3.4.15.1) has broad dipeptidyl carboxypeptidase and aminopeptidase activities and thus has other actions, for example the inactivation of bradykinin. Angiotensin II is ultimately metabolised to angiotensin III (angiotensin$_{2-8}$), angiotensin IV (angiotensin$_{3-8}$) and/or a variety of other fragments such as angiotensin$_{1-7}$, or angiotensin$_{2-7}$. Alternative, minor, metabolic pathways also exist whereby AI can be converted to angiotensin II by chymase; [des-ASP[1]] angiotensin I can be converted directly to angiotensin III by ACE; and angiotensin I can be converted to angiotensin$_{1-7}$ (see Wright and Harding, 1997) All of the angiotensins are pharmacologically active although they have significantly different potencies; the amino acids sequences of the human angiotensins are presented in figure 4.2.

	1 2 3 4 5 6 7 8 9 10 11 12 13 14
Angiotensinogen	Asp-Arg-Val-Tyr-Ile-His-Pro-Phe-His-Leu-Leu-Val-Tyr-Ser
Angiotensin I	Asp-Arg-Val-Tyr-Ile-His-Pro-Phe-His-Leu
Angiotensin II	Asp-Arg-Val-Tyr-Ile-His-Pro-Phe
Angiotensin-(2-8) (AIII)	Arg-Val-Tyr-Ile-His-Pro-Phe
Angiotensin-(1-7)	Asp-Arg-Val-Tyr-Ile-His-Pro
Angiotensin-(3-7}	Val-Tyr-Ile-His-Pro
Angiotensin-(3-8) (AIV)	Asp-Arg-Val-Tyr-Ile-His-Pro

Figure 4.2. Amino acid sequences of the angiotensin family

The renin-angiotensin system appears to have developed early in evolution with angiotensins, or angiotensin-like peptides, being identified in many species, for example the African locust (*Locusta migratoria*), leeches (*Theromyzon tessulatum, Erpobdella octocula, Hirudo medicinalis*), molluscs (eg *Aplysia californica),* crabs (*Chasmagnathus granulatus*), fish, alligators birds and mammals. Across these species the structures of the angiotensins are highly conserved, normally with 80-90% homology (Salzet et al., 2001).

3. The Angiotensin Receptors

The different rank order of potency of different angiotensin analogues in different tissues has indicated the existence of multiple angiotensin receptors (see de Gasparo et al., 2000). In humans and other mammals the most prevalent angiotensin receptor is the angiotensin type 1 receptor (AT$_1$), which is a G-protein coupled receptor. In rats and mice there are two subtypes of angiotensin AT$_1$ receptor, type 1$_A$ and type 1$_B$, which seem to be pharmacologically identical, but are coded by separate genes, whilst in humans there is a single receptor. Most of the physiological actions of angiotensin II are mediated via this receptor which has been identified in the gut, heart and vascular tissue, kidney, liver, uterus, ovaries, testes, adrenal gland and brain. In most cases the transduction process involves generation of inositol trisphosphate (IP$_3$) and the mobilisation of Ca^{++} ions, although other processes have also been identified. Angiotensin II and angiotensin III have almost equal potency at the AT$_1$ receptor whilst angiotensin IV has low affinity, but some efficacy.

Angiotensin $_{1-7}$ has affinity for the AT_1 receptor but little efficacy, thus in some systems it has been shown to act as an antagonist.

Angiotensin II is also the native ligand for the angiotensin type 2 receptor (AT_2). Like the AT_1 receptor, the AT_2 receptor is a G-protein coupled receptor with an amino acid sequence 34% identical to the AT_1 receptor. The AT_2 receptor is expressed widely in the foetus but densities decline rapidly after birth. AT_2 receptor expression, however, is maintained in the heart, non-pregnant uterus, adrenal glands, ovaries and brain and increases in tissues following injury or damage. Stimulation of AT_2 receptors induces an antiproliferative effect in damaged / regenerating tissues and, in some cases, apoptosis. AT_2 receptors have also been shown to have vasodilator effects thus in some tissues they appear to oppose the effects of AT_1 receptor stimulation. The signal transduction mechanism varies, but commonly involves K^+ and Ca^{++} ion channels and growth factor stimulation.

The existence of an angiotensin type 3 receptor, which is selective for angiotensin III has been proposed, but is, as yet, unproven, although angiotensin III is known to be active at the AT_1 receptor and may even be the endogenous agonist for that receptor in the brain.

Angiotensin type 4 receptors (AT_4), for which either angiotensin IV or an unrelated peptide, Leu Val Val-hemorphin-7 (LVV-hemorphin-7), isolated from sheep brain, may be endogenous ligands, have been clearly identified in the brain in areas distinct from those possessing AT_1 and AT_2 receptors, and also in the adrenal gland, heart, thymus, kidney, bladder and aorta. The binding site has been identified as an insulin-related amino peptidase (IRAP) also known as oxytocinase (Albiston et al.,2001), although other transduction processes may exist (Vauguelin et al., 2002). IRAP is known to cleave oxytocin, vasopressin, and other biologically active peptide such as angiotensin III and as angiotensin IV inhibits this enzyme it may potentiate their activity. Like the AT_2 receptor, the effect of AT_4 receptor stimulation may also oppose those of AT_1 receptor stimulation.

The identification of angiotensin receptors in the brain was of significance as neither renin nor the angiotensins cross the blood brain barrier. Only those brain areas unprotected by this barrier, for example the circumventricular organs (organum vasculosum of the lamina terminalis, the subfornical organ, the median eminence and the area postrema) are therefore sensitive to circulating angiotensins. It has now become apparent that the brain possesses a complete, and independent, renin-angiotensin system, although the details of its role have yet to be fully elucidated.

4. Brain Distributions

Brain concentrations of angiotensin II in the rat are approximately 50 fmol/g of brain tissue (range 590 fmol/g in hypothalamus – 15 fmol/g in cortex), compared with plasma concentrations of 17 fmol/ml (Hermann et al., 1984). Angiotensinogen, and its mRNA have been identified in the brain and found to be identical to those of the liver and renin and its mRNA are also present in the brain. The distribution angiotensinogen within the brain generally correlates with the distribution of the angiotensin receptors but there are also high concentrations within the choroid plexus and in astrocytes which constituitively secrete it. Disruption of astrocyte synthesis of angiotensinogen decreases brain concentrations of angiotensinogen and angiotensins I and II by over 90%. Angiotensinogen is a major component of cerebrospinal fluid. Concentrations of mRNA encoding for renin are low in the brain, with a distribution which is not closely associated with angiotensin II-containing neurones, nor angiotensin receptors. This finding may indicate that renin is not the only enzyme involved in the conversion of angiotensinogen to angiotensin I in the brain.

ACE is also widely distributed throughout the brain, and like angiotensinogen, it is found associated with the cerebral blood vessels, especially the choroid plexus, with astrocytes of the circumventricular organs; in brain areas with high concentrations of angiotensin receptors and, paradoxically, in areas such as the basal ganglia where there are low concentrations of angiotensin receptors. Angiotensin II itself is found within synaptic vesicles in nerve terminals in those areas with high angiotensin receptor concentrations. These nerve terminals either have synaptic contacts with other neurones or are associated with the blood vessels supplying the circumventricular organs. The enzymes responsible for breakdown of angiotensin II, aminopeptidase A and aminopeptidase N are also found within the brain (see Mendelsohn et al., 1990 and McKinley et al., 2003 for reviews).

The rat brain has high concentrations of angiotensin receptors in the septum with concentrations decreasing, in order, in the thalamus, midbrain, area postrema, medulla, hypothalamus, striatum, cerebellum, hippocampus and cortex. Septal concentrations are approximately 14 times higher than those of the cortex, but are half those found in the anterior pituitary gland and 12% of those of the adrenal glands, the highest concentration of angiotensin receptors (Sirett et al., 1977). Studies in adult human brain show that the receptors of the circumventricular organs are of the AT_1 subtype (Barnes et al., 1993; MacGregor et al., 1995) whilst in the basal ganglia 10-30% of the receptors are AT_2 (Barnes et al., 1993). Within the cerebellum the angiotensin II receptor subtype distribution was found to be approximately 50% AT_1 and 50% AT_2 subtype (Barnes et al., 1993; MacGregor et al., 1995). AT_4 receptors have been found in high concentrations in the cortex, cerebellum, thalamus and hippocampus (Wright and Harding, 1997).

5. Roles of Angiotensins in Cognition

Angiotensin II appears to have several roles as a neurotransmitter (for reviews see Ganong, 1984; Phillips 1987; Phillips and Sumners, 1998), it is involved with thirst, sodium appetite, drinking and antidiuretic hormone (ADH, arginine vasopressin) secretion; it has central pressor effects; it causes a decrease in body temperature; it facilitates secretion of adrenocorticotrophic hormone (ACTH) and it influences secretion of luteinizing hormone (LH), the nature of the influence being dependent upon the presence or absence of oestrogens and progesterone. There are also documented interactions between brain angiotensin II and other neurotransmitters such as noradrenaline and 5-hydroxytryptamine (5-HT) (Phillips, 1987). In the brain, angiotensin II potentiates the release of noradrenaline evoked by electrical stimulation or by application of K^+ and in cell culture angiotensin II increases neuronal concentrations of noradrenaline. Conversely noradrenaline inhibits angiotensin II release and decreases the number of angiotensin receptors. It therefore appears that there is a form of negative feedback relationship between noradrenaline and angiotensin II.

Angiotensin II also increases synthesis of 5-HT, an action that may be important in the dipsogenic effects of angiotensin II as 5-HT antagonists reduce the drinking response to angiotensin II in rats.

Studies of the physiological roles of the brain renin-angiotensin system have been facilitated by the development of drugs for its manipulation, drugs developed primarily for the control of blood pressure. Such drugs include saralasin, which is a peptide, nonselective antagonist of AT_1 and AT_2 receptors; losartan, a specific antagonist of AT_1 receptors and PD123319, an AT_2 receptor antagonist. Inhibitors of ACE include captopril and enalapril.

5.1. Cognitive Roles in Animals

One of the most prolific researchers of the roles of angiotensin in the brain is Braszko who has published extensively on the effects of angiotensin on learning and cognition. In rats, intracerebroventricular injection of angiotensin II has consistently been shown to increase the rate of acquisition of conditioned avoidance responses, recall of passive avoidance behaviour and object recognition (eg Braszko et al, 2002); the AT_1 receptor antagonist losartan was able to abolish the ability of angiotensin II to improve object recognition in rats, although it had no significant effect on angiotensin II-enhanced conditioned avoidance (Kulakowska et al., 1996). These effects probably involve noradrenaline and dopamine (Wisniewski & Braszko, 1984; Braszko & Wisniewski, 1990). The importance of angiotensin in normal learning is further highlighted by the demonstration that the ACE inhibitor Trandolapril can block conditioned avoidance, although it had no effect on passive avoidance nor object recognition (Braszko et al., 2000). Similar angiotensin-induced facilitation of learning has been seen in crabs where not only exogenous angiotensin, but also endogenous angiotensin synthesis, induced by water deprivation, has been shown to accelerate acquisition of an escape response to a bird-shaped shadow (Frenkel. et al 2002). These effects were blocked by prior administration of the non-selective angiotensin antagonist saralasin (ibid.)

The nature of the receptors involved in these responses to angiotensin administration has yet to be fully elucidated. The AT_1 receptor antagonist losartan was able to block the effect of the angiotensin II on object recognition and passive avoidance, but not conditioned avoidance, whilst the AT_2 receptor antagonist PD123319 blocked the effects of AII in both paradigms. When given together, losartan and PD123319 not only decreased the acquisition of conditioned avoidance in angiotensin II-treated rats, but also in control animals. These results suggested that angiotensin II is able to enhance passive avoidance, object recognition and conditioned avoidance but that the former two types of learning involve AT_1 receptors and possible AT_2 receptors whilst the latter type involves AT_2 receptors but not AT_1 receptors (Braszko 2002). The interplay between the receptor subtypes in influencing cognition, and the mechanisms underlying the observed effects of ACE inhibition still need to be characterized.

Angiotensin$_{3-7}$ was found to mimic angiotensin II in its ability to enhance passive avoidance, conditioned avoidance and object recognition in rats (Karwowska-Polecka et al.,

1997). Angiotensin$_{3-7}$ is a low affinity agonist at AT$_1$ receptors but binds with much higher affinity to AT$_4$ receptors; its effects on passive avoidance and object recognition were antagonized by losartan, suggesting the involvement of AT$_1$ receptors. The lack of effect of losartan on the enhancement of conditioned avoidance by angiotensin$_{3-7}$ suggests the involvement of AT$_4$ receptors in this latter form of memory (ibid.). These results are, however, difficult to reconcile with the earlier data obtained following the use of the ACE inhibitor Trandolapril, which was seen to block conditioned avoidance but not passive avoidance nor object recognition.

The difficulty lies in the fact that ACE is involved in the synthesis of angiotensin II, it can also be involved in the synthesis of angiotensin III via a route by-passing angiotensin I and angiotensin II (see earlier) and it is known to metabolise the endogenous AT$_4$ agonist LVV-hemorphin 7 (Hayakari et al., 2003). ACE inhibition would be expected to prevent the synthesis of angiotensin II, decreasing AT$_1$ and AT$_4$ receptor stimulation and increase concentrations of LVV-hemorphin-7, increasing AT$_4$ receptor stimulation. Why should Trandolapril therefore block conditioned avoidance, an AT$_4$ mediated effect, but not passive avoidance or object recognition, AT$_1$ receptor mediated effects?

A separate body of knowledge exists which apparently contradicts the research of Braszko and colleagues. In mice, Costall and colleagues reported that intraperitoneal administration of ACE inhibitors decreased the time taken to 'learn' to avoid a bright area – passive avoidance (Barnes et al., 1989). Furthermore, using the same methods, learning deficits in aged mice or those induced by scopolamine or lesion of the nucleus basalis were also reversed by ACE inhibitors. The ACE inhibitor ceronapril was also effective in improving learning in a water maze task (spatial memory) in rats. Furthermore Raghavendra et al. (1998) reported that the AT$_1$ receptor antagonist losartan was able to enhance memory in mice, as assessed by a passive avoidance task and by the elevated plus-maze. Losartan also reversed the cognitive deficits induced by scopolamine and itself was potentiated by co-administration of a cholinesterase inhibitor suggesting a cognitive-enhancing effect of angiotensin II suppression and indicating a mediating role of acetylcholine (ibid.). Manschot et al (2003), using a water maze, have similarly reported that the ACE inhibitor enalapril improved the impaired learning of stretozocin-induced diabetic rats, an effect attributed to maintenance of cerebral blood flow in these animals. The ACE inhibitor cilazapril and the AT$_1$ receptor antagonist E4177, at non-antihypertensive doses, have also been shown to improve memory function (passive avoidance) in aged, salt-sensitive, Dahl rats (Hirawa et al., 1999), and, in a maze task, losartan has been shown to increase performance in ethanol-impaired rats (Tracy et al., 1997). Pederson et al (2001) have also reported that the AT$_4$ receptor ligand norleucine-AIV is able to reverse scopolamine-induced spatial memory deficits in rats.

In addition to behavioural methods, learning and memory has been studied using electrophysiological techniques where long term potentiation (LTP) in brain slices, typically hippocampal, is seen as being fundamentally associated with memory acquisition and storage. Denny et al., (1991) reported that angiotensin II injected above the hippocampus in the intact rat blocked the induction of LTP in perforant path-stimulated dentate granule cells. That the effect was mediated by AT$_1$ receptors was later demonstrated by its antagonism by losartan (Wayner et al., 1993). Angiotensin II also suppresses LTP in the lateral nucleus of the amygdala (von Bohlen und Halbach et al., 1998). These effects of angiotensin II on LTP in the amygdala were also antagonised by losartan but not by PD123,319, the selective AT_2 receptor antagonist (ibid.). Such results suggest that suggest that angiotensin II acts on AT_1 receptors to suppress memory, and thus contradict the behavioural findings of Braszko and colleagues.

More recent evidence has highlighted the importance of the AT_4 receptors in learning and memory. AT_4 receptor agonists increase LTP, an effect blocked by AT_4 receptor antagonists (Wright et al., 2003). Importantly, the antagonist Nle^1, $Leual^3$-AngIV alone, reduces duration of the LTP suggesting that there may be an endogenous AT_4 receptor agonist involved in LTP (ibid.) or possibly that Nle^1, $Leual^3$-AngIV has some inverse agonist properties. Stimulation of AT_4 receptors has even been seen to overcome the inhibitory effects of acute and chronic ethanol on LTP (ibid.). The precise mechanism of angiotensin IV's effect on memory and learning remains to be clarified. As described previously the AT_4 receptor is believed to be an insulin-regulated amino peptidase that is associated with the GLUT4 glucose transporter and which degrades a variety of peptides including oxytocin and angiotensin III. Angiotensin IV inhibits the peptidase activity but enhances glucose uptake. Albiston et al (2003) suggest that, in the light of the knowledge that glucose enhances cognition in animals and humans and that mitogen-activated protein kinase (MAPK) is a signaling mechanism associated with memory processing, the memory/LTP enhancement induced by angiotensin IV may be a consequence of: (1) potentiation of the half-life of neuroactive peptides that potentiate memory; (2) increased glucose uptake; (3) direct activation of MAPK. Wright et al (2003), however, argue that the time course of the effect of AT_4 receptor agonists is too rapid for it to be associated with peptidase activity, furthermore they demonstrated that the effect appears to be associated with L-type calcium channels as it can be blocked using nimodipine, an L-type voltage gated calcium channel blocker. Another possibility is suggested by the report that angiotensin IV and LVV-hemorphin-7 potentiate the release of acetylcholine from rat hippocampal brain slices (Lee et al., 2001).

The results of animal studies are therefore confusing. Braszko's work suggests that angiotensin II enhances learning and memory, and that drugs which decrease angiotensin II function inhibit learning. Furthermore, different types of memory are mediated via different process with conditioned avoidance being mediated by AT_2 and AT_4 receptors but passive avoidance and object recognition involving AT_1 and AT_2 receptors. Other evidence, however, indicates that ACE inhibitors and Losartan enhance spatial memory and passive avoidance, suggesting a facilitatory involvement of AT_1 receptors and that AT_4 receptor stimulation enhances spatial memory. Importantly, the work of Braszko utilised 'normal, healthy animals', whilst many of the studies producing the opposing data utilise 'memory-impaired' animals. It is probable, however, that a normally functioning renin-angiotensin system is not necessary for normal learning and memory: memory is unchanged in mice lacking angiotensinogen (Walther et al., 1999), and in mice lacking AT_2 receptors (Sakagawa et al., 2000). This does not, of course, rule out a role for AT_4 receptors, for which the primary endogenous agonist may be LVV-hemorphin-7 rather than angiotensin IV. Abnormal brain angiotensin function may, however, impact on learning and memory in certain circumstances as evidenced by the report that m(Ren2)27 rats with increased brain angiotensin II due to over-expression of mouse renin in the brain had greater age-associated deficits in learning and that ASrAogen rats, with decreased brain angiotensin II maintained memory and learning into old age (Oden et al., 2002).

5.2. Cognitive Roles in Humans

The effects of ACE inhibitors and AT_1 receptor antagonists on cognitive function in humans have been investigated in a variety of settings. Until recently, studies which considered the effects of antihypertensive medication on cognitive function in humans looked only at their potential for adverse effects on performance but Amenta et al (2002) suggested that treatment of hypertensive patients with ACE inhibitors could produce positive cognitive outcomes. ACE inhibitors were significantly better than either diuretics or beta-blockers in improving cognitive function but no better than calcium channel blockers; all were equally effective in regulating hypertension. It is likely that these effects on cognition are consequential to actions on vascular damage, since the slowing of vascular cognitive impairment events runs in parallel with these cognitive changes, and this measure again differentiates ACE inhibitors from the other antihypertensive treatments. Amenta and colleagues (2002) even suggested that the ACE inhibitors may reverse vascular cognitive impairments associated with pre-existing hypertension. Muldoon et al., (2002) similarly reported that all of the antihypertensive therapies that they tested improved cognitive function, probably due to the decrease in blood pressure although Tzourio (2003) reported that ACE inhibition reduced cognitive decline to a greater extent than other antihypertensive treatments, but they took no account of differences in blood pressure. Looking at patients with diagnoses of Alzheimer's disease or dementia, Weiner et al (1992), for example, reported that four week administration of the ACE inhibitor ceranapril to a small sample of patients with dementia of Alzheimer's type and healthy controls was without effect on cognition, similar negative results were reported by Sudilovsky et al (1993). Another study by Louis et al (1999) tested effects of the ACE inhibitor perindopril (18 week cross-over study) on cognition in elderly hypertensives, and again reported no treatment-related changes in performance. The selective AT_1 receptor antagonist Candesartan also appears to be ineffective in improving cognitive function in Alzheimer's patients (Lithell et al., 2003).

In contrast, Tedesco et al (1999) reported a 26-month trial comparing the AT_1 antagonist losartan with hydrochlorothiazide, an antihypertensive diuretic, in matched samples of older and younger mild-moderate hypertensives. They reported a cognitive improvement in patients receiving losartan, which were paralleled by decreases in blood pressure. There were also significant improvements in 'Quality of Life'. The blood pressure and 'Quality of Life' scores were significantly improved in the hydrochlorothiazide groups, but there were no parallel improvements on the cognitive measures. More recently, Fogari et al (2002) have reported that Losartan produced positive effects on cognition in very elderly (75-89) mild-moderate hypertensives. These latter two studies suggest a potential dissociation between the ACE inhibitors and AT_1 receptor antagonists; ACE inhibitors appear to have no more than moderate benefits on cognition whereas the AT_1 receptor antagonist Losartan, in contrast, induces significant and absolute changes in objective measures of cognitive performance; the lack of any observed effect of the AT_1 receptor antagonist candesartan (Louis et al., 1999) may be due to the trial design, i.e. candesartan / placebo were used in combination with other active antihypertensives.

These results suggest that angiotensin may be important in human cognition, and that inhibition of angiotensin function is the key to improvement, a suggestion apparently contradictory to the findings of Braszko and colleagues in animals (see above). The differentiation between ACE inhibitors in the clinical studies is also important. ACE inhibitors prevent synthesis of AII and therefore reduce stimulation of AT_1 and AT_2 receptors, and potentially AT_4 receptors; AT_1 receptor antagonists, on the other hand, prevent AT_1 receptor stimulation, but may enhance AT_2 and AT_4 receptor stimulation due to increased availability of the agonist and its metabolites. Whether the losartan, however, is correcting some underlying abnormality in the brain RAS in patients with cognitive impairment is unlikely. Ge and Barnes (1996) reported a lack of association between Alzheimer's disease and brain AT_1 receptors although there was a substantial increase in AT_2 receptor density in the temporal cortices of such patients that may indicate involvement of AII in the degenerative process. Savaskan et al. (2001), however, reported increased ACE, angiotensin II and AT_1 receptor immunoreactivity in the cortices of Alzheimer's patients, particularly in association with the microvasculature. Whether changes such as those reported by Savaskan et al are the basis of the observed cognitive effects of losartan are unclear, but they would not explain the differential efficacy of ACE inhibitors and AT_1 receptor antagonists. Several studies have investigated possible links between renin-angiotensin system gene polymorphisms and dementias and Alzheimer's disease but as yet no robust associations have been identified (see Gard 2002).

6. Roles of Angiotensins in Mood Regulation

6.1. Anxiety

In addition to cognition, the brain renin-angiotensin system has also been implicated in the manifestation and potential treatment of anxiety. Georgiev and colleagues (1987) reported that angiotensin II influenced rat behaviour in an open field. The dose response relationship was non-linear and time-dependent with intracerebroventricular injection of angiotensin II reducing locomotion and rearing 5 min after administration, suggesting reduced anxiety, increasing rearing and grooming at 15 minutes, evidence of a possible rebound effect. These latter effects of angiotensin II could be antagonised by co-administration of saralasin, a non-selective angiotensin receptor antagonist; 15 min pretreatment with the antagonist alone gave effects opposite to those of angiotensin II, significantly reducing locomotion, rearing and grooming and suggesting possible antagonism of endogenous angiotensin II. The later (15 min) behavioural effects of angiotensin II were reported to be prevented by the dopamine antagonist haloperidol and potentiated by the dopamine agonist apomorphine and the dopamine reuptake inhibitor / receptor agonist nomifensin. This indicates that the 'rebound anxiolysis' may involve increased dopaminergic activity although the effects may have been dependent on the direct effects of haloperidol, apomorphine and nomifensin on the open field behaviour rather than any pharmacological interaction.

Further support for the proposal that brain angiotensin II is involved in anxiety-like behaviour was derived from the fact that administration of ACE inhibitors and losartan to rats and mice reduces behaviour normally susceptible to reduction by proven anxiolytic drugs; captopril, ceronapril and losartan have all been shown to exhibit anxiolytic properties commensurate with the a positive control such as diazepam (Costall et al., 1990; Barnes et al., 1990; Kaiser et al., 1992; Carbursano et al., 1997; Brasko et al, 2003; Srinivasan et al., 2003). Shepherd et al. (1996), however, were unable to replicate the anxiolytic-like effects of losartan in either rats or mice, possibly due to differences in the strain of animals tested, a feature highlighted by Costall et al. (1990), and Gard et al. (2001). Captopril and ceronapril also elicit anxiolytic-like responses in marmosets (Costall et al., 1990).

In another measure of behaviour associated with anxiety in rats, defensive burying of an aversive stimulus, 10-min pretreatment with angiotensin II or saralasin had anxiolytic-like effects (Tsuda et al., 1992), which give confusing messages about the role of angiotensin II in anxiety-like behaviours. In a more recent study combining elevated plus-maze and defensive burying in mice, however, it was revealed that losartan produced anxiolytic-like, and angiotensin II produced anxiogenic-like, responses 15 and 30 min after administration but opposite responses during the first 15 min with losartan causing anxiogenic-like burying and angiotensin II suppressing burying (Cresswell and Gard, 1998). The early anxiogenic-like effect of losartan was blocked by prior administration of the selective AT_2 receptor antagonist PD123319 (ibid.) suggesting that blocking AT_1 receptor activity initially unmasked a previously unreported, short-lived, AT_2 receptor-mediated anxiogenic-like response, but eventually resulted in reduced anxiety-related behaviours.

Taken together, the results suggest that central administration of angiotensin II causes anxiety-like behaviour and that reduction of the angiotensin II activity reduces anxiety. The timing of the treatment, and route of administration are however important, with peripheral administration of losartan giving early anxiogenic and later anxiolytic responses and central administration of angiotensin II giving similar early anxiogenic and later anxiolytic responses.

Despite these findings relating to perturbations of the brain renin-angiotensin system, the extent to which angiotensin II is involved in 'normal' anxiety is unclear as increases in endogenous angiotensin II synthesis by ligation of the renal artery has been associated with increase anxiety-like behaviour in the hypertensive rats produced (Srinivasan et al., 2003) and (mREN2)27 rats with increased brain formation of angiotensin II show increased anxiety-like behaviour (Wilson et al., 1996). Conversely, mice lacking angiotensinogen do not differ from control mice in a test of anxiety (Walther et al., 1999), but mice lacking AT_2 receptors display increased anxiety (Okuyama et al., 1999).

In clinical studies of drugs acting via the renin angiotensin system, the previously described improvements in 'Quality of Life' may reflect some anxiolysis but studies designed specifically to assess an effect on mood have failed to identify effects in healthy volunteers (Vanakoski et al., 2001) or in psychiatrically normal, hypertensive patients where neither ACE inhibitors nor AT_1 receptor antagonists affect anxiety scores (Muldoon et al., 2002; Lithell et al., 2003)

6.2. Depression

The brain renin-angiotensin system has also been implicated in the aetiology of depressive illness and its treatment. The earliest clues came from the finding that repeated administration of antidepressant drugs to rats reduced the fluid intake elicited by subcutaneous and intracerebroventricular isoprenaline (Goldstein et al., 1985; Przegalinski et al., 1988). The increased fluid intake is mediated by isoprenaline-induced stimulation of the renin-angiotensin system culminating in the production of angiotensin II. It was subsequently demonstrated that the antidepressant drugs desipramine, fluoxetine and tranylcypromine are all able to reduce angiotensin II-induced drinking in rats and to antagonise the contractile effects of angiotensin II in isolated smooth muscle (Gard & Mycroft, 1991; Gard et al., 1994). The antagonistic effect, however, is probably non-competitive as the antidepressant drugs do not displace radiolabelled angiotensin II from its receptors nor are they selective antagonists for angiotensin II, raising the possibility that they act on the post-receptor signal transduction processes (Gard & Barnes, 1994; Gard et al., 1999).

The suggestion that antidepressant drugs may disrupt angiotensin function was particulary interesting in the light of the report that, in mice, a single dose of captopril reduced immobility in the forced swim test to the same extent as the reduction produced by the proven antidepressants imipramine and mianserin (Giardina & Ebert, 1989); the forced swim test is a standard procedure for testing antidepressant activity. In another assessment of learned helplessness, 5 days treatment with captopril was as effective as imipramine (Martin et al., 1990). In both of these studies the effects of captopril could be reversed by naloxone, suggesting that the antidepressant-like effect of the ACE inhibitor involved opioid mediation. It is probable, however, that the antidepressant-like effects of captopril involve reduced angiotensin II function, as opposed to inhibition of any other actions of ACE, as losartan has also been shown to give positive antidepressant-like results in the mouse forced swim test (Gard et al., 1999). The animal studies therefore suggest that blockade of angiotensin II function is associated with antidepressant-like effects, but despite the finding that mice lacking angiotensinogen display reduced 'depressive-like' behaviour in the forced swim test (Okuyama et al.,1999) it is unlikely that the brain renin-angiotensin system is involved in the aetiology of depression in humans. No relationship was found between the number of receptors and the severity of the depressive symptoms in post-partum women (Gard et al., 1999) and studies of the relationship between genetic polymorphisms of the renin-angiotensin system and depression in humans have similarly failed to find a consistent link. The ACE D allele, which increases ACE activity was seen to be more frequent in Japanese patients with affective disorders (Arinami et al., 1996) but five studies have failed to replicate the association between ACE genotype and either unipolar or bipolar depression (Furlong et al., 2000; Meira-Lima et al., 2000; Pauls et al., 2000; Hong et al., 2002; Cataoluk et al., 2002), although one study found an increased frequency of the M allele of the M235T angiotensinogen gene, which raises plasma angiotensinogen, amongst bipolar depressive patients (Meira-Lima et al., 2000).

Apart from the anecdotal evidence of reduced depression amongst depressed hypertensives receiving ACE inhibitors (see Gard, 2002), there have been no systematic clinical studies of possible antidepressant effects of ACE inhibitors or AT_1 receptor antagonists in depressed subjects although clinical trials of antihypertensive agents such as ACE inhibitors show no effects on mood in psychiatric normal patients (Muldoon et al, 2002).

7. Conclusions

In conclusion, the body of knowledge relating to the roles of angiotensins in behaviour and cognition, and the potential for manipulation of the renin-angiotensin system for the treatment of cognitive and psychiatric disorders is both confusing and contradictory. A general overview suggests that reduction of brain angiotensin II function improves memory and learning, particularly in animals with disrupted cognitive function; decreases anxiety-like behaviour and mimics the effects of antidepressant drugs in animals. When considering animal data it is important to recognise, however, that there is an element of cross-contamination between the methods used (Braszko et al., 2003). Antidepressant drugs, for example, are assessed by means of learned helplessness and obviously drugs that affect learning will influence learned helplessness, similarly anxiety will influence animal behaviour within the mazes used to assess learning. The evidence in the human population, however, suggests that blockade of the AT_1 receptor has positive effects on cognitive function in the elderly, and that, as yet, there are no identified effects on other aspects of mood. A greater knowledge of the roles of the renin-angiotensin system in the brain, and the differential roles of the receptor subtypes will undoubtedly lead to the development of novel psychoactive agents and will increase our understanding of the aetiology of a range of psychological disorders.

References

Albiston AL, Mcdowall SG, Matsacos D, Sim P, Clune E, Mustafa T, Lee J, Mendelsohn FAO, Simpson RJ, Connolly LM, Chai SY. Evidence that the angiotensin IV (AT4) receptor is the enzyme insulin regulated aminopeptidase. *J. Biol. Chem.* **276**: 48623-48626, 2001.

Albiston AL, Mustafa T, McDowall SG, Mendelsohn FAO, Lee J, Chai SY. AT4 receptor is insulin-regulated membrane aminopeptidase: potential mechanisms of memory enhancement. *Trends in Endocrinology and metabolism* **14**: 72-77, 2003.

Amenta F, Mignini F, Rabbia F, Tomassoni D, Veglio F. Protective effect of anti-hypertensive treatment on cognitive function in essential hypertension: Analysis of published clinical data. *J. Neurol. Sci.* **203**: 147-151, 2002.

Arinami T, Li LM, Mitsushio H, Itokawa M, Hamaguchi H, Toru M. An insertion/deletion polymorphism in the angiotensin converting enzyme gene is associated with both brain substance P contents and affective disorders. *Biol. Psychiatry* **40**: 1122-1127, 1996.

Barnes JM, Barnes NM, Costall B, Coughlan J, Horovitz ZP, Kelly ME, Naylor RJ, Tomkins DM. ACE inhibition and cognition. In: MacGregor GA, Sever PS, editors. Current Advances in ACE inhibition, proceedings of an international symposium. Edinburgh: Churchill Livingstone, 1989 159-171.

Barnes NM, Costall B, Kelly ME, Murphy DA, Naylor RJ. Anxiolytic-like action of DuP753, a non-peptide angiotensin II receptor antagonist. *Neuroreport* **1:** 15-16, 1990.

Barnes JM, Steward LJ, Barber PC, Barnes NM. Identification and characterisation of angiotensin II receptor subtypes in human brain. *Eur. J. Pharmacol.* **230:** 251-258, 1993.

Braszko JJ. AT(2) but not AT(1) receptor antagonism abolishes angiotensin II increase of the acquisition of conditioned avoidance responses in rats. *Behav. Brain Res.* **131:** 79-86, 2002.

Braszko JJ, Kulakowska A, Winnicka MM. Effects of angiotensin-II and its receptor antagonists on motor activity and anxiety in rats. *J. Physiol. Pharmacol.* **54:** 271-281, 2003.

Braszko JJ, Paslawska L, Karwowska-Polecka W, Holowina A. Trandolapril attenuates acquisition of conditioned avoidance in rats. *Polish J. Pharmacol.*) **52:** 195-201, 2000.

Braszko JJ, Wisniewski K. α_1 and α_2 – adrenergic receptor blockade influences angiotensin II facilitation of avoidance behaviour and stereotypy in rats. *Psychoneuroendocrinology* **15:** 239-252, 1990.

Cambursano PT, Haigh SJ, Keightley J, Sutcliffe MA, Gard PR. Positive effects of losartan in laboratory tests indicative of anxiolytic-like activity and the importance of animal strain. *J. Pharm. Pharmacol.* **49 (suppl 4):** 64, 1997.

Cataloluk O, Nacak M, Savas HA, Tutkun H, Zoroglu SS, Herken H, Barlas O, Ozen ME, Arslan A. Angiotensin converting enzyme gene polymorphism and its association to bipolar affective disorder in Turkish population. *Neurol. Psychiat. Brain Res.* **10:** 129-132, 2002..

Costall B, Domeney AM, Gerrard PA, Horovitz ZP, Kelly ME, Naylor RJ, Tomkins DM. Effects of captopril and SQ29,852 on anxiety-related behaviours in rodent and marmoset. *Pharmacol., Biochem., Behav.* **36:** 13-20, 1990.

Cresswell AG, Gard PR. Behavioural evidence of a paradoxical anxiogenic effect of an angiotensin II (AT1) receptor antagonist. *J. Pharm. Pharmacol.* **50 (suppl):** 215, 1998.

de Gasparo M, Catt KJ, Inagami T, Wright, JW, Unger T. The angiotensin II receptors. *Pharmacol. Rev.* **52:** 415-472, 2000.

Denny JB, Polancurtain J, Wayner M, Armstrong DL. Angiotensin-II blocks hippocampal long-term potentiation. *Brain Res.* **567:** 321-324. 1991.

Fogari R, Mugellini A, Zoppi A, Derosa G, Pasotti C, Fogari E, Preti P Influence of losartan and atenolol on memory function in very elderly hypertensive patients. *J. Hum. Hypertension* **17**: 781-785, 2003.

Frenkel L, Freudenthal R, Romano A, Nahmod VE, Maldonado H, Delorenzi A. Angiotensin II and the transcription factor Rel/NF-kappaB link environmental water shortage with memory improvement. *Neuroscience* **115:**1079-1087, 2002.

Furlong RA, Keramatipour M, Ho LW, Rubinsztein JS, Michael A, Walsh C, Paykel ES, Rubinsztein DC. No association of an insertion/deletion polymorphism in the angiotensin I converting enzyme gene with bipolar or unipolar affective disorders. *Am. J. Med. Genet.* **96:** 733-735, 2000.

Ganong WF. The brain renin-angiotensin system. *Ann. Rev. Physiol.* **46:** 17-31, 1984.

Gard PR. The role of angiotensin in cognition and behaviour. *Eur. J. Pharmacol.* **438**: 1-14, 2002.

Gard PR, Barnes NM. The effects of desipramine and fluoxetine on responses to angiotensin and angiotensin receptors. *Can. J. Physiol. Pharmacol.* **72 (Suppl. 1):** 439, 1994.

Gard PR, Haigh SJ, Cambursano PT, Warrington CA. Strain differences in the anxiolytic effects of losartan in the mouse. *Pharmacol. Biochem. Behav.* **69:** 35-40. 2001.

Gard PR, Mandy A, Sutcliffe, MA. Evidence of a possible role of altered angiotensin function in the treatment, but not aetiology, of depression. *Biol. Psychiatry* **45:** 1030-1034, 1999.

Gard PR, Mandy A, Whiting JM, Nickels DPD, Meakin AJLS. Reduction of responses to angiotensin II by antidepressant drugs. *Eur. J. Pharmacol.* **264:** 295-300, 1994.

Gard PR, Mycroft N. Reduction of angiotensin II-induced drinking in rats by 21 hour pretreatment with desipramine. *J. Pharm. Pharmacol.* **43 (suppl):** 1, 1991.

Ge JA, Barnes NM. Alterations in angiotensin AT_1 and AT_2 receptor subtype levels in brain regions from patients with neurodegenerative disorders. *Eur. J. Pharmacol.* **297:** 299-306, 1996.

Georgiev V, Getova D, Opitz M.; Mechanisms of the angiotensin II effects on the exploratory behaviour of rats in open field. 1. Interaction of angiotensin II with saralasin and catecholamine drugs. *Find. Exp. Clin. Pharmacol.* **9:** 297-301, 1987.

Giardina WJ, Ebert DM. Positive effects of captopril in the behavioural despair swim test. *Biol. Psychiatry* **25:** 697-702, 1989.

Goldstein JM, Knobloch-Litwin LC, Malick JB. Behavioural evidence for β-adrenoceptor subsensitivity after subacute antidepressant / $α_2$-adrenoceptor antagonist treatment. *Naunyn-Schmiedebergs Arch. Pharmacol.* **329:** 355-358, 1985.

Hayakari M, Satoh K, Izumi H, Kudoh T, Asano J, Yamazaki T, Tsuchida, S. Kinetic-controlled hydrolysis of Leu-Val-Val-hemorphin-7 catalyzed by angiotensin-converting enzyme from rat brain. *Peptides* **24:** 1075-1082, 2003.

Hermann K, Lang RE, Unger T, Bayer C, Ganten D. Combined high-performance liquid chromatography – radioimmunoassay for the characterization and quantitative measurement or neuropeptides. *J. Chromatog.* **312:** 273-284, 1984.

Hirawa N, Uehara Y, Kawabata Y, Numabe A, Comi T, Ikeda T, Suzuki T, Goto A, Toyo-Oka T, Omata M. Long-term inhibition of renin-angiotensin system sustains memory function in aged Dahl rats. *Hypertension* **34:** 496-502,1999

Hong CJ, Wang YC, Tsai SJ.Association study of angiotensin-I-converting enzyme polymorphism and symptomatology and antidepressant response in major depressive disorder. *J. Neural. Transm.* **109:** 1209-1214, 2002.

Kaiser FC, Palmer GC, Wallace AV, Carr RD, Fraserrae L, Hallam C. Antianxiety properties of the angiotensin-II antagonist, DuP753, in the rat using the elevated plus-maze. *Neuroreport* **3:** 922-924, 1992.

Karwowska-Polecka W, Kulakowska K, Wisniewski K, Braszko JJ. Losartan influences behavioural effects of angiotensin II (3-7) in rats. *Pharmacol. Res.* **36:** 275-283, 1997.

Kulakowska A, Karwowska W, Wisnieski K, Braszko JJ. Losartan influences behavioural effects of angiotensin II in rats. *Pharmacol. Res.* **34:** 109-115, 1996.

Lee J, Chai, S-Y, Mendelsohn FAO, Morris MJ, Allen AM. Potentiation of cholinergic transmission in the rat hippocampus by angiotensin IV and LVV-hemorphin-7. *Neuropharmacology* **40**: 618-623, 2001.

Lithell H, Hansson L, Skoog I, Elmfeldt D, Hofman A, Olofsson B, Trenkwalder P, Zanchetti A. The Study on cognition and prognosis in the elderly (SCOPE): principal results of a randomized double-blind intervention trial. *J Hypertens.* **21**: 875-886, 2003.

Louis WJ, Mander AG, Dawson M, O'Callaghan C, Conway EL. Use of computerised neuropsychological test (CANTAB) to assess cognitive effects of antihypertensive drugs in the elderly. *J. Hypertens.* **17**: 1813-1819, 1999).

MacGregor DP, Murone C, Song K, Allen AM, Paxinos G, Mendelsohn FAO. Angiotensin II receptor subtypes in the human central nervous system. *Brain Res.* **675**: 231-240, 1995.

Manschot SM, Biessels GJ, Cameron NE, Cotter MA, Kamal A, Kappelle LJ, Gispen WH. Angiotensin converting enzyme inhibition partially prevents deficits in water maze performance, hippocampal synaptic plasticity and cerebral blood flow in streptozocin-diabetic rats. *Brain Res.* **966**: 274-282, 2003.

Martin P, Massol J, Puech AJ. Captopril as an antidepressant? Effects on the learned helplessness paradigm in rats. *Biol. Psychiatry*, **27**: 968-974. 1990.

McKinley MJ, Albiston AL, Allen AM, Mathai ML, May CN, McAllen RM, Oldfield BJ, Mendelsohn FAO, Chai SY. The brain renin-angiotensin system: location and physiological roles. *Int. J. Biochem. Cell Biol.* **35**: 901-918, 2003.

Miera-Lima IV, Pereira AC, Mota GFA, Krieger JE, Vallada H. Angiotensinogen and angiotensin converting enzyme gene polymorphisms and the risk of bipolar affective disorders in humans. *Neurosci. Lett.,* **293**: 103-106, 2000.

Mendelsohn FAO, Allen AM, Chai S-Y, McKinley MJ, Oldfield BJ, Paxinos G. The brain angiotensin system – insights from mapping its components. *Trends Endocrin. Met.* **1**: 189-198, 1990.

Muldoon MF Waldstein SR, Ryan CM, Jennings JR, Polefrone JM, Shapiro AP, Manuck SB. Effects of six anti-hypertensive medications on cognitive performance. *J. Hypertens.* **20**: 1643-1652, 2002.

Oden SD, Carter C, Farrario CM, Ganten D, Basso N, Ferder LF, Sonntag WE, Diz DI. Influence of the brain renin-angiotensin system on cognitive ability during aging. *Hypertension* **40**: 381, 2002.

Okuyama S, Sakagawa T, Chaki S, Imagawa Y, Ichiki T, Inagami T. Anxiety-like behaviour in mice lacking the angiotensin II type-2 receptor. *Brain Research* **821**: 150-159, 1999.

Okuyama S, Sakagawa T, Sugiyama F, Fukamizu A, Murakami K. Reduction of depressive-like behaviour in mice lacking angiotensinogen. *Neuroscience Letters* **261**: 167-170, 1999.

Pauls J, Bandelow B, Ruther E, Kornhuber J. Polymorphism of the gene of angiotensin converting enzyme: lack of association with mood disorder. *J. Neural. Transm.* **107**: 1361-1366, 2000.

Pederson ES, Krishnan R, Harding JW, Wright JW. A role for the angiotensin AT(4) receptor subtype in overcoming scopolamine-induced spatial memory deficits. *Regulatory Peptides* **102**: 147-156, 2001.

Phillips MI. Functions of angiotensin in the central nervous system. *Annu. Rev. Physiol.* **49**: 413-435, 1987.

Phillips MI, Sumners C, Angiotensin II in central nervous system physiology. *Regul. Pept.* **78**: 1-11, 1998.

Przegalinski E, Siwanowicz J, Baran L, Effect of repeated administration of antidepressant drugs on the isoprenaline-induced drinking in rats. *Pol. J. Pharmacol.* **40**: 251-258, 1988.

Raghavendra V, Chopra K, Kulkarni SK, Involvement of cholinergic system in losartan-induced facilitation of spatial and short-term working memory. *Neuropeptides* **32**: 417-421, 1998.

Sakagawa T, Okuyama S, Kawashima N, Hozumi S, Nakagawasai O, Tadano T, Kisara K, Ichiki T, Inagami, T. Pain threshold, learning and formation of brain edema in mice lacking the angiotensin II type-2 receptor. *Life Sciences* **67**: 2577-2585, 2000.

Salzet M, Deloffre L, Breton C, Vieau D, Schoofs L. The angiotensin system elements in invertebrates. *Brain Research Reviews.* **36**: 35-45, 2001.

Savaskan E, Hock C, Olivieri G, Bruttel S, Rosenberg C, Hulette C, Muller-Spahn F. Cortical alterations of Angiotensin converting enzyme, angiotensin II and AT_1 receptor in Alzheimer's dementia. *Neurobiol. Aging* **22**: 541-546, 2001.

Shepherd J, Bill DJ, Dourish CY, Grewal SS, McLenachan A, Stanhope KJ. Effects of the selective angiotensin II receptor antagonists losartan and PD123177 in animal models of anxiety and memory. *Psychopharmacology* **126**: 206-218, 1996.

Sirett NE, McLean AS, Bray JJ, Hubbard JI. Distribution of angiotensin II receptors ion the rat brain. *Brain Res.* **122**: 299-312, 1977.

Srinivasan J, Suresh B, Ramanathan M. Differential anxiolytic effect of enalapril and losartan in normotensive and renal hypertensive rats. *Physiol Behav.* **78**: 585-591, 2003.

Sudilovsky A, Cutler NR, Sramek JJ, Wardle T, Veroff AE, Mickelson W, Markowitz J, Repetti S. A pilot clinical-trial of the angiotensin-converting enzyme-inhibitor ceranapril in Alzheimer-disease. *Alzheimer Dis. Assoc. Disord.* **7**: 105-111, 1993.

Tedesco MA, Ratti G, Mennella S, Manzo G, Grieco M, Rainone AC, Iarussi D, Iacono A. Comparison of losartan and hydrochlorthiazide on cognitive function and quality of life in hypertensive patients. *Am. J. Hypertens.* **12**: 1130-1134, 1999.

Tracy HA, Wayner MJ, Armstrong DL. Losartan improves the performance of ethanol-intoxicated rats in an eight-arm radial maze. *Alcohol* **14**: 511-517, 1997.

Tsuda A, Tanaka M, Georgiev V, Emoto H, Effects of angiotensin II on behavioral responses of defensive burying paradigm in rats. *Pharmacol. Biochem. Behav.* **43**: 729-732, 1992.

Tzourio C. Vascular factors and cognition: toward a prevention of dementia? *J. Hypertens.* **21**: Suppl 5: S15-S19, 2003.

von Bohlen und Halbach O, Albrecht D, Halbach OVU. Angiotensin II inhibits long-term potentiation within the lateral nucleus of the amygdala through AT(1) receptors. *Peptides* **19**: 1031-1036, 1998.

Vanakoski J, Seppala T, Stromberg C, Naveri L, Hammett J, Ford N. Effects of ceronapril alone or in combination with alcohol on psychomotor performance in healthy volunteers: a placebo-controlled crossover study. *Current Therapeutic Research* **62**: 699-708, 2001.

Vauquelin G, Michotte Y, Smolders I, Sarre S, Ebinger G, Dupont A, Vanderheyden P Cellular targets for angiotensin II fragments: pharmacological and molecular evidence. *JRAAS* **3**: 195-204, 2002.

Walther T, Voigt JP, Fukamizu A, Fink H, Bader M. Learning and anxiety in angiotensin-deficient mice *Behav. Brain Res,* **100**: 1-4, 1999.

Wayner MJ, Armstrong DL, Polancurtain JL, Denny JB. Role of angiotensin-II and AT_1 receptors in hippocampal LTP. *Pharmacol. Biochem. Behav.* **45**: 455-464, 1993.

Weiner MF, Bonte FJ, Tintner R, Ford N, Svetlik D, Riall T. ACE inhibitor lacks acute effect on cognition or brain blood-flow in Alzheimer's disease. *Drug Devel. Res.* **26**: 467-471, 1992.

Wisniewski K, Braszko JJ. The significance of central monoamine systems in the angiotensin II (AII) improvement of learning. *Clin. Exp. Hypertension.* **6**: 2127-2131, 1984.

Wilson W, Voigt P, Bader M, Marsden CA, Fink H. Behaviour of the transgenic (mREN2) 27 rat. *Brain Res.* **729**: 1-9, 1996.

Wright JW, Harding JW. Important roles for angiotensin III and IV in the brain renin-angiotensin system. *Brain Res. Rev.* **25**: 96-124, 1997.

Wright JW, Kramar EA, Myers DT, Davis CJ, Harding JW. Ethanol-induced suppression of LTP can be attenuated with an angiotensin IV analog. *Regulatory Peptides* **113**: 49-56, 2003.

In: Cognition and Mood Interactions
Editor: Miao-Kun Sun, pp. 89-103

ISBN 1-59454-229-5
2005 © Nova Science Publishers, Inc.

Chapter V

Mouse Models of Alzheimer Disease: Beyond Cognitive Impairments

*Robert Gerlai**

Department of Psychology, University of Hawaii, USA

Several reviews and book chapters have been published on animal models of human dementia of the Alzheimer type. They attest that the functional endpoint of the models concerns cognition and memory related impairments. Similarly, clinical studies of Alzheimer's Disease (AD) also focus on cognition. However, numerous other behavioral phenotypes, for example abnormal emotion or anxiety related traits, are also characteristic aspects of AD. Here some of the available animal models of AD are reviewed. In addition to the traditionally quantified traits, an empirical example is presented showing that AD mouse models can exhibit alterations not only in learning and memory but also in other behavioral characteristics including fear and exploratory behavior. It is argued that similarly to the human condition the behavioral changes elicited in mouse models of AD are complex and a spectrum of changes may be revealed if properly investigated. It is concluded that thorough behavioral characterization of mouse models of human dementia with the use of test batteries tapping into multiple domains of behavior is needed. This will significantly facilitate drug screening efforts in the models and will ultimately allow better development of pharmacotherapies in the human clinic.

1. Introduction

As the chapters of this book show, numerous types of human dementia exist. Similarly, many attempts have been made to model these diseases in animals. Without trying to be exhaustive the animal models may be grouped into four main categories: (i) natural processes models (e.g. aging models), (ii) spontaneously occurring mutants or inbred strains with idiosyncratic genetic characteristics (e.g. the senescence accelerated mouse or the DBA/2 mouse strain), (iii) pharmacological models (e.g. scopolamine induced impairment), and (iv) transgenic models. The latter will be the focus of the present review.

Transgenic mice are genetically engineered animals that carry an artificially modified "foreign" gene, the transgene. These animals are thought to be particularly useful for modeling human diseases in which the genetic underpinnings of the disease are known. Perhaps one of the most devastating human diseases that has also been found to have a tractable genetic origin (in the familial form of the disease) is Alzheimer's Disease (AD), a neurodegenerative brain disorder that affects approximately 15-20 % of the elderly population worldwide [Breteler et al., 1992]. The mechanisms underlying AD are hotly debated but one of the most widely accepted hypotheses concerns the expression and processing of the amyloid precursor protein, APP (e.g. [Johnson et al., 1997]). Mutations within exons 16 and 17 of the beta-amyloid precursor protein (APP) gene are known to cause familial Alzheimer's disease (for review see [Goate, 1998]). Each of these mutations alters proteolytic processing of APP, resulting in an increase in the production of $A\beta_{1-42}$, a highly fibrillogenic peptide, that spontaneously aggregates and deposits in the brain. Similarly, overexpression of APP, for example as a result of trisomy of Chromosome 21 seen in Down's Syndrome (DS), has been implicated as a causal factor in AD because DS patients develop AD by their age of 40 [Wisniewski et al., 1985]. In addition to APP, other major genes have also been identified whose mutations, or allelic variants, may cause AD or predispose the carriers to AD. They are the presenilins (PS1 and PS2) and the apolipoprotein-E4 (APOE4) allele. It must be mentioned that in addition to these molecular players, numerous other genes may be involved in AD, some of which may be functionally associated with the above known molecular targets and others may work through so far unrevealed biochemical pathways.

2. Concerns about Transgene Design in AD Models

Transgenic models of Alzheimer's Disease may be classified into three main categories according to the methods of their production (Duff, 1999): cDNA transgenics, whole-gene transgenics, and gene knock out mice. cDNA based transgenic mice were the first to be generated, however, the earlier models had a significant problem: as the transgene was based on expressed mRNA sequences it lacked several intronic regions and regulatory elements that are present in the endogenous gene of interest and are thought to be required for proper gene expression. Later cDNA based transgenic models attempted to correct this and had transgenes that contained some intronic and/or regulatory sequences. Another solution attempted has been to use the whole gene as transgene. However, these transgenes were too large for pronuclear injection, the usual method of transgene delivery, and therefore an alternative technique, artificial chromosomes (e.g. the Yeast Artificial Chromosome, or YAC) system was used. YAC could carry longer DNA sequences and thus was capable of delivering the transgene to Embryonic Stem (ES) cells that could then be screened for DNA incorporation and used for the generation of germ-line transmitting ES cell chimeras.

It is important to note, however, that both the cDNA and the YAC based transgenic mice suffer from a potentially important disadvantage: insertion of the transgene into the host genome occurs randomly. This leads to three potential problems. One, if the insertion site is in a functionally important gene or in its control elements, the transgene may disrupt the endogenous gene leading to a phenotypical alteration that is not related to the transgene itself. Two, the functioning of the transgene may be influenced by neighboring regulatory elements, which may be different depending on landing site. Three, the transgene is expressed in addition to the expression of its endogenous homolog and thus the normally expressed endogenous gene may mask the effects of the mutant transgene, a definite problem in APP transgenics where the endogenous (non-mutant) APP, which is neuroprotective, may reduce the pathologic effects of the mutant APP transgene. To circumvent these problems, the use of gene targeting has been proposed. In this approach one designs a transgene that replaces the endogenous gene using the methodologies developed for gene targeting (homologous recombination in ES cells). Because the endogenous gene gets replaced by the mutant transgene and the mutant transgene is inserted at the exact locus of its endogenous homolog none of the above problems occur.

Although all above considerations are valid, whether the generated transgenic mice exhibited phenotypical alterations (e.g. amyloid deposits, or age dependent progressive behavioral defects) relevant for Alzheimer's Disease could not be predicted solely based on the transgenic techniques employed, a finding that may be due to the large number of differences in how the mice were bred (host genotype) and tested (for recent review see [Higgins and Jacobsen, 2003]).

3. Transgenic Mouse Models of AD

The most well studied transgenic mouse strains developed for modeling AD had some form of mutation in their APP transgene [Games et al., 1995, Hsiao et al., 1995, Sturchler-Pierrat et al., 1997, Nalbantoglu et al., 1997]. The APP^{V717F} mouse, also known as the PDAPP mouse model [Games et al., 1995], was the first successful model and it will be described in more detail later in this chapter. The Tg2576 mouse model [Hsiao et al., 1996] followed shortly. This mouse expresses a human APP695 gene harboring the "Swedish" double mutation (K670N/M671L, APPsw) driven by the hamster prion protein promoter. These mice exhibit amyloid deposits, astrocytic gliosis and neuritic dystrophy, as well as age-dependent alterations in synaptic transmission. Cognitive impairment originally reported in this mouse model was questioned but later confirmed.

The APP23 mouse model expresses a human APP751 transgene that harbors the "Swedish" double mutation. Transgene expression in this mouse is driven by a neuron specific murine Thy-1 promoter. These transgenic mice develop cortical Aβ deposits by 6 months of age and also show activated microglia and astrocytes. Interestingly, APP23 mice have significantly more, not less, cortical neurons compared to age-matched control mice, and these animals also show neurofibrillary pathology similar to what is seen in the early stages of AD [Sturchler-Pierrat et al., 1997].

Given that the pathological hallmarks of AD include not only extracellular amyloid plaques comprised of β-amyloid protein but also intracellular neurofibrillary tangles comprised of hyperphosphorylated tau protein (reviewed in [Selkoe, 2001]), attempts have been made to mimic tau pathology in transgenic mice. JNPL3 mouse reported by Lewis et al.

(2000) is one example. The transgene in these mice contains the most common tau mutation associated with frontotemporal dementia and Parkinsonism (FTDP-17 mutation P301L) and is driven by the mouse prion promoter. Pathological and neurological changes observed in these mice (from ages 6-7 months onward) include delayed righting reflex, hypolocomotion and reduced muscle strength [Lewis et al., 2000] as well as development of neurofibrillary tangles (NFT) as confirmed by tau immunostaining, silver staining and electron microscopy. However, unlike in APP transgenics, amyloid plaques have not been found in these mice. Astrogliosis is seen in regions containing NFTs in areas spanning the spinal cord pons, and also to a certain degree the amygdala, cortex and hippocampus [Lewis et al., 2000, 2001]. Given the severity of phenotypical changes affecting important performance characteristics such as motor function, analysis of cognitive traits has not been completed for the JNPL3 mouse.

Another important player in AD is Apolipoprotein E. Among the four allelic variants of the ApoE gene, ApoE4 has been found to predispose patients to AD. ApoE knockout mice show no pathological alterations [e.g. Anderson et al., 1998; Hartman et al., 2001], but when crossed with the PDAPP mouse, the resulting double transgenics do not develop thioflavin-positive amyloid plaques and astrogliosis [Bales et al., 1997, 1999] despite the elevated Aβ levels typical of the PDAPP mouse. Thus absence of the ApoE product appears to protect against deposition of amyloid plaques in the mouse brain a conclusion that is in accordance with what has been inferred from human clinical observations [Corder et al., 1993]. Conversely, the crossing of the PDAPP mouse with mice expressing the ApoE4 isoform results in higher Aβ plaque burden compared to mice carrying other alleles of the ApoE gene, e.g. the ApoE3 [Fagan et al., 2002].

The role of presenilins has also been investigated with transgenesis. Mice overexpressing a mutant form of PS1 [Duff et al., 1996] developed elevated levels of Aβ42(43), a hallmark feature of AD. Furthermore, crossing these PS1 mice to APP overexpressor animals (e.g. the Tg2576 mice) led to an accelerated appearance of pathological changes. Another PS1 mutant transgenic mouse generated carries the L235P mutation (substitution of leucine by proline at codon 235) in the human PS1 gene, a mutation that has been linked to a form of early-onset Alzheimer's disease. These transgenic mice showed a significant increase in the production of Aβ42 but the mutant mice did not exhibit plaque formation, changes in choline acetyltransferase activity, or somatostatin content in the brain. The L235P PS1 transgenic mice also showed normal acquisition or reversal of a spatial reference memory in the water maze and had unaltered spatial working memory as well. However, they exhibited a significant impairment in a test of spontaneous object recognition suggesting a potential impairment of the extrahippocampal memory system.

Several other transgenic lines that express mutant human APP transgenes alone [Hsiao et al., 1999; Moechars et al., 1999; Chishti et al., 2001] or in combination with mutant human PS genes [Borchelt et al., 1997; Holcomb et al., 1998] have also been created. These mice show numerous neuropathological features similar to the previously described APP based mouse models, however, the abnormalities appear earlier. Another double transgenic example is the mouse generated by Lewis et al. (2000) who crossed the Tg2576 mice with JNPL3 mice. These mice were found to develop both amyloid deposits as well as neurofibrillary tangles, the two most important hallmarks of human AD. But the occurrence of neurofibrillary tangles in brain regions (e.g. spinal cord and pons) other than those typically affected in human AD, and the fact that these regions are involved in motor function, among other functions, has made it difficult to analyze cognitive traits of these mice.

Investigators have also started to analyze the role of genes whose proteins may interact with the major molecular players of AD discussed above. For example, in a recent study Lilliehook et al., (2003) analyzed the effects of silencing the calsenilin gene in mice. Calsenilin is a presenilin interacting protein that coimmunoprecipitates with both PS1 and PS2. It also increases presenilin-dependent γ- cleavage of the amyloid precursor protein, APP leading to elevated Aβ42 levels (Jo et al., 2003). In the null mutant mice Lilliehook et al. found reduced Aβ levels, a finding that was expected based on the known role of calsenilin. However, the authors also discovered that the lack of calsenilin expression led to increased long-term potentiation (LTP) recorded from the dentate gyrus, a finding that they believe is independent of Aβ but is due to the downregulation of Kv4 channel-dependent A-type current in the neurons.

Calsenilin belongs to a family of neuronal calcium sensors that bind Ca^{2+} with high affinity and thus appear to be ideal for responding to minor and fast changes in Ca^{2+} intracellular concentrations. Calcium is a key player in intracellular signaling and thus synaptic plasticity. In a recent study Palop et al. (2003) found a strong correlation between AD-related cognitive deficits and decreased levels of the calcium binding protein, calbindin-D_{28k} and the calcium-dependent immediate early gene product, c-fos. The investigators studied transgenic mice expressing the Swedish and the Indiana familial AD mutations in the APP transgene and found that calbindin-D_{28k} and c-fos were downregulated in the dentate gyrus of the transgenic mice and the changes were age-dependent and correlated with Aβ1-42 levels but not with Aβ amyloid plaques, supporting the notion that the pathological effects of Aβ are perhaps mediated via disrupted synaptic physiology rather than plaque induced neuronal death.

4. Cognition vs. Other Domains of Behavior: The Example of the APP^{V717F} Mouse

In most of the above transgenic mice the impairments revealed in behavioral analyses fell in the category of cognition or mnemonic characteristics, which is not surprising because the focus of the behavioral studies was exactly this. The narrow focus represents a potential problem as it may result in failure to identify the possibly broad range of phenotypical changes a mutation generates. In the following pages, an experimental example is presented [Gerlai et al., 2002] in which the analysis has gone beyond the characterization of cognitive traits. The mouse model investigated was one of the first AD mouse models generated, the APP^{V717F} mouse [Games et al., 1995].

APP^{V717F} mice express the human APP gene carrying a mutation leading to substitution of valine by phenylalanine at amino acid residue 717, the first mutation found in humans which leads to an early onset familial AD [Goate et al., 1991]. The expression of the APP transgene was driven by the platelet derived growth factor, PD, promoter in these transgenic mice. AD associated neuropathological changes including the appearance of neurofibrillary tangles and neuritic plaques containing the Aβ peptide have been thoroughly investigated in the APP^{V717F} mice and they were found to exhibit the latter only (i.e. Aβ neuritic plaques). In addition, the mice showed astrocytosis and microgliosis [e.g. Games et al., 1995; also see Dodart et al., 1999], pathological alterations observed in human AD. At the behavioral level, APP^{V717F} mice have been found to exhibit impaired performance in spatial learning paradigms in the water maze [Chen et al., 2000] or radial maze [Dodart et al., 1999] as well as in object recognition tasks [Dodart et al., 1999, Chen et al., 2000]

However, as argued above, impaired cognitive abilities are not the only concern in AD patients. Complex disturbances of emotion and behavior have been recognized as part of the syndrome since Dr. Alzheimer reported his original observation in 1907 (for review see [Gilley, 1993]). The behavioral disturbances include psychosis, depression, aphasia, agnosia, apraxia, and personality disorders [Ferris & Kluger, 1997; Perry & Hodges, 1999; Collie & Maruff, 2000; Cummings, 2000]. Analysis of the APP^{V717F} mice has now confirmed that changes other than cognitive ones may occur in mouse models of AD too.

5. Fear Conditioning with Event Recording: A Tool for Behavioral Profiling

APP^{V717F} mice were tested in a learning paradigm, context and cue dependent fear conditioning [see e.g. Gerlai 2001], which not only allowed the investigators to study memory performance but also made it possible for them to analyze several other aspects of behavior, including behavioral posture patterns associated with motor activity, fear, and emotionality [Gerlai et al., 2002]. The study included comparative quantification of motor and posture patterns that were exhibited by the APP^{V717F} mice and their wild type control counter parts in fear conditioning. The principle of this approach, which is often called "event recording", is that the behavioral patterns, just like gestures or facial expressions in human communication, reveal fundamental characteristics of the psychological/behavioral status of the experimental animal. The results of event recording analysis in the fear conditioning paradigm showed that although memory performance of APP^{V717F} mice appeared impaired this was associated with alterations in fear responses and modified exploratory behavior.

Briefly, fear conditioning entailed placing the mice into a chamber in which they received three electric shocks during a short (6 min) training session. The shocks were paired with a tone cue. In subsequent tests, the mice were studied for their responses to the tone cue (the associative stimulus) and to the shock chamber itself (the so called context). Traditionally, the behavioral response to pain or fear in rodents is tested by measuring immobility, or freezing [e.g. Gerlai, 2001]. This reaction is a natural behavior that is elicited by predators but can also be observed under artificial laboratory conditions. In addition to this behavior numerous other behavioral patterns may be tested in the paradigm. These included several motor/posture patters (see below; for detailed definitions also see [Gerlai et al., 2002; Gerlai et al., 1993]). What was found was somewhat surprising. APP^{V717F} transgenic mice exhibited significant alterations in freezing in the cue test only, which may at first sight suggest impaired elemental learning, i.e. reduced ability to make association between two stimuli (figure 5.1). However, the reduction of freezing in the cue test could be seen even before the tone cue was presented. Thus it could not have been related to elemental learning but perhaps was due to a generalized alteration of fear. The pattern of changes across all three phases of the fear conditioning paradigm (Fig. 5.1 A, B, C) also suggests a consistent, albeit not always significant, reduction of freezing, a result that is indeed compatible with altered fear.

Nevertheless, as fear cannot be measured *per se*, one could also argue that reduction of freezing was perhaps due to altered motor performance, e.g., increased general activity. Quantification of locomotion revealed that APP^{V717F} mice did not exhibit more locomotion compared to their wild type counterparts during training. In fact these mice showed a modest reduction of locomotory activity. Similarly, locomotion of APP^{V717F} mice was not increased in the context test compared to control. Thus elevation of general activity could be ruled out. The increased locomotion of APP^{V717F} mice found in the cue test may be due to factors other than general activity levels. A potential factor may be emotionality or fear.

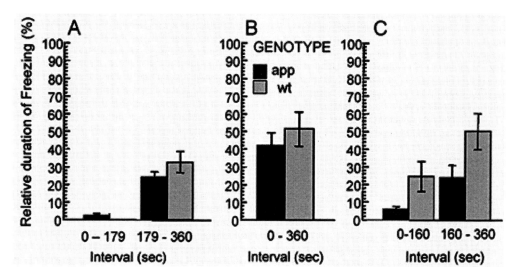

Figure 5.1. APP^{V717F} transgenic mice (gray) exhibit reduction of freezing compared to wild type control (black) in the cue test of the fear conditioning paradigm. (**A**) Training. (**B**) Context test. (**C**) Cue test. Means ± SEM are indicated. Relative duration of freezing is calculated for different periods of the three phases of the paradigm. (**A**) Training, pre-shock period (0 – 179 sec), shock period (179 – 360 sec). (**B**) Context test, entire period (0 – 360 sec). (**C**) Cue test, pre-tone cue period (0 – 160 sec), tone cue period (160 – 360 sec). Note the trend for reduced freezing in APPV717F transgenic mice as compared to wild type control mice in the context test (**B**) and the second half of training (**A**). Also note the significantly reduced freezing throughout the entire cue test (**C**). Observe the increase of freezing in the context test (**B**) compared to pre-shock baseline of the training in both genotypes, indicating context induced fear. Also observe the increase of freezing in both genotypes in response to tone cue presentation in the cue test (**C**).

Several behavioral elements have been previously shown to correlate with fear (see e.g. [Fitch et al., 2002, Gerlai et al., 1999]). One of them, grooming, has been shown to decrease in response to electric shocks or presentation of stimuli that were previously associated with shocks. Grooming was found decreased in APP^{V717F} mice during the training phase of fear conditioning and a similar trend was observed in the context test suggesting that the transgenic mice were more responsive (fearful) to the training environment and the shock.

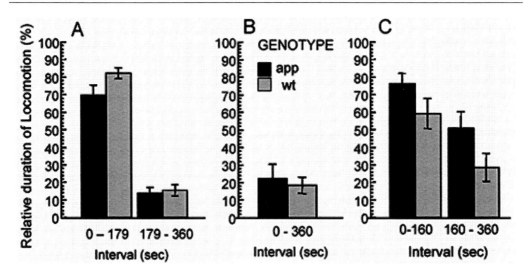

Figure 5.2. APP^{V717F} transgenic mice (gray) do not exhibit increased general activity levels (locomotion) compared to wild type control (black) in fear conditioning. Relative duration of locomotion is calculated for different periods of the three phases of the paradigm. (**A**) Training, pre-shock period (0 – 179 sec), shock period (179 – 360 sec). (**B**) Context test, entire period (0 – 360 sec). (**C**) Cue test, pre-tone cue period (0 – 160 sec), tone cue period (160 – 360 sec). Means $\pm$ SEM are indicated. Note the non-significant reduction of locomotion of APPV717F transgenic mice compared to wild type control in the pre-shock interval (0 – 179 sec), and the very similar locomotion levels during the shock phase (interval 179 – 360 sec) of training (**A**). Also note the lack of difference between genotypes in the context test (**B**) and an increase of locomotion in APP^{V717F} transgenic mice compared to wild type control in the pre-cue (interval 0 – 160 sec) and cue phase (interval 160 – 360) of the cue test (**C**).

This conclusion was supported by the analysis of another behavioral element, long-body posture. Increased amount of long-body posture was found in APP^{V717F} mice compared to control during training and the context test and a similar trend was also seen during the cue test. Long-body, or stretch attend posture as it is known in the literature, has been observed under aversive conditions in mice (and rats) when cues associated with natural predators are present [Blanchard et al., 1991]. This behavior is also evoked in mice by other fear inducing stimuli including electric shocks or the context in which the shocks were delivered [Fitch et al., 2002, Gerlai et al., 1999]. Thus, long-body posture has been interpreted as a sign of fear [Blanchard et al., 1991, Fitch et al., 2002, Gerlai et al., 1999]. Accordingly, increased long-body posture suggests increased fear in APP^{V717F} mice.

It is also notable that long-body posture may represent a type of fear that is <u>qualitatively</u> different from the behavioral state associated with freezing. While the latter behavior can be seen in the case of clear presence of danger or pain [Blanchard and Blanchard, 1969], long-body posture is usually observed when a rodent is ambivalent with regard to the nature or degree of danger [Blanchard et al., 1991.]

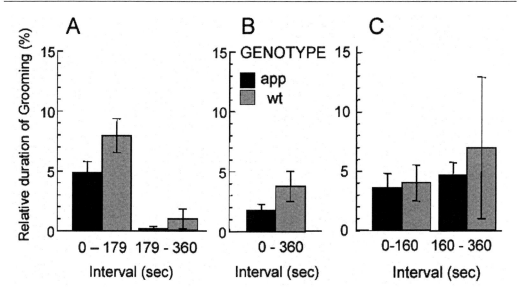

Figure 5.3. APP^{V717F} transgenic mice (gray) groom significantly less compared to wild type control (black) in the training phase of fear conditioning. Relative duration of grooming is calculated for different periods of the three phases of the paradigm. (**A**) Training, pre-shock period (0 – 179 sec), shock period (179 – 360 sec). (**B**) Context test, entire period (0 – 360 sec). (**C**) Cue test, pre-tone cue period (0 – 160 sec), tone cue period (160 – 360 sec). Means ± SEM are indicated. Note that the differences between the genotypes are significant only for the training phase (**A**) of fear conditioning but a similar trend is also seen in the context test (**B**). For detailed statistical analysis see Results.

The above study uncovered yet another previously not described alteration. Analysis of spontaneous activity of APP^{V717F} mice before shocks were delivered in the training session showed that these mice exhibited significantly reduced number of leaning.

This behavior is thought to represent exploratory activity [Cabib et al., 1990, van Abeelen and van den Heuvel, 1982; van Daal et al., 1991]. It has been suggested to be associated with gathering information about the surroundings of the experimental subjects. The robust reduction of leaning frequency seen in APP^{V717F} mice compared to wild type control implies that these mice exhibited reduced exploratory behavior, which in turn might have led to an impaired ability of these mice to gather information about their environment. This hypothesis is in accordance with previous findings showing impaired object recognition [Dodart et al., 1999], and spatial learning [Chen et al., 2000] in APP^{V717F} mice, and it may also explain why APP^{V717F} mice behaved like experimental subjects with incomplete information about the contextual cues of the fear conditioning chamber.

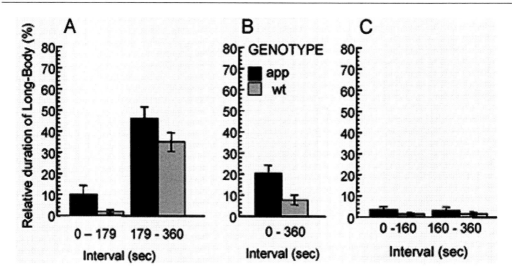

Figure 5.4. APP^{V717F} transgenic mice (gray) exhibit long-body posture significantly more compared to wild type control (black) in fear conditioning. Relative duration of long-body posture is calculated for different periods of the three phases of the paradigm. (**A**) Training, pre-shock period (0 – 179 sec), shock period (179 – 360 sec). (**B**) Context test, entire period (0 – 360 sec). (**C**) Cue test, pre-tone cue period (0 – 160 sec), tone cue period (160 – 360 sec). Means ± SEM are indicated. Note the significant differences between genotypes during training (**A**) and the context test (**B**) and also a similar trend in the cue test (**C**). Also note that while this behavior is almost completely absent in the cue test (**C**), it is more observable in the context test (**B**) especially in the APP^{V717F} transgenic mice.

6. Conclusions

In summary, the profile of behavioral abnormalities of APP^{V717F} mice revealed by the quantification of motor and posture patterns suggests that these mice may suffer from alterations in fear and exploratory behaviors. What was previously thought to be impaired cognition *per se* may actually be due, at least in part, to alterations in these characteristics, a working hypothesis whose validity will be ascertained in the future. A recent study has already confirmed that behavioral abnormalities lying outside of the domain of cognition are evident in APP^{V717F} mice. Huitron-Resendiz et al (2002) showed that the transgenic mice suffer from abnormalities in sleep–wake patterns, thermoregulation, and motor activity.

Clearly, these findings may be important for the proper interpretation of performance changes one may observe in cognitive tasks. Discovery of such findings is strongly facilitated by conducting a thorough behavioral analysis that may start with detailed descriptive analysis of behavior such as employed in the present study but perhaps even better by a study that employs a battery of tests that allows one to tap into multiple domains of behavior in a systematic manner.

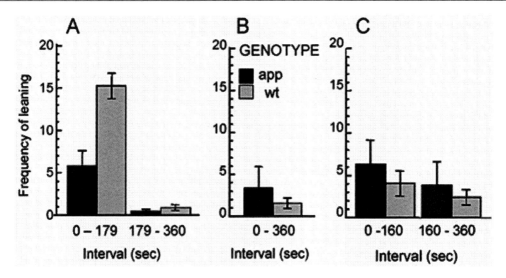

Figure 5.5. APP^{V717F} transgenic mice (gray) exhibit significantly smaller number of leaning compared to wild type control (black) during spontaneous exploration of the shock chamber in fear conditioning. Frequency of leaning is calculated for different periods of the three phases of the paradigm. (**A**) Training, pre-shock period (0 – 179 sec), shock period (179 – 360 sec). (**B**) Context test, entire period (0 – 360 sec). (**C**) Cue test, pre-tone cue period (0 – 160 sec), tone cue period (160 – 360 sec). Means ± SEM are indicated. Note the robust difference between genotypes of mice before shock presentation (interval 0 – 179 sec) during training (**A**). Also note the dramatic decrease of leaning in both genotypes in response to shock delivery (interval 179 – 360 sec of training). Finally observe the apparent increase of leaning in the APP^{V717F} transgenic mice compared to control in both the context (**B**) and the cue (**C**) tests.

Proper characterization and discovery of changes in non-cognitive traits in animal models may have crucial relevance for drug development and thus for the human clinic. Disturbances including affective and emotional behavioral abnormalities and sleep related problems are common among AD patients (for review see [Gilley, 1993]) and these alterations are often more debilitating than memory loss itself. Also important to note that numerous drugs have already been or are being developed for psychiatric diseases whose symptoms include some of the above mentioned disturbances. Animal models such as the APP^{V717F} mouse may thus allow investigators to screen existing and novel drugs for their ability to alter non-cognitive traits including anxiety in a preclinical setting, which will significantly accelerate the development of pharmacotherapies for the patient.

Acknowledgments

This work was supported by Eli Lilly and Company. I also thank my previous colleagues Bruce Gitter, Kelly Bales, Thomas Fitch, Benjamin Adams and Stephen Chaney for their thoughts and help.

References

Anderson R, Barnes JC, Bliss TVP, Cain DP, Cambon K, Davies HA, et al. Behavioural, physiological and morphological analysis of a line of apolipoprotein E knockout mouse. *Neuroscience* (1998) 85:93–110.

Bales KR, Verina T, Dodel RC, Du Y, Altsteil L, Bender M, et al. Lack of apolipoprotein E dramatically reduces amyloid b-peptide deposition. *Nat Genet* (1997) 17:263–264.

Bales KR, Verina T, Cummins DJ, Du Y, Dodel RC, Saura J, et al. Apolipoprotein E is essential for amyloid deposition in the APPV717F transgenic mouse model of Alzheimer's disease. *Proc Natl Acad Sci USA* (1999) 96:15233–15238.

Blanchard BC, Blanchard RJ, Rogers RJ. Risk assessment and animal models of anxiety. In: Olivier B, Mos J, Slangen JL (eds.) *Animal models in psychopharmacology. Advances in pharmacological sciences.* Basel: Birkhauser Verlag. 1991;117-134.

Blanchard RJ, Blanchard DC. Crouching as an index of fear. *Journal of Comparative Physiology and Psychology* 1969;81:281-290.

Borchelt, D.R., Ratovitski, T., van Lare, J., Lee, M.K., Gonzales, V., Jenkins, N.A., Copeland, N.G., Price, D.L. & Sisodia, S.S. Accelerated amyloid deposition in the brains of transgenic mice coexpressing mutant presenilin 1 and amyloid precursor proteins. *Neuron* 1997; 19: 939-945.

Breteler MMB, Claus JJ, Van Duijn CM, Launer LJ, Hofman A. Epidemology of Alzheimer's Disease. *Epidemol. Rev* 1992;14:59-82.

Cabib S, Algeri S, Perego C, Puglisi-Allegra S. Behavioral and biochemical changes monitored in two inbred strains of mice during exploration of an unfamiliar environment. *Physiology & Behavior* 1990;47:749-753.

Chen G, Chen KS, Knox J, Inglis J, Bernard A, Martin SJ, Justice A, McConlogue L, Games D, Freedman SB, Morris RGM. A learning deficit related to age and beta-amyloid plaques in a mouse model of Alzheimer's disease. *Nature* 2000;408:975-979.

Chishti, M.A., Yang, D.S., Janus, C., Phinney, A.L., Horne, P., Pearson, J., Strome, R., Zuker, N., Loukides, J., French, J., Turner, S., Lozza, G., Grilli, M., Kunicki, S., Morissette, C., Paquette, J., Gervais, F., Bergeron, C., Fraser, P.E., Carlson, G.A., George-Hyslop, P.S. & Westaway, D. Early-onset amyloid deposition and cognitive deficits in transgenic mice expressing a double mutant form of amyloid precursor protein 695. *J Biol Chem* 2001; 276: 21562-21570.

Collie, A. & Maruff, P. The neuropsychology of preclinical Alzheimer's disease and mild cognitive impairment. *Neurosci Biobehav Rev* 2000; 24: 365-374.

Corder EH, Saunders AM, Strittmatter WJ, Schmechel DE, Gaskell PC, Small GW, et al. Gene dose of apolipoprotein E type 4 allele and the risk of Alzheimer's disease in late onset families. *Science* (1993) 261:921–923.

Cummings, J.L. Cognitive and behavioral heterogeneity in Alzheimer's disease: seeking the neurobiological basis. *Neurobiol Aging* 2000; 21: 845-861

Dodart JC, Meziane H, Mathis C, Bales KR, Paul SM, Ungerer A. Behavioral disturbances in transgenic mice overexpressing the V717F beta-amyloid precursor protein. *Behavioral Neuroscience* 1999;113:982-990.

Duff, K. Transgenic mouse models of Alzheimer's disease. In: (Crusio WE, Gerlai RT Eds) *Handbook of Molecular-Genetic Techniques for Brain and Behavior Research.* Elsevier, Amsterdam (1999), pp 880-894.

Duff K, Eckman C, Zehr C, Yu X, Prada CM, Perez-tur J, Hutton M, Buee L, Harigaya Y, Yager D, Morgan D, Gordon MN, Holcomb L, Refolo L, Zenk B, Hardy J, Younkin S. Increased amyloid-β42(43) in brains of mice expressing mutant presenilin 1. *Nature*, 383: 710-713.

Fagan AM,Watson M, Paradanian M, Bales KR, Paul SM, Holtzman DM. Human and murine ApoE markedly alters Aβ metabolism before and after plaque formation in a mouse model of Alzheimer's disease. *Neurobiol Dis* (2002) 9:305–318

Ferris, S.H. & Kluger, A. Assessing cognition in Alzheimer disease research. *Alzheimer Dis Assoc Disord* 1997; 11: 45-49.

Fitch T, Adams B, Chaney S, Gerlai R. Force transducer based movement detection in fear conditioning in mice: A comparative analysis. *Hippocampus* 2002;12:4-17.

Games D, Adams D, Alessandrini R, Barbour R, Berthelette P, Blackwell C, Carr T, Clemens J, Donaldson T, Gillespie F. Alzheimer-type neuropathology in transgenic mice overexpressing V717F beta-amyloid precursor protein. *Nature* 1995;373:523-527.

Gerlai R. Behavioral tests of hippocampal function: Simple paradigms, complex problems. *Behav. Brain Res* 2001;125:269-277.

Gerlai, R., Fitch T, Bales, K, Gitter B. (2002). Behavioral impairment of APP[V717F] mice in fear conditioning: Is it only cognition? *Behav. Brain Res.* **136:503-509**

Gerlai R, Clayton NS. Analysing hippocampal function in transgenic mice: An ethological perspective. *Trends Neurosci* 1999;22:47-51.

Gerlai R, Shinsky N, Shih A, Williams P, Winer J, Armanini M, Cairns B, Winslow J, Gao W-Q, Phillips HS. Regulation of learning by EphA receptors: A protein targeting study. *J. Neuroscience* 1999;19:9538-9549.

Gerlai R, Friend W, Becker L, O'Hanlon R, Marks A, Roder J. Female transgenic mice carrying the human gene for S100ß are hyperactive. *Behavioural Brain Research* 1993;55:51-55

Gilley DW. Behavioral and affective disturbances in Alzheimer's Disease. In: Parks RW, Zec RF, Wilson RS (Eds.) *Neuropsychology of Alzheimer's Disease and Other Dementias.* Oxford University Press. Oxford 1993;112-137.

Goate AM. Monogenetic determinants of Alzheimer's disease: APP mutations. *Cellular & Molecular Life Sciences* 1998;54:897-901

Goate A, Chartier-Harlin MC, Mullan M, Brown J, Crawford F, Fidani L, Giuffra L, Haynes A, Irving N, James L. Segregation of a missense mutation in the amyloid precursor protein gene with familial Alzheimer's disease. *Nature* 1991;349:704-706.

Higgins GA, Jacobsen H. Transgenic mouse models of Alzheimer's disease: phenotype and application. *Behavioural Pharmacology* (2003) 14:419–438.

Holcomb, L., Gordon, M.N., McGowan, E., Yu, X., Benkovic, S., Jantzen, P., Wright, K., Saad, I., Mueller, R., Morgan, D., Sanders, S., Zehr, C., O'Campo, K., Hardy, J., Prada, C.M, Eckman, C., Younkin, S., Hsiao, K. & Duff, K. Accelerated Alzheimer-type phenotype in transgenic mice carrying both mutant amyloid precursor protein and presenilin 1 transgenes. *Nat Med* 1998; 4: 97-100.

Hsia, A.Y., Masliah, E., McConlogue, L., Yu, G.Q., Tatsuno, G., Hu, K., Kholodenko, D., Malenka, R.C., Nicoll, R.A. & Mucke, L. Plaque-independent disruption of neural circuits in Alzheimer's disease mouse models. *Proc Natl* Acad Sci USA 1999; 96: 3228-3233.

Hsiao, K.K., Chapman, P., Nilsen, S., Eckman, C., Harigaya, Y., Younkin, S., Yang, F. & Cole, G. Correlative memory deficits, Aβ elevation, and amyloid plaques in transgenic mice. *Science* 1996; 274: 99-102.

Hsiao KK, Borchelt DR, Olson K, Johannsdottir R, Kitt C, Yunis W, Xu S, Eckman C, Younkin S, Price D. Age-related CNS disorder and early death in transgenic FVB/N mice overexpressing Alzheimer amyloid precursor proteins. *Neuron* 1995;15:1203-1218.

Huang XG, Yee BK, Nag S, Chan ST, Tang F. Behavioral and neurochemical characterization of transgenic mice carrying the human presenilin-1 gene with or without the leucine-to-proline mutation at codon 235. *Exp Neurol.* (2003) 183:673-681.

Huitron-Resendiz S, Sanchez-Alavez M, Gallegos R, Berg G, Crawford E, Giacchino JL, et al. Age-independent and age-related deficits in visuospatial learning, sleep–wake states, thermoregulation and motor activity in PDAPP mice. *Brain Res* (2002) 928:126–137.

Jo DG, Chang JW, Hong HS, Mook-Jung I, Jung YK. Contribution of presenilin/gamma-secretase to calsenilin-mediated apoptosis. *Biochem Biophys Res Commun.* 2003; 305:62–66.

Johnson-Wood K, Lee M, Motter R, Hu K, Gordon G, Barbour R, Khan K, Gordon M, Tan H, Games D, Lieberburg I, Schenk D, Seubert P, McConlogue L. Amyloid precursor protein processing and Aβ42 deposition in a transgenic mouse model of Alzheimer's disease. *Proc. Natl. Acad. Sci* 1997;94:1550-1555.

Lewis J, Dickson DW, Lin W-L, Chisholm L, Corral A, Jones G, et al.. Enhanced neurofibrillary degeneration in transgenic mice expressing mutant tau and APP. *Science* (2001) 293:1487–1491

Lewis, J., McGowan, E., Rockwood, J., Melrose, H., Nacharaju, P., Van Slegtenhorst, M., Gwinn-Hardy, K., Paul Murphy, M., Baker, M., Yu, X., Duff, K., Hardy, J., Corral, A., Lin, W.L., Yen, S.H., Dickson, D.W., Davies, P. & Hutton, M. Neurofibrillary tangles, amyotrophy and progressive motor disturbance in mice expressing mutant (P301L) tau protein. *Nat Genet* 2000; 25: 402-405.

Lilliehook, C., Bozdagi, O., Yao, J., Gomez-Ramirez, M., Zaidi,N., F., Wasco, W., Gandy,S., Santucci, A., C., Haroutunian, V., Huntley, G. W., Buxbaum, J., D. Altered A□ Formation and Long-Term Potentiation in a Calsenilin Knock-Out. *The Journal of Neuroscience,* 2003; 23: 9097–9106.

Moechars, D., Dewachter, I., Lorent, K., Reverse, D., Baekelandt, V., Naidu, A., Tesseur, I., Spittaels, K., Haute, C.V., Checler, F., Godaux, E., Cordell, B. & Van Leuven, F. Early phenotypic changes in transgenic mice that overexpress different mutants of amyloid precursor protein in brain. *J Biol Chem* (1999) 274: 6483-6492.

Nalbantoglu J, Tirado-Santiago G, Lahsaini A, Poirier J, Goncalves O, Verge G, Momoli F, Welner SA, Massicotte G, Julien JP, Shapiro ML. Impaired learning and LTP in mice expressing the carboxy terminus of the Alzheimer amyloid precursor protein. *Nature* 1997;387:500-505.

Palop J., J., Jones, B., Kekonius, L., Chin, J., Yu, G-Q., Raber, J., Masliah, E., Mucke, L. Neuronal depletion of calcium-dependent proteins in the dentate gyrus is tightly linked to Alzheimer's disease-related cognitive deficits. *Proc. Natl. Acad. Sci.* 2003; 100: 9572-9577.

Perry, R.J. & Hodges, J.R. Attention and executive deficits in Alzheimer's disease. A critical review. *Brain* 1999; 122: 383-404.

Selkoe DJ. Alzheimer's disease: genes, proteins, and therapy. *Physiol Rev* (2001) 81:741–766.

Sturchler-Pierrat C, Abramowski D, Duke M, Wiederhold KH, Mistl C, Rothacher S, Ledermann B, Burki K, Frey P, Paganetti PA, Waridel C, Calhoun ME, Jucker M, Probst A, Staufenbiel M, Sommer B. Two amyloid precursor protein transgenic mouse models with Alzheimer disease-like pathology. *Proceedings of the National Academy of Sciences of the United States of America* 1997;94:13287-13292.

van Abeelen JH, van den Heuvel CM. Behavioural responses to novelty in two inbred mouse strains after intrahippocampal naloxone and morphine. *Behavioural Brain Research* 1982;5:199-207.

van Daal JH, Herbergs PJ, Crusio WE, Schwegler H, Jenks BG, Lemmens WA, van Abeelen JH. A genetic-correlational study of hippocampal structural variation and variation in exploratory activities of mice. *Behavioural Brain Research* 1991;43:57-64.

Wisniewski KE, Wisniewski HM, Wen GY. Occurrence of neuropathological changes and dementia of Alzheimer's disease in Down's syndrome. *Ann. Neurol* 1985;17: 278–282.

In: Cognition and Mood Interactions
Editor: Miao-Kun Sun, pp. 105-115

ISBN 1-59454-229-5
2005 © Nova Science Publishers, Inc.

Chapter VI

Alzheimer's Dementia and Mood

M. Cristina Polidori, Elena Mariani[#],*
Antonio Metastasio[#] and Patrizia Mecocci[#]

Institut für Biochemie und Molekularbiologie I, Heinrich-Heine Universität Düsseldorf,
Düsseldorf, Germany
[#]Sezione di Gerontologia e Geriatria, Dipartimento di Medicina Clinica e Sperimentale,
Università degli Studi di Perugia, Perugia, Italy

The diagnosis of mood disorders in dementia is a complex task because of the overlap in symptomatology between the two diseases. In this chapter, epidemiological, neurochemical, and clinical issues related to the presence of behavioral and psychological symptoms of dementia (BPSD) in Alzheimer's disease (AD) – with particular attention to depression – are presented. Physicians should use the available tools for the diagnosis of BPSD in AD, be aware of preventive strategies against the onset/worsening of cognitive and noncognitive symptoms, and take into account nonpharmarmacological options especially in the management of newly diagnosed AD patients with BPSD.

1. Introduction

Behavioral and psychological symptoms frequently accompanying AD are generally indicated with the acronym BPSD (Behavioral and Psychological Symptoms of Dementia). They include **disorders of mood** – depression, anxiety, euphoria/mania-, **psychosis** – delusions and hallucinations-, **agitation** – physical aggression, verbal outburst, psychomotor restlessness including wandering-, **personality changes** – apathy, irritability, disinhibition as well as changes for that the AD patient becomes ureasonable, demanding, suspicious-, **neurovegetative changes** including sleep disturbances and disorders of diurnal variation – insomnia, sundowning, eating disorders, sexual disturbances-, and **psychomotor changes**.

The reciprocal influence between cognitive and noncognitive symptoms is not a trivial issue in patients with AD. This is mainly due to the fact that the definition of specific behaviors varies considerably among studies; furthermore, most of the existing studies report altered behaviors only as occurring when they are identified as problems (Rabins, 1999). Nevertheless, it has been estimated that BPSD frequently occur in this disease. At least 50% (Steele et al., 1990) and up to 88% (Kunik et al., 1994) of outpatients with dementia have at least one behavioral disturbance. As summarized by Rabins (1999), the reported prevalence of specific common noncognitive symptoms in representative AD studies including reviews varies between 16% and 28% for hallucinations, between 22% and 56% for delusions, and between 23% and 90% for depression (Reisberg et al., 1987; Merriam et al., 1988; Swearer et al., 1988; Teri et al., 1989; Burns et al., 1990a; Burns et al., 1990b; Wragg and Jeste, 1989).

BPSD can occur at any point of the disease process in AD, and are often the presenting symptom (Swearer et al., 1996). In a recent study, 43% of patients with mild cognitive impairment (MCI) were shown to exhibit neuropsychiatric symptoms in the month preceding the evaluation (20% with depression, 15% with apathy, 15% with irritability) (Lyketsos et al., 2002). The neuropsychological differentiation between very mild AD and major depression is a very critical and sensitive task (desRosiers et al., 1995), and what for many years has been called "pseudodementia" – i.e., depression mimicking memory dysfunction - (Kiloh, 1981) is being currently largely seen as a pre-dementia condition (Reifler, 2000). Interestingly, not all abormal behaviors occur with increasing frequency or severity with progression of the disease. Rather, certain behaviors occur more frequently at different stages of disease (Mega et al., 1996). The number and severity of behavioral problems, however, appear to increase with worsening cognitive impairment (Teri et al., 1988; Devanand et al., 1992). On the other hand, both depressed mood and subjective bradyphrenia seem to indicate subclinical AD at least in some subgroups of patients, such as older people with higher levels of education (Geerlings et al., 2000a; Geerlings et al., 2000b).

Behavioral changes are disturbing not only to patients, but also to their caregivers (Rabins et al., 1982; Deimling and Bass, 1986; Mace and Rabins, 1991; Cummings, 1996; Teri et al., 2002; Mittelman et al., 2004) and have been associated with increased likelihood of institutionalization (Morriss et al., 1990; Steele et al., 1990; Cummings, 1996; Gaugler et al., 2003). Furthermore, nursing home residents have a higher incidence of behavioral changes than patients with AD residing in the community (Steele et al., 1990). In the former group of individuals, 90% manifest a minimum of one behavioral problem (Ballard and Oyebode, 1995) and 50% have at least four (Tariot et al., 1993). This is in contrast to the degree of cognitive impairment, which is not greater in nursing home residents compared to those dwelling in the community (Steele et al., 1990).

For these reasons, and due to the fact that dementia and depression - together with parkinsonism - represent the most prevalent and disabling pathologies in the elderly (Polidori et al., 2001), BPSD in AD may pose the greatest challenge to caregivers, physicians, and other health care professionals. This chapter will focus on biological and clinical aspects of mood disorders in AD, with particular attention to depression.

2. Mood Disorders in AD: Neuroradiologic, Genetic and Biologic Perspectives

The study of the relationship between dementia and mood disorders in late life is facilitated by neuroimaging investigations. In general, the neurobiological basis for the clinical heterogeneity of cognitive and behavioral features in AD is rather unclear, but corresponding abnormalities on functional imaging show that this variability is correlated with disturbances on positron emission tomography and single photon emission computerized tomography (Cummings, 2000). Cerebral atrophy and ventricular enlargement are almost universal findings in dementia, with a similar but weaker association with depression (Alexopoulos et al., 1992). A prominent feature of AD is the atrophy of temporal structures (Laakso et al., 1995). Few studies have examined these structures in late life depression with conflicting results (Rabins et al., 1991; Coffey et al., 1993; Pantel et al., 1997; Bremner et al., 2000; Steffens et al., 2000). Cerebral magnetic resonance imaging in patients with severe depression shows a higher frequency of white-matter hyperintensities (Soares and Mann, 1997); the severity of the deep white matter lesions and the deterioration of cognitive functions appear to be more pronounced in patients with late onset compared to those with early onset depression.

In order to explain the relationship between depression and dementia, it was hypothesized that they share the same genetic risk factors. The search for the specific susceptibility loci for depression in dementia has previously focused on the apolipoprotein E ε4 allele (ApoE ε4), a well established risk factor for AD. An association between ApoE ε4 and late-onset depression was found (Krishnan et al., 1996; Rigaud et al., 2001). While a higher frequency of the ApoE ε4 allele has been reported in depressed AD women but not in men (Muller-Thomsen et al., 2002), other studies failed to find a difference in ApoE ε4 allele frequency between depressed AD subjects and healthy controls (Forsell et al., 1995; Zubenko et al., 1996). In a recent longitudinal study on the association between ApoE genotype and psychopathological symptoms in AD, Scarmeas (Scarmeas et al., 2002) found that the presence of ε4 allele is not related with depression but strongly predicts the incidence of delusions. In summary, current evidences indicate that there is not a relationship between late-onset depression and ApoE ε4 allele, and suggest that both variables contribute independently to the development of dementia.

Atrophy and neuronal loss in AD is most prominent in association cortex, hippocampus, entorhinal cortex, locus ceruleus, and nucleus basalis. The most profound neurochemical deficit is that of acetylcholine. The activity of choline acetyltransferase has been found to be lower in AD patients compared to controls as well as in demented patients with hyperactivity and aggressive behavior (Minger et al., 2000). A decrease of neurotransmitters other than acetylcholine, however, occurs: most notably somatostatin, serotonin, norepinephrine, GABA, and indoleamines (Sky and Grossberg, 1994). Depletion of some of these transmitters has been specifically related to particular behavior abnormalities in animal and human studies. For example, reductions in serotonin and GABA have been associated with aggressive behavior (Sky and Grossberg, 1994). As far as depression is concerned, the mechanisms of its pathophysiology in AD are still largely unknown. A recent neuropathologic study demonstrated that in AD neuronal loss is more prominent in the locus coeruleus than in the nucleus basalis (Zarow et al., 2003), and several studies found that depression is associated with selective loss of noradrenergic cells in the locus coeruleus and is therefore linked to deficiencies in serotonin and norepinephrine (Zweig et al., 1988; Zubenko et al., 1992; Forstl et al., 1994), but causality has not been shown yet.

Nevertheless, pharmacological manipulations which enhance functions in particular neurotransmitter systems have led to improvement in certain behaviors. It is important to underline that some behavioral changes are more responsive to pharmacological intervention, while others are not. Those which tend to respond to medication include: depression, anxiety, agitation, delusions, and hallucinations. In contrast, behavioral disturbance less prone to response to medical treatment include disinhibited behaviors (like public undressing, social inappropriateness), wandering, hoarding or concealing objects, social withdrawal, and repetitive questioning.

The high prevalence of depression together with its treatability, frequency of occult onset and caregiver burden in AD warrant a careful consideration of critical issues that may help the characterization of this highly disabling noncognitive symptom. Several aspects of the relationship between depression and dementia is discussed in the following section.

3. Mood Disorders in AD: Focus on Depression

The diagnosis of depression in dementia is a complex task because of the overlap in symptomatology between the two diseases: decreased energy, apathy, gradual loss of interest, difficulties with concentration, psychomotor slowing, emotional lability, insomnia, weight loss, and inability to verbalize affective state, in fact, occur in both depressed and non depressed demented patients. Since the patient is often unable to communicate distress coherently, and usually perceives to be less depressed than caregivers or clinicians do, diagnosis is often based on the observation of patient's behavior and caregiver's report (Teri and Wagner, 1991). Assessment tools of depression in AD such as the Neuropsychiatric Inventory (NPI) (Cummings, 1997) have been reviewed in detail by Lyketsos and Lee (2004). The presence of depression has negative consequences on demented patients and their caregivers. Depression in dementia, in fact, is associated with impairment in quality of life (Gonzalez-Salvador et al., 2000), excess disability (Lyketsos et al., 1997), increased caregiver's depression and burden (Gonzalez-Salvador et al., 1999), and earlier placement in nursing homes (Steele et al., 1990).

Concerning AD, previous studies in clinical settings suggested that the prevalence of depression (major and minor) is between 30% and 50% (Lee and Lyketsos, 2003). Recently, several studies showed that depressive symptoms in the elderly are predictive of subsequent cognitive decline (Devanand et al., 1996; Bassuk et al., 1998; Yaffe et al., 1999). It has been found that the risk for AD in depressed subjects is inversely related to the temporal gap between dementia onset and depression onset: the risk ratio was particularly strong when depression occurred in the two years prior the diagnosis of AD, supporting the hypothesis that depression is a prodromal condition for AD (Steffens et al., 1997). Also a large community-based prospective study concluded that depressive symptoms appeared to be an early manifestation rather than a predictor of AD (Chen et al., 1999). On the contrary, Speck (Speck et al., 1995) reported that depressive symptoms occurring more than 10 years before the onset of dementia represent a risk factor for AD. Jorm and colleagues (Jorm et al., 1991) found that episodes of depression were a risk factor for AD when the onset of dementia was after the age of 70 years. A recent meta-analysis concluded that patients with dementia have more frequently a history of depression and that both early and midlife depression are risk factors for dementia (Jorm, 2000). In a longitudinal study, depressive symptoms at baseline were associated both with risk of AD and with the severity of cognitive decline in patients who became cognitively impaired but not demented at follow up (Wilson et al., 2002). Recently, the MIRAGE, a large cross-sectional, family-based, case control study, showed that depressive symptoms are associated with the development of AD, and this association is much stronger among families in which the onset of depressive symptoms occurred in the year before the onset of AD. However, there was a significant association even when the onset of depression preceded the onset of AD by 25 or more years (Green et al., 2003). Importantly, the high rate of major depressive episodes that have been shown to occur after the onset of cognitive impairment among AD patients does suggest that the major depressive syndrome of AD may be among the most common mood disorders of older adults (Zubenko et al., 2003).

4. Practical Approaches

The presence of BPSD in AD patients is extremely frequent, and a wide range of dementia-associated mental and behavioral disturbances may develop in the majority of community dwellers with dementia. Screening programmes aimed to the early identification of behavioral problems in demented patients should be available to physicians (Ikeda et al., 2004). In this regard, simple tools like the 5-item Geriatric Depression Scale have been proven useful in the clinical practice (Rinaldi et al., 2003). In spite of the high frequency of the co-presence depression/AD, there is a lack of data on the natural course, etiology, and treatment of depression in AD. The National Institute of Mental Health has recently proposed provisional diagnostic criteria for the *depression of Alzheimer's disease* and has started a longitudinal cohort study of depression in incident AD cases which may help clarifying these unsolved issues (Lee and Lyketsos, 2003). Furthermore, additional studies are necessary to better understand the pathophysiological role of genetic and biochemical factors of depression in AD, including those mentioned above and potentially relevant others such as immunological changes (Leonard, 2001), estrogen depletion (Schupf et al., 2003), brain energy alterations and oxidative stress (Pettegrew et al., 2000).

Physical exercise, social support, instrumental assistance, emotional support and social integration are all important protective factor for depression in later life (Alexopoulos et al., 2002). Setting the environment, determining the cause, observing new behaviors and monitoring behavioral disorders are obligatory steps in the management of the AD patient with behavioral disturbances (Yeager et al., 1995). A psychotherapeutic approach has to be considered for AD patients presenting mild symptoms of depression and anxiety, or for AD patients with moderate or severe depression in combination with antidepressants. This latter approach does depend on the patient's intellectual abilities and capacity for insight. For more cognitively impaired patients, behavioral strategies including pleasant activities may be more helpful. The use of pharmacologic agents in the treatment of BPSD should be considered once environmental and psychological strategies have been proven ineffective. Especially in the elderly, in fact, the benefits of managing agitation, depression or anxiety with medications should be carefully weighed against the risks of adverse effects (sedation, incontinence, confusion, etc). Benzodiazepines are effective in AD for the treatment of anxiety, non-aggressive agitation and insomnia; lithium has been helpful in some patients for the treatment of acute agitation, mania and explosive rage (Bauer et al., 2003). The best available evidence-based therapeutic approaches for the treatment of depression in AD have been elegantly overviewed and commented by Lyketsos and Lee (2004) and include the initiation of citalopram and sertraline as the first step; two trials comparing the efficacy of selective serotonin reuptake inhibitors (SSRIs) with that of tricyclic antidepressants (TCAs) in the treatment of depression in dementia (Taragano et al., 1997; Katona et al., 1998) have both reported comparable efficacy without suggesting superiority of either class of drugs. AD patients, however, appear to tolerate SSRIs better than TCAs (Taragano et al., 1997; Katona et al., 1998). On the other hand, well controlled studies on the pharmacotherapeutic management of depression in AD are rendered difficult by the high placebo response. In addition, no single clinical characteristic clearly predicts the response to treatment of major depression in AD (Steinberg et al., 2004). Nevertheless, beneficial treatment modalities are available for depression in AD, and these have been shown to reduce its adverse impact on patients and caregivers.

Thus, physicians should use the available tools for the diagnosis of mood disorders in AD, be aware of preventive strategies against the onset/worsening of cognitive and noncognitive symptoms, and take into account nonpharmarmacological options especially in the management of newly diagnosed AD patients with mood disorders.

References

Alexopoulos GS, Young RC, Shindledecker RD. Brain computed tomography findings in geriatric depression and primary degenerative dementia. *Biol Psychiatry* **31**: 591-599, 1992.

Alexopoulos GS, Buckwalter K, Olin J, Martinez R, Wainscott C, Krishnan KR. Comorbidity of late life depression: an opportunity for research on mechanisms and treatment. *Biol Psychiatry* **52**: 543-558, 2002.

Ballard C, Oyebode F. Psychotic symptoms in patients with dementia. *Int J Geriatr* **142**: 202-211, 1995.

Bassuk SS, Berkman LF, Wypij D. Depressive symptomatology and incident cognitive decline in an elderly community sample. *Arch Gen Psychiatry* **55**: 1073-1081, 1998.

Bauer M, Alda M, Priller J, Young LT; International Group For The Study Of Lithium Treated Patients (IGSLI). Implications of the neuroprotective effects of lithium for the treatment of bipolar and neurodegenerative disorders. *Pharmacopsychiatry* **36**: 250-254, 2003.

Bremner JD, Narayan M, Anderson ER, Staib LH, Miller HL, Charney DS. Hippocampal volume reduction in major depression. *Am J Psychiatry* **157**: 115-118, 2000.

Burns A, Jacoby R, Levy R. Psychiatric phenomena in Alzheimer's disease. III: Disorders of mood. *Br J Psychiatry* **157**: 81-86, 1990a.

Burns A, Jacoby R, Levy R. Psychiatric phenomena in Alzheimer's disease. IV: Disorders of behaviour. *Br J Psychiatry* **157**: 86-94, 1990b.

Chen P, Ganguli M, Mulsant BH, DeKosky ST. The temporal relationship between depressive symptoms and dementia: a community-based prospective study. *Arch Gen Psychiatry* **56**: 261-266, 1999.

Coffey CE, Wilkinson WE, Weiner RD, Parashos IA, Djang WT, Webb MC, Figiel GS, Spritzer CE. Quantitative cerebral anatomy in depression. A controlled magnetic resonance imaging study. *Arch Gen Psychiatry* **50**: 7-16, 1993.

Cummings JL. Neuropsychiatric assessment and intervention in Alzheimer's disease. *International Psychogeriatrics* **8**: 25-30, 1996.

Cummings JL. The Neuropsychiatric Inventory: assessing psychopathology in dementia patients. *Neurology* **48**: S10-16, 1997.

Cummings JL. Cognitive and behavioral heterogeneity in Alzheimer's disease: seeking the neurobiological basis. *Neurobiol Aging* **21**: 845-861, 2000.

Deimling GT, Bass DM. Symptoms of mental impairment among elderly adults and their effects on family caregivers. *J Gerontol* **41**: 778-784, 1986.

DesRosiers G, Hodges JR, Berrios G. The neuropsychological differentiation of patients with very mild Alzheimer's disease and/or major depression. *J Am Geriatr Soc* **43**: 1256-1263, 1995.

Devanand DP, Miller L, Richards M, Marder K, Bell K, Mayeux R, Stern Y. The Columbia University scale for psychopathology in Alzheimer's disease. *Arch Neurol* **49**: 371-376, 1992.

Devanand DP, Sano M, Tang MX, Taylor S, Gurland BJ, Wilder D, Stern Y, Mayeux R. Depressed mood and the incidence of Alzheimer's disease in the elderly living in the community. *Arch Gen Psychiatry* **53**: 75-182, 1996.

Forsell Y, Jorm AF, von Strauss E, Winblad B. Prevalence and correlates of depression in a population of nonagenarians. *Br J Psychiatry* **167**: 61-64, 1995.

Forstl H, Levy R, Burns A, Luthert P, Cairns N. Disproportionate loss of noradrenergic and cholinergic neurons as cause of depression in Alzheimer's disease--a hypothesis. *Pharmacopsychiatry* **27**: 11-15, 1994.

Gaugler JE, Zarit SH, Pearlin LI. The onset of dementia caregiving and its longitudinal implications. *Psychol Aging* **18**: 171-180, 2003.

Geerlings MI, Schoevers RA, Beekman AT, Jonker C, Deeg DJ, Schmand B, Ader HJ, Bouter LM, Van Tilburg W. Depression and risk of cognitive decline and Alzheimer's disease. Results of two prospective community-based studies in The Netherlands. *Br J Psychiatry* **176**: 568-575, 2000a.

Geerlings MI, Schmand B, Braam AW, Jonker C, Bouter LM, van Tilburg W. Depressive symptoms and risk of Alzheimer's disease in more highly educated older people. *J Am Geriatr Soc* **48**: 1092-1097, 2000b.

Gonzalez-Salvador MT, Arango C, Lyketsos CG, Barba AC. The stress and psychological morbidity of the Alzheimer patient caregiver. *Int J Geriatr Psychiatry* **14**: 701-710, 1999.

Gonzalez-Salvador T, Lyketsos CG, Baker A, Hovanec L, Roques C, Brandt J, Steele C. Quality of life in dementia patients in long-term care. *Int J Geriatr Psychiatry* **15** : 181-189, 2000.

Green RC, Cupples LA, Kurz A, Auerbach S, Go R, Sadovnick D, Duara R, Kukull WA, Chui H, Edeki T, Griffith PA, Friedland RP, Bachman D, Farrer L. Depression as a risk factor for Alzheimer disease: the MIRAGE Study. *Arch Neurol* **60**: 753-759, 2003.

Ikeda M, Fukuhara R, Shigenobu K, Hokoishi K, Maki N, Nebu A, Komori K, Tanabe H. Dementia associated mental and behavioural disturbances in elderly people in the community: findings from the first Nakayama study. *J Neurol Neurosurg Psychiatry* **75**: 146-148, 2004.

Jorm AF, van Duijn CM, Chandra V, Fratiglioni L, Graves AB, Heyman A, Kokmen E, Kondo K, Mortimer JA, Rocca WA, et al. Psychiatric history and related exposures as risk factors for Alzheimer's disease: a collaborative re-analysis of case-control studies. EURODEM Risk Factors Research Group. *Int J Epidemiol* **20**: S43-S47, 1991.

Jorm AF. Is depression a risk factor for dementia or cognitive decline? A review. *Gerontology* **46**: 219-227, 2000.

Katona CL, Hunter BN, Bray J. A double-blind comparison of the efficacy and safely of paroxetine and imipramine in the treatment of depression with dementia. *Int J Geriatr Psychiatry* **13**: 100-108, 1998.

Kiloh LG. Depressive illness masquerading as dementia in the elderly. *Med J Aust* **14**: 550-553, 1981.

Krishnan KR, Tupler LA, Ritchie JC Jr, McDonald WM, Knight DL, Nemeroff CB, Carroll BJ. Apolipoprotein E-epsilon 4 frequency in geriatric depression. *Biol Psychiatry* **40**: 69-71, 1996.

Kunik ME, Yudofsky SC Silver JM, Hales RE. Pharmacologic approach to management of agitation associated with dementia. *J Clin Psychiatry* **55 (S2)**: 13-17, 1994.

Laakso MP, Soininen H, Partanen K, Helkala EL, Hartikainen P, Vainio P, Hallikainen M, Hanninen T, Riekkinen PJ Sr. Volumes of hippocampus, amygdala and frontal lobes in the MRI-based diagnosis of early Alzheimer's disease: correlation with memory functions. *J Neural Transm Park Dis Dement Sect* **9** : 73-86, 1995.

Lee HB, Lyketsos CG. Depression in Alzheimer's disease: heterogeneity and related issues. *Biol Psychiatry* **54**: 353-362, 2003.

Leonard BE. Changes in the immune system in depression and dementia: causal or co-incidental effects? *Int J Dev Neurosci* **19**: 305-312, 2001.

Lyketsos CG, Steele C, Baker L, Galik E, Kopunek S, Steinberg M, Warren A. Major and minor depression in Alzheimer's disease: prevalence and impact. *J Neuropsychiatry Clin Neurosci* **9**: 556-561, 1997.

Lyketsos CG, Lopez O, Jones B, Fitzpatrick AL, Breitner J, DeKosky S. Prevalence of neuropsychiatric symptoms in dementia and mild cognitive impairment: results from the cardiovascular health study. *JAMA.* **288:** 1475-1483, 2002.

Lyketsos CG, Lee HB. Diagnosis and treatment of depression in Alzheimer's disease. *Dement Geriatr Cogn Disord* **17:** 55-64, 2004.

Mace, N.L., Rabins, P.V. The 36-hour-day. Maryland: Johns-Hopkins University Press, 1981.

Mega MS, Cummings JL, Fiorello T, Gornbein J. The spectrum of behavioral changes in Alzheimer's disease. *Neurology* **46:** 130-135, 1996.

Merriam AE, Aronson MK, Gaston P, Wey SL, Katz I. The psychiatric symptoms of Alzheimer's disease. *J Am Geriatr Soc* **36:** 7-12, 1988.

Minger SL, Esiri MM, McDonald B, Keene J, Carter J, Hope T, Francis PT. Cholinergic deficits contribute to behavioral disturbance in patients with dementia. *Neurology* **55:** 1460-1467, 2000.

Mittelman MS, Roth DL, Haley WE, Zarit SH. Effects of a caregiver intervention on negative caregiver appraisals of behavior problems in patients with Alzheimer's disease: results of a randomized trial. *J Gerontol B Psychol Sci Soc Sci* **59:** P27-34, 2004.

Morriss RK, Rovner BW, Folstein MF, German PS. Delusions in newly admitted residents of nursing homes. *Am J Psychiatry* **147:** 299-302, 1990.

Muller-Thomsen T, Arlt S, Ganzer S, Muller-Thomsen T, Arlt S, Ganzer S. Depression in Alzheimer's disease might be associated with apolipoprotein E epsilon 4 allele frequency in women but not in men. *Dement Geriatr Cogn Disord* **14:** 59-63, 2002.

Pantel J, Schroder J, Schad LR, Friedlinger M, Knopp MV, Schmitt R, Geissler M, Bluml S, Essig M, Sauer H. Quantitative magnetic resonance imaging and neuropsychological functions in dementia of the Alzheimer type. *Psychol Med* **27:** 221-229, 1997.

Pettegrew JW, Levine J, McClure RJ. Acetyl-L-carnitine physical-chemical, metabolic, and therapeutic properties: relevance for its mode of action in Alzheimer's disease and geriatric depression. *Mol Psychiatry* **5:** 616-632, 2000.

Polidori MC, Menculini G, Senin U, Mecocci P. Dementia, depression and parkinsonism: a frequent association in the elderly. *J Alzheimers Dis* **3:** 553-562, 2001.

Rabins PV, Mace NL, Lucas MJ. The impact of dementia on the family. *JAMA* **248:** 333-335, 1982.

Rabins PV, Pearlson GD, Aylward E, Kumar AJ, Dowell K. Cortical magnetic resonance imaging changes in elderly inpatients with major depression. *Am J Psychiatry* **148:** 148: 617-620, 1991.

Rabins PV. The treatment of noncognitive symptoms. In: Terry RD, Katzman R, Bick KL, Sisodia SS, editors. *Alzheimer Disease.* 2nd ed. Philadelphia: Lippincott Williams & Wilkins, 1999, pp. 415-421.

Reifler BV. A case of mistaken identity: pseudodementia is really predementia. *J Am Geriatr Soc* **48:** 593-594, 2000.

Reisberg B, Borenstein J, Salob SP, Ferris SH, Franssen E, Georgotas A. Behavioral symptoms in Alzheimer's disease: phenomenology and treatment. *J Clin Psychiatry* **48:** 9-15, 1987.

Rigaud AS, Traykov L, Caputo L, Coste J, Latour F, Couderc R, Moulin F, Boller F, Forette F. Association of the apolipoprotein E epsilon4 allele with late-onset depression. *Neuroepidemiology* **20**: 268-272, 2001.

Rinaldi P, Mecocci P, Benedetti C, Ercolani S, Bregnocchi M, Menculini G, Catani M, Senin U, Cherubini A. Validation of the five-item geriatric depression scale in elderly subjects in three different settings. *J Am Geriatr Soc* **51**: 694-698, 2003.

Scarmeas N, Brandt J, Albert M, Devanand DP, Marder K, Bell K, Ciappa A, Tycko B, Stern Y. Association between the APOE genotype and psychopathologic symptoms in Alzheimer's disease. *Neurology* **58**: 1182-1188, 2002.

Schupf N, Pang D, Patel BN, Silverman W, Schubert R, Lai F, Kline JK, Stern Y, Ferin M, Tycko B, Mayeux R. Onset of dementia is associated with age at menopause in women with Down's syndrome. *Ann Neurol* **54**: 433-438, 2003.

Sky AJ, Grossberg GT. The use of psychotropic medication in the management of problem behaviors in the patient with Alzheimer's disease. *Med Clin North America* **78**: 811-822, 1994.

Soares JC, Mann JJ. The anatomy of mood disorders-review of structural neuroimaging studies. *Biol Psychiatry* **41** : 86-106, 1997.

Speck CE, Kukull WA, Brenner DE, Bowen JD, McCormick WC, Teri L, Pfanschmidt ML, Thompson JD, Larson EB. History of depression as a risk factor for Alzheimer's disease. *Epidemiology* **6**: 366-369, 1995.

Steele C, Rovner B, Chase GA, Folstein M. Psychiatric symptoms and nursing home placement of patients with Alzheimer's disease. *Am J Psychiatry* **147**: 1049-1051, 1990.

Steffens DC, Plassman BL, Helms MJ, Welsh-Bohmer KA, Saunders AM, Breitner JC. A twin study of late-onset depression and apolipoprotein E epsilon 4 as risk factors for Alzheimer's disease. *Biol Psychiatry* **41**: 851-856, 1997.

Steffens DC, Byrum CE, McQuoid DR, Greenberg DL, Payne ME, Blitchington TF, MacFall JR, Krishnan KR. Hippocampal volume in geriatric depression. *Biol Psychiatry* **48** : 301-309, 2000.

Steinberg M, Munro CA, Samus Q, V Rabins P, Brandt J, Lyketsos CG. Patient predictors of response to treatment of depression in Alzheimer's disease: the DIADS study. *Int J Geriatr Psychiatry* **19** : 144-150, 2004.

Swearer JM, Drachman DA, O'Donnell BF, Mitchell AL. Troublesome and disruptive behaviors in dementia. Relationships to diagnosis and disease severity. *J Am Geriatr Soc* **36** : 784-790, 1988.

Swearer JM. Predicting aberrant behavior in Alzheimer's disease. *Neuropsychiatry, Neuropsychology and Behavioral Neurology* **9**: 162-170, 1996.

Taragano FE, Lyketsos CG, Mangone CA, Allegri RF, Comesana-Diaz E. A double-blind, randomized, fixed-dose trial of fluoxetine vs. amitriptyline in the treatment of major depression complicating Alzheimer's disease. *Psychosomatics* **38**: 246-252, 1997.

Tariot PN, Podgorski CA, Blazina L, Leibovici A. Mental disorders in the nursing home: another perspective. *Am J Psychiatry* **150**: 1063-1069, 1993.

Teri L, Larson EB, Reifler BV. Behavioral disturbance in dementia of the Alzheimer's type. *J Am Geriatr Soc* **36**: 1-6, 1988.

Teri L, Borson S, Kiyak HA, Yamagishi M. Behavioral disturbance, cognitive dysfunction, and functional skill. Prevalence and relationship in Alzheimer's disease. *J Am Geriatr Soc* **37**: 109-116, 1989.

Teri L, Wagner AW. Assessment of depression in patients with Alzheimer's disease: concordance among informants. *Psychol Aging* **6**: 280-285, 1991.

Teri L, Logsdon RG, McCurry SM. Nonpharmacologic treatment of behavioral disturbance in dementia. *Med Clin North Am* **86**: 641-656, 2002.

Wilson RS, Barnes LL, Mendes de Leon CF, Aggarwal NT, Schneider JS, Bach J, Pilat J, Beckett LA, Arnold SE, Evans DA, Bennett DA. Depressive symptoms, cognitive decline, and risk of AD in older persons. *Neurology* **59**: 364-370, 2002.

Wragg RE, Jeste DV. Overview of depression and psychosis in Alzheimer's disease. *Am J Psychiatry* **146**: 577-587, 1989.

Yaffe K, Blackwell T, Gore R, Sands L, Reus V, Browner WS. Depressive symptoms and cognitive decline in nondemented elderly women: a prospective study. *Arch Gen Psychiatry* **56**: 425-430, 1999.

Yeager BF, Farnett LE, Ruzicka SA. Management of the behavioral manifestations of dementia. *Arch Intern Med* **155**: 250-260, 1995.

Zarow C, Lyness SA, Mortimer JA, Chui HC. Neuronal loss is greater in the locus coeruleus than nucleus basalis and substantia nigra in Alzheimer and Parkinson diseases. *Arch Neurol* **60**: 337-341, 2003.

Zubenko GS. Biological correlates of clinical heterogeneity in primary dementia. *Neuropsychopharmacology* **6**: 77-93, 1992.

Zubenko GS, Henderson R, Stiffler JS, Stabler S, Rosen J, Kaplan BB. Association of the APOE epsilon 4 allele with clinical subtypes of late life depression. *Biol Psychiatry* **40**: 1008-1016, 1996.

Zubenko GS, Zubenko WN, McPherson S, Spoor E, Marin DB, Farlow MR, Smith GE, Geda YE, Cummings JL, Petersen RC, Sunderland T. A collaborative study of the emergence and clinical features of the major depressive syndrome of Alzheimer's disease. *Am J Psychiatry* **160**: 857-866, 2003.

Zweig RM, Ross CA, Hedreen JC, Steele C, Cardillo JE, Whitehouse PJ, Folstein MF, Price DL. The neuropathology of aminergic nuclei in Alzheimer's disease. *Ann Neurol* **24**: 233-242, 1988.

In: Cognition and Mood Interactions
Editor: Miao-Kun Sun, pp. 117-135

ISBN 1-59454-229-5
2005 © Nova Science Publishers, Inc.

Chapter VII

Neural Atrophy in Major Depression and Alzheimer's Disease

Safa Elgamal and Glenda MacQueen *

Dept of Psychiatry and Behavioral Neurosciences, McMaster University, Canada

The neuropathological mechanisms underlying major depressive disorder include several morphological changes. Atrophy of the hippocampal formation, reduction of caudate and globus pallidus, and change in the volume of amygdala have been reported by a number of magnetic resonance imaging studies. Histopathological reports describing the changes in major depressive disorder are few, but suggest the involvement of both neuronal and glial cells in frontal and temorolimbic regions. While global cerebral atrophy is not consistently reported in patients with major depression, it is a prominent brain change among patients with Alzheimer's dementia, which is characterized by the presence of neurofibrillary tangles and neuritic plaques besides the neuronal atrophy and synaptic loss. Volume loss is apparent in the entorhinal cortex and the hippocampus early in Alzheimer's disease; temporal, parietal, frontal cortex, and cingulate gyrus appear affected later. In this chapter, we will review the studies describing gross and microscopic correlates of neural atrophy in depression and Alzhemier's disease, and briefly consider whether the current postmortem or neuroimaging literature can explain the relatively robust and provocative clinical data that suggest major depressive disorder is a risk factor for development of Alzheimer's disease.

1. Neural Atrophy in Dementia and Depression

Recent clinical evidence suggests that major depression and dementia may be associated or have a common underlying neuropathological mechanism. Major depressive disorder (MDD) is often associated with impaired cognitive function, particularly memory deficits, and depression occurs in approximately one-quarter of patients with Alzheimer's disease (AD; Lyketsos et al., 2000). Depression, even when onset is early in life, appears to be a risk factor for the development of Alzheimer's disease. These associations raise an interesting question: does recurrent depression indeed predispose individuals to Alzheimer's disease? Or is there a common factor between the two conditions that leads to the high co-occurrence of these illnesses? The answers to these questions are unknown, but examining the underlying neuropathological mechanism for each disorder may uncover links or dissimilarities between the disorders that provide a partial answer to the question of the relation between unipolar MDD and AD.

2. Neuropathology of Major Depression

Although MDD is the most prevalent psychiatric disorder (Kessler et al., 1994), the etiology and time course of the neuropathological abnormalities in mood disorder are largely unknown. Stress, genetic and environmental factors influence the development of MDD (Duman et al., 1999). Occurrence of depression may be related to stress exposure; and cortisol levels are elevated in 40-50% of patients with depressive episodes (Carroll et al., 1976). Depression may lead to dysfunction in the hypothalamo-pituitary-adrenal axis (HPA) that is believed to cause both structural and functional brain changes. Stress induced dysfunction of the hypothalamo-pituitary-adrenal axis can cause reduction in neurotrophic factors, reduction in neurogenesis, and glial cell loss (Sheline, 2003). Depression induced hypercortisolemia results in neurotoxicity and atrophy of the affected structures that have a high density of glucocorticoid receptors such as the hippocampus, amygdala, and prefrontal cortex resulting in volume loss of these brain regions; however, the structural changes may be driven by excitatory amino acids and facilitated by glucocorticoids (Sapolsky, 2000).

Global cerebral atrophy is not consistently reported in patients with MDD (Soares and Mann, 1997); rather the histology and apparent specificity for areas implicated in the modulation of emotional behaviour suggest the regions most strongly involved in the pathogenesis of this disorder. A limbic-thalamic-cortical branch composed of the amygdala and hippocampus, mediodorsal nucleus of the thalamus, and medial and ventrolateral prefrontal cortex has been proposed as one circuit and a limbic-striatal-pallidal-thalamic branch constitutes another circuit. The caudate and putamen (striatum) and globus pallidus (pallidum) are organized in parallel to connect with limbic and cortical regions. Several brain areas, as well as multiple neurotransmitter systems, and multiple neural circuits are implicated in the neuropathology of MDD. Recent imaging studies provide evidence for involvement of the prefrontal cortex (Kumar et al., 1997; Drevets et al., 1997; Drevets, 2000; Soares and Mann, 1997; Öngür et al., 1998), hippocampus (Mervaala et al., 2000; Sheline et al., 1996; Sheline et al., 1999; Posener et al., 2003), basal ganglia (Husain et al., 1991; Krishnan et al., 1992; Parashos et al., 1998; Lacerda et al., 2003), and amygdala (Frodl et al., 2002; Drevets et al., 1992; Drevets et al., 2002; Sheline et al., 1998; Mervaala et al., 2000) in MDD and these will be given particular attention in the following sections.

3. Prefrontal Cortex

The prefrontal cortex has extensive interconnections with several cortical-subcortical structures such as the basal ganglia and the limbic regions. Areas of prefrontal cortex implicated in MDD include the dorsolateral prefrontal cortex (involved in working memory) and medial prefrontal cortex (mediating emotion), which consists of several related areas, including orbitofrontal cortex (Bremner et al., 2003), anterior cingulate (area 25, subcallosal gyrus; area 24, subgenual gyrus; and area 32, the Stroop area), and anterior prefrontal cortex (area 9) (Bremner et al., 2003; Botteron et al., 2002; Drevets et al., 1997).

Several brain stem nuclei including the dorsal raphe, locus coeruleus and ventral tegmental area give origin to extensive monoamine projections that terminate in the prefrontal cortex and which are implicated in MDD; for example, SERT (serotonin transporter) binding is reduced in patients with a history of MDD in a number of Brodmann areas throughout the dorsal-ventral extent of the prefrontal cortex (Austin et al., 2002; Mann et al., 2000; Arango et al., 1995).

Both neurons and glial cells appear involved in the histopathology of MDD in the prefrontal cortex. Various prefrontal cortical regions and layers are differentially affected (Rajkowska et al., 1999). Rajkowska and colleagues reported that reductions in neuronal size and density are most prominent in the rostral orbitofrontal cortex; decreases in glial cell density were greatest in more caudally located regions of the prefrontal cortex, including the caudal orbitofrontal cortex and dorso-lateral prefrontal cortex (Rajkowska et al., 1999). Glial density reductions have been reported in the orbital cortex, the anterior cingulate cortex (ACC), and the dorso-lateral prefrontal cortex (Rajkowska et al., 1999; Cotter et al., 2001; Öngür et al., 1998). Glial changes are most prominent in the deeper cortical layers and are accompanied by reduced neuronal size (Cotter et al., 2001). Glia are known to affect several processes that are essential for normal neuronal integrity, including regulation of extracellular potassium, glucose storage and metabolism, and glutamate uptake which may be dysregulated in MDD (Öngür et al., 1998). Subgenual prefrontal cortex glial cell loss is also reported in MDD (Öngür et al., 1998). Only the rostral and medial orbitofrontal cortices have been reported to have significant reduction in cortical thickness in MDD (Rajkowska et al., 1999).

Functional imaging studies in adult patients with MDD have shown dysfunction in the dorsolateral prefrontal, anterior cingulate, and orbitofrontal cortex. In MDD, there is reduced metabolism in the anterior cingulate cortex (Roger et al., 1998) particularly on the left (Bench et al., 1995; Drevets et al., 1997; Hirayasu et al., 1999). In depression, findings consist largely of increased ventral and decreased dorsal activity in prefrontal and anterior cingulate cortex (Baxter et al., 1989; Bench et al., 1992; Cohen et al., 1992; Biver et al., 1994; Drevets, 1999). The hemispheric lateralization of abnormalities has consisted primarily of relative reductions in left hemisphere activity in depression (Baxter et al., 1989; Bench et al., 1992; Biver et al., 1994; Drevets, 1999). These data are consistent with other literature suggesting that left hemisphere lesions are more frequently associated with depression, while right hemisphere lesions are more commonly associated with mania (Soares and Mann, 1997). Decreased cortical volume and resting cerebral glucose metabolism have been reported in the subgenual cortex, again, particularly in the left hemisphere (Drevets et al., 1997; Öngür et al., 1998). In geriatric major depression, functional imaging studies have reported decreased blood flow in the orbitofrontal cortex (lesser et al., 1994) and ACC (Awata et al., 1998; de Asis et al., 2001) as well as biochemical abnormalities in frontal white matter (Kumar et al., 2002). Normalized prefrontal lobe volumes show a significant linear trend with severity of depression, with volumes decreasing with illness severity (Kumar et al. 1998).

Pronounced gray matter deficits are observed in three brain regions, including the orbitofrontal cortex as well as the anterior cingulate and the gyrus rectus (Ballmaier et al., 2004). Prominent frontal lobe white matter hyperintensities are particularly apparent in older individuals with late-onset MDD (Krishnan, 1991; Coffey et al., 1989; O'Brien et al. 2000) particularly those with underlying cerebrovascular disease originating from atherosclerotic disease (Coffey et al., 1989; Awad et al., 1986; Lesser et al., 1991; Krishnan and McDonald, 1995; Schirmer and Fels, 1999).

4. Hippocampus

Considerable correlative evidence implicates glucocorticoid action on hippocampal cells in the pathogenesis of MDD (Sapolsky, 2001). Elevated levels of glucocorticoids may result in damage of hippocampal neurons, and reduction of hippocampal volume. The hippocampus is particularly sensitive to signs of atrophy as a result of elevated glucocorticoids, and tends to show greater changes than other brain areas in recurrent depressive illness (McEwen, 2001). The effect of increased glucocorticoid levels on the hippocampus includes retraction of dendritic processes, inhibition of neurogenesis, and neurotoxicity (Sapolsky, 1999; Thomas and Peterson, 2003). Elevation of cortisol levels in elderly patients correlates with reduced hippocampal volume and is associated with memory deficits (Lupien et al., 1998). As McEwen has outlined (2001), hippocampal atrophy in stress related disorders may be due to one of at least four different processes: (1) a reduced volume of Ammon's horn or dentate gyrus due to reduced dendritic branching; (2) a reduction in dentate gyrus neuron number due to a suppression of neurogenesis; (3) a decreased rate of neuron survival; (4) permanent neuron loss. Despite a wealth of preclinical data suggesting that the hippocampus may be altered in MDD, there remains a lack of direct postmortem studies reporting significant pathological changes in this region in patients with MDD (Harrison, 2002). Few studies, heterogenous patient populations, and small overall sample sizes in studies to date have probably contributed to the paucity of direct data examining the effect of recurrent MDD on the hippocampus.

A number of studies have examined gross hippocampal changes using imaging techniques, however, and most, although not all, MRI studies have found smaller hippocampal volumes in MDD (Sheline et al., 1996; Sheline et al., 1998; Shah et al., 1998; Bremner et al., 2000; MacQueen et al., 2003). A recent meta-analysis (Campbell et al., 2004) confirmed that when examined in the aggregate, the imaging data support a decrease in hippocampal volume of approximately 14% in patients with recurrent MDD. Left hippocampal volumes may be more reliably reduced than right hippocampal volumes. A preliminary report has suggested that antidepressants may protect against hippocampal volume loss associated with cumulative episodes of MDD as hippocampal volume was significantly predicted by duration of untreated, but not treated, MDD (Sheline et al., 2003).

5. Amygdala

The amygdala plays a crucial role in the regulation of mood and affect (Aggleton, 1993). Glial density and the glia/neuron ratio are substantially reduced in the amygdala in patients with MDD. The reduction is mainly accounted for by counts in the left hemisphere. A 53% reduction in the glia to neuron ratio has been reported in MDD, with no change is found in neuronal number or structure overall (Bowley et al., 2002). This provocative finding requires replication as to date it remains the only neuropathological report of abnormality in the amygdala among patients with a history of MDD.

With respect to volumetric imaging studies, the amygdala is a difficult structure to measure, since in many areas the cortical amygdala merges with surrounding cortex, and specific boundaries selected vary greatly in different studies; this may partially account for the inconsistent results found in amygdala volumes in studies involving MDD (Sheline, 2003). In general, however, it appears that depressed patients showed increased amygdala volumes in both hemispheres. Enlarged amygdala volumes in patients with a first episode of MDD might be due to enhanced blood flow in the amygdala rather than to a neurodevelopmental structural predisposition to MDD (Frodl et al., 2002). Other studies reported increased volume in the right amygdala (Bremner et al., 2000), significant asymmetry of the amygdala volumes (right smaller than left) (Mervaala et al, 2000), or reduction in the bilateral core nuclei (which is composed of the lateral, basal, and accessory basal nuclei) in patients with recurrent MDD with no significant change of the amygdala total volume (Sheline et al., 1998). Increases in resting cerebral blood flow and glucose metabolism have been reported in the left amygdala of depressed patients with familial pure depressive disease (Drevets et al., 1992; Drevets, 2000) and these are positively correlated with severity of illness (Drevets et al., 1992). Individuals with MDD who have greater baseline right amygdala glucose metabolism experience more severe negative affect (Abercrombie et al., 1998). Treatment with antidepressants appears to reduce amygdala metabolism to normative levels, consistent with preclinical evidence that chronic antidepressants administration has inhibitory effects on amygdala function (Drevets, 1999).

6. Basal Ganglia

The caudate and putamen receive input from the medial temporal structures involved in regulation of emotions, and they have connections to the prefrontal cortex. Thus, these structures may be relevant for mood regulation, and lesions affecting these circuits may contribute to the pathogenesis of mood disorders (Soares and Mann, 1997). Notably, degenerative diseases of the basal ganglia, such as Huntington's disease (HD), Parkinson's disease (PD), and Wilson's disease are associated with high prevalence of MDD (Rosenblatt and Leroi, 2000). A postmortem study of basal ganglia structures in idiopathic MDD reported a focally accentuated volume reduction of the left nucleus accumbens, the external pallidum bilaterally, and the right putamen (Baumann et al., 1999), but there are no other postmortum data currently to suggest that the basal ganglia are structurally altered in the neuropathology of MDD unrelated to another degenerative disorder.

Neuroimaging studies have suggested that structural abnormalities exist in basal ganglia of patients with mood disorders. Magnetic resonance imaging of the caudate nuclei in MDD found that right and left caudate nucleus volumes were smaller in depressed patients compared with controls (Krishnan et al., 1992; Parashos et al., 1998). In other studies, depressed patients also had significantly smaller putamen nuclei (Husain et al., 1991; Parashos et al., 1998), but the previous findings were not supported by Pillay et al. (1998) who found no statistically significant difference in caudate and lentiform nucleus grey matter volumes between patients and comparison subjects. Lenze and Sheline (1999) also reported no volumetric differences in caudate and putamen in depressed women. Furthermore, another MRI study did not find significant differences between patient and control groups in basal ganglia volumetric measures (Lacerda et al., 2003). MDD patients did have decreased asymmetry in globus pallidus volumes in comparison with healthy controls, however, while left putamen volume correlated inversely with length of illness, and left globus pallidus volume correlated directly with number of prior depressive episodes. These findings suggest that abnormalities in lateralization and possibly neurodegenerative changes in basal ganglia structures participate in the pathophysiology of MDD (Lacerda et al., 2003).

In summary, the most extensive postmortem data support changes in frontal cortex and associated regions in patients with MDD. Postmortem data supporting changes in the hippocampus, amygdala and basal ganglia are relatively sparse, but there are a number of imaging studies that report volumetric and functional changes consistent with atrophy in these regions. Previous reviews (see Harrison, 2002) have emphasized the shortcomings of many of the postmortem studies to date. Some of the most obvious limitations of past studies are that patients' histories of illness and treatment are rarely controlled or accounted for, despite the fact that MDD is thought to be heterogenous, a long or recurrent form of MDD may be necessary to observe substantive structural changes in key brain regions, and treatment may exert as yet poorly understood neuroprotective effects that could minimize or even eliminate the atrophy associated with untreated disease. Furthermore, patients with onset of MDD late in life secondary to a recognized or unrecognized degenerative neurological disease, or secondary to cerebrovascular disease, may demonstrate a very different pathological pattern than patients with recurrent MDD with onset in adolescence or early adulthood.

It is notable that, other than a commonality of brain regions involved, there is little in the neuropathological studies of patients with MDD that suggests a process similar to the early stages of Alzheimer's disease; the neuropathology of this much more extensively studied disorder is briefly reviewed below.

7. Neuropathology of Alzheimer's Disease

Alzheimer's disease (AD) is a progressive, neurodegenerative disease characterized by loss of functioning and death of neurons in several areas of the brain (Selkoe, 1999). Some regions of the brain are affected early in the course of the disease while others remain unaffected until advanced stages. Staging of AD is determined by the extent and severity of the affected neurons. The disease remains dormant for several years after the development of the neuropathology with the clinical symptoms observed only late in the course of the disease when the pathological changes reach the neocortical association areas (Braak et al., 1999).

Alzheimer's disease is characterized by degenerative changes in selected brain regions, including the temporal and parietal lobes and restricted regions within the frontal cortex and cingulate gyrus. The degeneration of these systems may underlie specific aspects of the dementia associated with AD (Wenk, 2003). Alzheimer's disease has a particular pattern of distribution of the neuropathological changes among different brain regions including the entorhinal cortex, the hippocampus and the medial temporal lobe (MTL; Braak and Braak, 1991). Alzheimer pathology typically starts in the entorhinal cortex before affecting the hippocampus, probably for several years, before spreading cortically (Braak et al., 1993). The pathologic hallmarks of AD (e.g., neurofibrillary tangles and neuritic plaques) are evident in the entorhinal cortex in the earliest phase of disease (Gomez-Isla et al., 1996; Braak et al., 1993).

Alzheimer's disease is characterized by degenerative changes in a variety of neurotransmitter systems (Wenk, 2003). Neuronal loss or atrophy in the nucleus basalis of Meynert, locus ceruleus, and raphe nuclei of the brainstem are found and lead to deficits in cholinergic, noradrenergic, and serotonergic transmitters, respectively (Cummings and Cole, 2002). Marked reductions in cholinergic markers have been found in the cerebral cortex among AD patients even at an early stage of the disease (Bowen et al., 1982). Moreover, the number of neurons containing choline acetyltransferase (ChAT) and the vesicular acetylcholine transporter correlates significantly with the severity of dementia, as determined by the Mini-Mental State Examination (Gilmor et al., 1999). The neurodegenerative changes required for the diagnosis of Alzheimer's disease include neuritic plaques (NPs), neurofibrillary tangles (NFTs), as well as neuronal loss, and each neurodegnerative feature has been extensively examined in pathological studies that are beyond the scope of this review. They are briefly outlined below.

8. Neuritic Plaques

Neuritic (NPs) plaques consist of a central core of amyloid protein surrounded by astrocytes, microglia, and dystrophic neurites often containing paired helical filaments (Cummings et al., 1998). NPs alone are a fairly good indicator of the presence of dementia, in that normal older individuals have few or none, whereas patients with AD have many. NPs are among the earliest neuropathological lesions in AD. Even very mild or questionable dementia is associated with increased density of neocortical NPs (Haroutunian et al., 1998). Neuritic plaque density correlates with age at death (Bierer et al., 1995), but there appears to be little correlation between NP count and dementia severity (Bierer et al., 1995).

Three stages in the evolution of plaque deposition have been described. Stage A is characterized by deposition in the basal temporal neocortex, or entorrhinal cortex. There then is extension through the hippocampal formation in stage B, eventually leading to deposits in virtually all cortical areas, including the highly myelinated primary areas of the neocortex in stage C (Braak and Braak, 1999b). Temporal and occipital lobes have the highest NPs densities, limbic and frontal lobes have the lowest, and the parietal lobe is intermediate (Arnold et al., 1991).

9. Neurofibrillary Tangles

Neurofibrillary tangles are the second major histopathological feature of AD. They contain paired helical filaments of abnormally phosphorylated tau protein that occupy the cell body and extend into the dendrites (Cummings and Cole, 2002). "The density of NFTs in AD is as follows: periallocortex (area 28) greater than allocortex (subiculum/CA1 zones of hippocampal formation, area 51) greater than corticoid areas (accessory basal nucleus of amygdala, nucleus basalis of Meynert) greater than proisocortex (areas 11, 12, 24, 23, anterior insula, 38, 35) greater than nonprimary association cortex (32, 46, superior temporal sulcus, 40, 39, posterior parahippocampal cortex, 37, 36) greater than primary sensory association cortex (7, 18, 19, 22, 21, 20) greater than agranular cortex (44-5, 8, 6, 4) greater than primary sensory cortex (41-2, 3-1- 2, 17)" (Arnold et al., 1991). The laminar distribution of NFTs tends to be selective; starts by affecting layers III and V of cortical association areas as well as layers II and IV of limbic periallocortex. Higher density of NFTs is observed in both limbic and temporal lobes than in frontal, parietal, and occipital lobes (Arnold et al., 1991).

Six stages are described in the evolution of neurofibrillary tangles. The intraneural formation of neurofibrillary tangles in the transentorhinal region occurs in the early stage of the disease (stage I); this is followed by progressive appearance of NFTs in the entorhinal region and the hippocampal formation in stage II. Extensive involvement of the entorhinal cortex, amygdala, and hippocampal formation occurs in stages III and IV. At this level, the limbic loop is affected with disruption of the transfer of data between the neocortex and hippocampal formation. The nucleus basalis of Meynert, among other subcortical nuclei is also affected at this stage leading to dysfunction of the cholinergic system of the basal forebrain. Primary and association areas of the cerebral cortex are involved in stage V. Finally, involvement of the sensory area with relative sparing of motor area occurs in stage VI. Stages I and II represent the preclinical phase of the disease before any cognitive deterioration can be detected. Stages III and IV represent mild clinical phase, while stages V and VI are associated with severe cognitive impairment (Braak and Braak, 1999b).

Much of the existing literature suggests that the NFTs of AD have a closer correlation with cognitive function than do amyloid plaques. Large numbers of NFTs and amyloid plaques are diagnostic markers for AD, but lesser numbers of these lesions may also be observed in nondemented older individuals (Guillozet et al., 2003). Neurofibrillary tangles are more numerous in medial temporal lobe regions associated with memory function in AD and also have a relation to performance on memory tests in nondemented individuals. These results suggest that NFTs may constitute a pathological substrate for memory loss not only in AD but also in normal aging and *cases of* mild cognitive impairment (Guillozet et al., 2003). NFTs are observed in the hippocampus and entorhinal cortex of most nondemented older subjects (>94%) suggesting that some NFTs pathological features in these regions may be relatively benign, occurring as a consequence of advanced age without causing discernable cognitive impairments (Haroutunian et al., 1999). In the neocortex, NFTs are absent in nonimpaired subjects, but increasing cognitive impairment is associated with the appearance of NFTs with densities that are in the sparse to moderate range (Haroutunian et al., 1999). Densities of neocortical neurofibrillary tangles are related to degree and duration of dementia (Berg et al., 1993). NFTs densities in the superior temporal cortex are most strongly correlated with dementia severity, followed by those in the inferior parietal and mid frontal cortex. No such correlations are apparent for the amygdala, hippocampus, or entorhinal cortex. Medial temporal lobe structures display high NFTs scores, even in cases of mild dementia (Bierer et al., 1995). No significant left- right hemispheric differences for NFTs or NPs densities in AD are found (Arnold et al., 1991).

10. Neuronal Loss

Early neuronal loss occurs in the entorhinal, parahippocampal and temporo-parietal cortex in AD, consistent with the spatial pattern of early perfusion deficits and metabolic changes (Thompson et al., 2001). These deficits mirror the time course of cognitive impairment, proceeding from the entorhinal, temporal and perisylvian association cortices into more anterior regions as the disease progresses. Severe reductions in gray matter (up to 30% loss) are observed across the lateral temporal surfaces in the AD patients (Thompson et al., 2001). These deficits are clearly found in the temporo-parietal cortices bilaterally (Thompson et al., 2001). In a neuropathologic study, Gomez-Isla et al. reported specific neuronal loss in the entorhinal cortex in persons with very mild AD (Gomez-Isla et al., 1996). Patterns of left greater than right gray matter loss are reported in *one study*, with severe gray matter loss observed bilaterally in the vicinity of Brodmann areas 9 and 46, regions of increased synaptic loss and ß-amyloid protein deposition (Clinton et al., 1994). Immunocytochemical studies have reported between 11 and 50% synaptic loss in the superior temporal and inferior parietal cortices, with a comparative sparing of occipital cortices (Thompson et al, 2001). In the amygdala, total numbers of neurons and glia are significantly reduced; medium and large neurons are preferentially affected (Scott et al., 1992).

11. White Matter

White matter changes in AD are characterized by partial loss of myelin, axons, and oligodendroglial cells; mild reactive astrocytic gliosis; sparsely distributed macrophages as well as stenosis resulting from hyaline fibrosis of arterioles and smaller vessels was observed in 60% of patients in one study (Brun and Englund, 1986). Histopathologically, the denudation of the ventricular ependyma and gliosis are more severe in AD, and there may be greater loss of myelinated axons in the deep white matter in AD than in normal aging (Scheltens et al., 1995). The MRI abnormalities correlate with the loss of myelinated axons in the deep white matter and with the denudation of the ventricular lining (Scheltens et al., 1995). A greater extent of periventricular hyperintensities in AD patients is observed than in controls (Fazekas et al., 1996). Periventricular hyperintensities may represent denudation of the ventricular lining, while deep white matter hyperintensities probably represent loss of myelinated axons. Subcortical hyperintensities do not appear to have marked effects on individual clinical symptoms (Sultzer et al, 2002).

12. MRI Findings in AD

Cortical atrophy is widespread apart from in the primary motor and sensory cortices and cerebellum, reflecting the clinical phenomenology of AD (Fox et al., 2001). Increased global atrophy occurs with advancing disease (Scahill et al., 2002). Progressive atrophy is apparent in presymptomatic individuals, with posterior cingulate and neocortical temporoparietal cortical losses, and medial temporal-lobe atrophy (Fox et al., 2001). Significantly increased rates of hippocampal atrophy are seen in presymptomatic and mildly affected patients. There is a shift in the distribution of temporal lobe atrophy with advancing disease; the inferolateral regions of the temporal lobes show the most significantly increased rates of atrophy by the time the patients are mildly or moderately affected (Scahill et al., 2002). Significantly increased rates of medial parietal lobe atrophy are seen at all stages, with frontal lobe involvement occurring later in the disease (Scahill et al., 2002).

Patients with AD show significant reduction of gray matter volumes in the medial temporal structure, hippocampal formation, entorhinal cortex, and parahippocampal gyrus (Ohnishi et al., 2001). In patients with histopathologically-confirmed Alzheimer's disease the size of the medial temporal lobe is almost half that in age-matched controls and the rate of atrophy shown by yearly scans (15% per year) is 10-fold greater (Smith and Jobst, 1996). The degree of medial temporal lobe atrophy is related to the density of NFTs in the hippocampus (Smith and Jobst, 1996).

Hippocampal atrophy occurs early in Alzheimer's disease (Laakso et al, 1998); hippocampal and entorhinal cortex volumes reflect disease severity in AD (Jack et al., 1997; Du et al., 2001) and measures of both the entorhinal cortex and the hippocampus are correlated with tests of memory (Killiany et al, 2002). Volumetric measures of the hippocampus may be useful in identifying nondemented individuals at risk for AD, as the volume of the entorhinal cortex can differentiate individuals with memory problems who are going to develop AD from those who will not with considerable accuracy (84%; Killiany et al., 2002). Overall, total hippocampal volume measurements are best at discriminating patients with AD from normal control subjects (Jack et al., 1997). In one study, an MRI measure of the entorhinal cortex showed an average 37% decrease in those destined to develop AD in comparison with control subjects (Killiany et al., 2000). Magnetic resonance imaging measurements of hippocampal atrophy correlate with clinical measurements of disease severity, pathological disease stage, neuropsychological performance, and disease progression (Jack et al., 2000; Petersen et al., 2000). This makes volumetric MRI potentially useful in the early diagnosis of AD (Bobinski et al., 1999; Gosche et al., 2002), but whether there is added diagnostic value to volumetric assessment given the high correlation with clinical function, is not well established. Hippocampal volumes are strongly correlated with both mean NFT and senile plaque counts in the CA-1 region of the hippocampus and the subiculum, although volumes were best correlated with the severity of NFTs degeneration (Gosche et al., 2001).

Patients with AD also have atrophy in the parietal, precuneus, and posterior cingulate cortices compared to normal controls (Boxer et al., 2003). Cinguloparietal atrophy is a feature of presymptomatic patients with familial AD (Scahill et al., 2002) and cinguloparietal hypometabolism found on positron emission tomography with [18]fluorodeoxyglucose may be the earliest metabolic abnormality in AD (Minoshima et al., 1997). The superior central and post-central gyri and occipital poles show very little reduction in gray matter but the adjacent posterior temporal cortex and the parietal operculum are severely affected (Thompson et al., 2001). Significant amygdala atrophy can be detected in patients with early AD (Cuenod et al., 1993). It is apparent, therefore, that several of the same regions that appear critically involved in MDD are also involved early in AD. Whether the pathological processes that lead to neural atrophy in MDD and AD share common features is not well-established, but the studies to date do not suggest the presence of the characteristic pathological processes of AD that are reviewed here even in patients with long histories of severe MDD.

11. Conclusions

Neural atrophy is reliable and profound in AD and is observed to a lesser extent in patients with MDD, probably those who have had a long or recurrent form of illness. The illnesses share common regions, with the medial-temporal region implicated as a region showing early changes in AD and also showing volume reductions in MDD. The pathognomonic changes of AD, however, have not been reported in an early form in studies of patients with MDD, although to date these studies are limited.

Clinically, however, there is overlap with symptoms of AD and presence of MDD is a risk factor for development of AD. Depression frequently occurs before the onset of AD and is associated with the development of AD, even in patients where first depressive symptoms occurred more than 25 years before the onset of AD (Green et al., 2003). Given the available literature on both illnesses, the most parsimonious explanation for this association currently is probably that patients with MDD have vulnerable hippocampi, with discernable volumetric reductions, and probable functional impairment, based on neuropsychological studies examining hippocampal-dependent memory performance in MDD. It may be that as a consequence of the hippocampal compromise, AD – with its early impact on the hippocampal formation and related structures - is observed earlier or appears to have a more rapid course when the patholophysiology of this separate disease is superimposed on an individual with a pre-existing history of MDD. That is, when AD begins, the individual with previous depressive episodes may have less hippocampal reserve and may express clinical symptoms of AD earlier as an additive effect of early AD and long-standing atrophy associated with depression. This hypothesis is speculative, but currently there is little in our understanding of the processes that underlie the atrophy associated with MDD or AD that would more specifically link the two illnesses from a neuropathological perspective. Future studies may, however, uncover a common thread that links MDD and AD more substantively; such a study could contribute much to our understanding of both these common and severely disabling illnesses.

References

Abercrombie HC, Schaefer SM, Larson CL, Oakes TR, Lindgren KA, Holden JE, Perlman SB, Turski PA, Krahn DD, Benca RM, Davidson RJ. Metabolic rate in the right amygdala predicts negative affect in depressed patients. *Neuroreport* 9(14): 3301-3307, 1998.

Aggleton JP. The contribution of the amygdala to normal and abnormal emotional states. *Trends Neurosci* 16(8): 328-333, 1993.

Arango V, Underwood MD, Gubbi AV, Mann JJ. Localized alterations in pre- and postsynaptic serotonin binding sites in the ventrolateral prefrontal cortex of suicide victims. *Brain Res* 688(1-2): 121-133, 1995.

Arnold SE, Hyman BT, Flory J, Damasio AR, Van Hoesen GW. The topographical and neuroanatomical distribution of neurofibrillary tangles and neuritic plaques in the cerebral cortex of patients with Alzheimer's disease. *Cereb Cortex* 1(1): 103-116, 1991.

Austin MC, Whitehead RE, Edgar CL, Janosky JE, Lewis DA. Localized decrease in serotonin transporter-immunoreactive axons in the prefrontal cortex of depressed subjects committing suicide. *Neuroscience* 114 (3): 807-815, 2002.

Awad IA, Spetzler RF, Hodak JA, Awad CA, Carey R. Incidental subcortical lesions identified on magnetic resonance imaging in the elderly: correlation with age and cerebrovascular risk factors. *Stroke* 17(6): 1084-1089, 1986.

Awata S, Ito H, Konno M, Ono S, Kawashima R, Fukuda H, Sato M. Regional cerebral blood flow abnormalities in late-life depression: relation to refractoriness and chronification. *Psychiatry Clin Neurosci* 52(1): 97–105, 1998.

Ballmaier M, Toga AW, Blanton RE, Sowell ER, Lavretsky H, Peterson J, Pham D, Kumar A. Anterior cingulate, gyrus rectus, and orbitofrontal abnormalities in elderly depressed patients: an MRI-based parcellation of the prefrontal cortex. *Am J Psychiatry* 161(1): 99-108, 2004.

Baumann B, Danos P, Krell D, Diekmann S, Leschinger A, Stauch R, Wurthmann C, Bernstein HG, Bogerts B. Reduced volume of limbic system–affiliated basal ganglia in mood disorders: preliminary data from a postmortem study. *J Neuropsychiatry Clin Neurosci* 11(1): 71 – 78, 1999.

Baxter LR Jr, Schwartz JM, Phelps ME, Mazziotta JC, Guze BH, Selin CE, Gerner RH, Sumida RM. Reduction of prefrontal cortex glucose metabolism common to three types of depression. *Arch Gen Psychiatry* 46(3): 243-250, 1989.

Bench CJ, Frackowiak RS, Dolan RJ. Changes in regional cerebral blood flow on recovery from depression. *Psychol Med* 25(2): 247-261, 1995.

Bench CJ, Friston KJ, Brown RG, Scott LC, Frackowiak RS, Dolan RJ. The anatomy of melancholia: focal abnormalities of cerebral blood flow in major depression. *Psychol Med* 22(3): 607-615, 1992.

Berg L, McKeel DW Jr, Miller JP, Baty J, Morris JC. Neuropathologic indexes of Alzheimer's disease in demented and nondemented people aged 80 years and older. *Arch Neurol.* 50(4): 349-358, 1993.

Bierer LM, Hof PR, Purohit DP, Carlin L, Schmeidler J, Davis KL, Perl DP. Neocortical neurofibrillary tangles correlate with dementia severity in Alzheimer's disease. *Arch Neurol* 52(1): 81-88, 1995.

Biver F, Goldman S, Delvenne V, Luxen A, De Maertelaer V, Hubain P, Medlewicz J, Lotstra F. Frontal and parietal metabolic disturbances in unipolar depression. *Biol Psychiatry* 36(6): 381-388, 1994.

Bobinski M, de Leon MJ, Convit A, De Santi S, Wegiel J, Tarshish CY, Saint Louis LA, Wisniewski HM. MRI of entorhinal cortex in mild Alzheimer's disease. *Lancet* 353 (9146): 38-40, 1999.

Botteron KN, Raichle ME, Drevets WC, Heath AC, Todd RD. Volumetric reduction in left subgenual prefrontal cortex in early onset depression. *Biol Psychiatry* 51(4): 342–344, 2002.

Bowen DM, Najlerahim A, Procter AW, Francis PT, Murphy E. Circumscribed changes of the cerebral cortex in neuropsychiatric disorders of later life. *Proc Natl Acad Sci USA* 86(23): 9504–9508, 1989.

Bowen, DM, Benton JS, Spillane JA, Smith CC, Allen SJ. Choline acetyltransferase activity and histopathology of the frontal neocortex from biopsies of demented patients. *J Neuro. Sci.* 57(2-3): 191-202, 1982.

Bowley MP, Drevets WC, Öngür D, Price JL. Low glial numbers in the amygdala in major depressive disorder. *Biol Psychiatry* 52(5): 404-412, 2002.

Boxer AL, Rankin KP, Miller BL, Schuff N, Weiner M, Gorno-Tempini ML, Rosen HJ. Cinguloparietal atrophy distinguishes Alzheimer disease from semantic dementia. *Arch Neurol.* 60(7): 949-956, 2003.

Braak E, Griffing K, Arai K, Bohl J, Bratzke H, Braak, H. Neuropathology of Alzheimer's disease: what is new since A. Alzheimer? *Eur Arch Psychiatry Clin Neurosci* 249(3): 14-22, 1999.

Braak H, Braak E, Bohl J. Staging of Alzheimer-related cortical destruction. *Eur Neurol* 33(6): 403–408, 1993.

Braak H, Braak E. Neuropathological staging of Alzheimer-related changes. *Acta Neuropathol* 82(4): 239-259, 1991.

Braak H, Braak E. Neuropathological stages of Alzheimer's disease. In: de Leon MJ, editor. *An atlas of Alzheimer's disease.* New York, NY: Parthenon, 1999b; pp. 57-74.

Bremner JD, Narayan M, Anderson ER, Staib LH, Miller HL, Charney DS. Hippocampal volume reduction in major depression. *Am J Psychiatry* 157(1): 115-118, 2000.

Bremner JD, Randall P, Scott TM, Bronen RA, Seibyl JP, Southwick SM, Delaney RC, McCarthy G, Charney DS, Innis RB. MRI-based measurement of hippocampal volume in patients with combat-related posttraumatic stress disorder. *Am J Psychiatry* 152(7): 973–981, 1995.

Bremner JD, Vythilingam M, Ng CK, Vermetten E, Nazeer A, Oren AD, Berman RM, Charney DS. Regional brain metabolic correlates of {alpha}-methylparatyrosine-induced depressive symptoms: Implications for the neural circuitry of depression. *JAMA* 289 (23): 3125–3134, 2003.

Bremner JD. Does stress damage the brain? *Biol Psychiatry* 45: 797–805, 1999.

Brun A, Englund E. A white matter disorder in dementia of the Alzheimer type: a pathoanatomical study. *Ann Neurol* 19(3): 253-262, 1986.

Campbell S, Marriott M, Nahmias C, MacQueen GM. Hippocampal volume reduction in patients with major depressive disorder: A meta-analysis. *American Journal of Psychiatry,* 2004.

Carroll BJ, Curtis GC, Davies BM, Mendels J, Sugarman AA. Urinary free cortisol excretion in depression. *Psychol Med* 6(1): 43–50, 1976.

Clinton J, Blackman SE, Royston MC, Roberts GW. Differential synaptic loss in the cortex in Alzheimer's disease: a study using archival material. *Neuroreport* 5(4): 497-500, 1994.

Coffey CE, Figiel GS, Djang WT, Saunders WB, Weiner RD. White matter hyperintensity on magnetic resonance imaging: clinical and neuroanatomic correlates in the depressed elderly. J *Neuropsychiatry Clin Neurosci* 1(2): 135-144, 1989.

Cohen RM, Gross M, Nordahl TE, Semple WE, Oren DA, Rosenthal N. Preliminary data on metabolic brain patterns of patients with winter seasonal affective disorder. *Arch Gen Psychiatry* 49(7): 545-552, 1992.

Cotter D, Mackay D, Landau S, Kerwin R, Everall I. Reduced glial cell density and neuronal size in the anterior cingulate cortex in major depressive disorder. *Arch Gen Psychiatry* 58(6): 545-553, 2001.

Cuenod CA, Denys A, Michot JL, Jehenson P, Forette F, Kaplan D, Syrota A, Boller F. Amygdala atrophy in Alzheimer's disease. An in vivo magnetic resonance imaging study. *Arch Neurol* 50(9): 941–945, 1993.

Cummings JL, Cole G. Alzheimer Disease. *JAMA* 287(18): 2335-2338, 2002.

Cummings JL, Vinters HV, Cole GM, Khachaturian ZS. Alzheimer's disease: etiologies, pathophysiology, cognitive reserve, and treatment opportunities. *Neurology* 51(1): S2-S17, 1998.

de Asis JM, Stern E, Alexopoulos GS, Pan H, Van Gorp W, Blumberg H, Kalayam B, Eidelberg D, Kiosses D, Silbersweig DA. Hippocampal and anterior cingulate activation deficits in patients with geriatric depression. *Am J Psychiatry* 158(8): 1321–1323, 2001.

Drevets WC, Price JL, Simpson JR Jr, Todd RD, Reich T, Vannier M, Raichle ME. Subgenual prefrontal cortex abnormalities in mood disorders. *Nature* 386(6627): 824-827, 1997.

Drevets WC, Videen TO, Price JL, Preskorn SH, Carmichael ST, Raichle M.E. A functional anatomical study of unipolar depression. J *Neurosci* 12(9): 3628-3641, 1992.

Drevets WC. Neuroimaging studies of mood disorders. Biol Psychiatry 48(8): 813:829, 2000.

Drevets WC. Prefrontal-amygdalar metabolism in major depression. *Ann N Y Acad Sci* 877: 614-637, 1999.

Drevets, WC, Price JL, Bardgett ME, Reich T, Todd RD, Raichle ME. Glucose metabolism in the amygdala in depression: relationship to diagnostic subtype and plasma cortisol levels. *Pharmacol Biochem Behav* 71(3): 431-447, 2002.

Du AT, Schuff N, Amend D, Laakso MP, Hsu YY, Jagust WJ, Yaffe K, Kramer JH, Reed B, Norman D, Chui HC, Weiner MW. Magnetic resonance imaging of the entorhinal cortex and hippocampus in mild cognitive impairment and Alzheimer's disease. J *Neurol Neurosurg Psychiatry* 71(4): 441-447, 2001.

Duman RS, Malberg J, Thome J. Neural plasticity to stress and antidepressant treatment. *Biol Psychiatry* 46(9): 1181-1191, 1999.

Fazekas F, Kapeller P, Schmidt R, Offenbacher H, Payer F, Fazekas G. The relation of cerebral magnetic resonance signal hyperintensities to Alzheimer's disease. *J Neurol Sci* 142(1-2): 121- 125, 1996.

Fox NC, Crum WR, Scahill RI, Stevens JM, Janssen JC, Rossor MN. Imaging of onset and progression of Alzheimer's disease with voxel-compression mapping of serial magnetic resonance images. *Lancet* 358(9277): 201-205, 2001.

Frodl T, Meisenzahl E, Zetzsche T, Bottlender R, Born C, Groll C, Jager M, Leinsinger G, Hahn K, Moller HJ. Enlargement of the amygdala in patients with a first episode of major depression. *Biol Psychiatry* 51(9): 708-714, 2002.

Gilmor ML, Erickson JD, Varoqui H, Hersh LB, Bennett DA, Cochran EJ, Mufson EJ, Levey AI. Preservation of the nucleus basalis neurons containing choline acetyltransferase and the vesicular acetylcholine transporter in the elderly with mild cognitive impairment and early Alzheimer disease. *J Comp Neurol* 411(4): 693-704, 1999.

Gomez-Isla T, Price JL, McKeel DW Jr, Morris JC, Growdon JH, Hyman BT. Profound loss of layer II entorhinal cortex neurons occurs in very mild Alzheimer's disease. *J Neurosci* 16(14): 4491–4500, 1996.

Gosche KM, Mortimer JA, Smith CD, Markesbery WR, Snowdown DA. An automated technique for measuring hippocampal volumes for MR imaging studies. *Am J Neuroradiol* 22(9): 1686-1689, 2001.

Gosche KM, Mortimer JA, Smith CD, Markesbery WR, Snowdown DA. Hippocampal volume as an index of Alzheimer neuropathology: findings from the nun study. *Neurology* 58(10): 1476-1482, 2002.

Green RC, Cupples LA, Kurz A, Auerbach S, Go R, Sadovnick D, Duara R, Kukull WA, Chui H, Edeki T, Griffith PA, Friedland RP, Bachman D, Farrer L. Depression as a risk factor for Alzheimer disease: the MIRAGE Study. *Arch Neurol* 60(5): 753-759, 2003.

Guillozet AL, Weintraub S, Mash DC, Mesulam MM. Neurofibrillary tangles, amyloid, and memory in aging and mild cognitive impairment. *Arch Neurol* 60(5): 729-736, 2003.

Halgren E, Walter RD, Cherlow DG, Crandall PH. Mental phenomena evoked by electrical stimulation of the human hippocampal formation and amygdala. *Brain* 101(1): 83-117, 1978.

Haroutunian V, Perl DP, Purohit DP, Marin D, Khan K, Lantz M, Davis KL, Mohs RC. Regional distribution of neuritic plaques in the nondemented elderly and subjects with very mild Alzheimer disease. *Arch Neurol* 55(9): 1185-1191, 1998.

Haroutunian V, Purohit DP, Perl DP, Marin D, Khan K, Lantz M, Davis KL, Mohs RC. Neurofibrillary Tangles in Nondemented Elderly Subjects and Mild Alzheimer Disease. *Arch Neurol* 56(6): 713-718, 1999.

Harrison PJ. The neuropathology of primary mood disorder. *Brain* 125(7): 1428-1449, 2002.

Hirayasu Y, Shenton ME, Salisbury DF, Kwon JS, Wible CG, Fischer IA, Yurgelun-Todd D, Zarate C, Kikinis R, Jolesz FA, McCarley RW. Subgenual cingulate cortex volume in first-episode psychosis. *Am J Psychiatry* 156(7): 1091-1093, 1999.

Husain MM, McDonald WM, Doraiswamy PM, Figiel GS, Na C, Escalona PR, Boyko OB, Nermeroff CB, Krishnan KR. A magnetic resonance imaging study of putamen nuclei in major depression. *Psychiatry Res* 40 (2): 95-99, 1991.

Jack CR Jr, Petersen RC, Xu Y, O'Brien PC, Smith GE, Ivnik RJ, Boeve BF, Tangalos EG, Kokmen E. Rates of hippocampal atrophy correlate with change in clinical status in aging and AD. *Neurology* 55(4): 484-489, 2000.

Jack CR Jr, Petersen RC, Xu YC, Waring SC, O'Brien PC, Tangalos EG, Smith GE, Ivnik RJ, Kokmen E. Medial temporal atrophy on MRI in normal aging and very mild Alzheimer's disease. *Neurology* 49(3): 786-794, 1997.

Kessler R, McGonagle K, Zhao S, Nelson C, Hughes M, Eshleman S, Wittchen H, Kendler K. Lifetime and 12-month prevalence of DSM-III-R psychiatric disorders in the United States. Results from the National Comorbidity Survey. *Arch Gen Psychiatry* 51(1): 8-19, 1994.

Killiany RJ, Hyman BT, Gomez-Isla T, Moss MB, Kikinis R, Jolesz F, Tanzi R, Jones K, Albert MS. MRI measures of entorhinal cortex vs hippocampus in preclinical AD. *Neurology* 58(8): 1188-1196, 2002.

Killiany, RJ, Gomez-Isla T, Moss M, Kikinis R, Sandor T, Jolesz F, Tanzi R, Jones K, Hyman BT, Albert MS. Use of structural magnetic resonance imaging to predict who will get Alzheimer's disease. *Ann Neurol* 47(4): 430–439, 2000.

Krishnan KR, McDonald WM, Escalona PR, Doraiswamy PM, Na C, Husain MM, Figiel GS, Boyko OB, Ellinwood EH, Nemeroff CB. Magnetic resonance imaging of the caudate nuclei in depression. Preliminary observations. *Arch Gen Psychiatry* 49 (7): 553-557, 1992.

Krishnan KR, McDonald WM. Arteriosclerotic depression. *Med Hypotheses* 44(2): 111-115, 1995.

Krishnan KR. Organic bases of depression in the elderly. *Annu Rev Med* 42: 261-266, 1991.

Kumar A, Jin Z, Bilker W, Udupa J, Gottlieb G. Late-onset minor and major depression: early evidence for common neuroanatomical substrates detected by using MRI. *Proc Natl Acad Sci U S A* 95(13): 7654-7658, 1998.

Kumar A, Miller D, Ewbank D, Yousem D, Newberg A, Samuels S, Cowell P, Gottlieb G. Quantitative anatomic measures and comorbid medical illness in late- life major depression. *Am J Geriatr Psychiatry* 5(1): 15-25, 1997.

Kumar A, Thomas A, Lavretsky H, Yue K, Huda A, Curran J, Venkatraman T, Estanol L, Mintz J, Mega M, Toga A. Frontal white matter biochemical abnormalities in late-life major depression detected with proton magnetic resonance spectroscopy. *Am J Psychiatry* 159(4): 630–636, 2002.

Laakso MP, Soininen H, Partanen K, Lehtovitra M, Hallikainen M, Hanninen T, Helkala EL, Vainio P, Riekkinen PJ Sr. MRI of the Hippocampus in Alzheimer's Disease: Sensitivity, Specificity, and Analysis of the Incorrectly Classified Subjects. *Neurobiol Aging* 19 (1): 23-31, 1998.

Lacerda AL, Nicolettia MA, Brambilla P, Sassi RB, Mallinger AG, Frank E, Kupfer DJ, Keshavana MS, Soares JC. Anatomical MRI study of basal ganglia in major depressive disorder. *Psychiatry Res* 124 (3): 129-140, 2003.

Lenze EJ, Sheline YI. Absence of striatal volume differences between depressed subjects with no comorbid medical illness and matched comparison subjects. *Am J Psychiatry* 156(12): 1989-1991, 1999

Lesser IM, Mena I, Boone KB, Miller BL, Mehringer CM, Wohl M. Reduction of cerebral blood flow in older depressed patients. *Arch Gen Psychiatry* 51(9): 677–686, 1994.

Lesser IM, Miller BL, Boone KB, Hill-Gutierrez E, Mehringer CM, Wong K, Mena I. Brain injury and cognitive function in late-onset psychotic depression. *J Neuropsychiatry Clin Neurosci.* 3(1): 33-40, 1991.

Lupien SJ, de Leon M, de Santi S, Convit A, Tarshish C, Nair NP, Thakur M, McEwen BS, Hauger RL, Meaney MJ. Cortisol levels during human aging predict hippocampal atrophy and memory deficits. *Nat Neurosci* 1(1): 69-73, 1998.

Lyketsos CG, Steinberg M, Tschantz JT, Norton MC, Steffens DC, Breitner JCS. Mental and behavioral disturbances in dementia: Findings from the Cache County Study on Memory in Aging. *Am J Psychiatry* 157 (5): 708-714, 2000.

MacQueen GM, Campbell S, McEwen BS, MacDonald K, Amano S, Joffe RT, Nahmias C, Young LT. Course of illness, hippocampal function and volume in major depression. *Proc Natl Acad Sci U S A* 100(3): 1387-1392, 2003.

Mann JJ, Huang YY, Underwood MD, Kassir SA, Oppenheim S, Kelly TM, Dwork AJ, Arango V. A serotonin transporter gene promoter polymorphism (5-HTTLPR) and prefrontal cortical binding in major depression and suicide. *Arch Gen Psychiatry* 57(8): 729-738, 2000.

McEwen BS. Plasticity of the hippocampus: adaptation to chronic stress and allostatic load. *Ann N Y Acad Sci* 933: 265-277, 2001.

Mervaala E, Fohr J, Kononen M, Valkonen-Korhonen M, Vainio P, Partanen K, Partanen J, Tiihonen J, Viinamki H, Karjalainen AK, Lehtonen J. Quantitative MRI of the hippocampus and amygdala in severe depression. *Psychol Med* 30(1): 117-125, 2000.

Minoshima S, Giordani B, Berent S, Frey KA, Foster NL, Kuhl DE. Metabolic reduction in the posterior cingulate cortex in very early Alzheimer's disease. *Ann Neurol* 42(1): 85-94, 1997.

O'Brien J, Perry R, Barber R, Gholkar A, Thomas A. The association between white matter lesions on magnetic resonance imaging and noncognitive symptoms. *Ann N Y Acad Sci* 903: 482-489, 2000.

Ohnishi T, Matsuda H, Tabira T, Asada T, Uno M. Changes in brain morphology in Alzheimer disease and normal aging: is Alzheimer disease an exaggerated aging process? *Am J Neuroradiol* 22(9): 1680-1685, 2001.

Öngür D, Drevets WD, Price JL. Glial reduction in the subgenual prefrontal cortex in mood disorders. *Proc Natl Acad Sci U S A* 95 (22): 13290-13295, 1998.

Parashos IA, Tupler LA, Blitchington T, Krishnan KR. Magnetic-resonance morphometry in patients with major depression. *Psychiatry Res* 84 (1): 7-15, 1998.

Petersen RC, Jack CR Jr, Xu YC, Waring SC, O'Brian PC, Smith GE, Ivnik RJ, Tangalos EG, Boeve BF, Kokmen E. Memory and MRI-based hippocampal volumes in aging and Alzheimer's disease. *Neurology* 54(3): 581-587, 2000.

Pillay SS, Renshaw PF, Bonello CM, Lafer BC, Fava M, Yurgelun-Todd D. A quantitative magnetic resonance imaging study of caudate and lenticular nucleus gray matter volume in primary unipolar major depression: relationship to treatment response and clinical severity. *Psychiatry Res* 84(2-3): 61-74, 1998.

Posener JA, Wang L, Price JL, Gado MH, Province MA, Miller MI, Babb CM, Csernansky JG. High-dimentional mapping of the hippocampus in depression. *Am J Psychiatry* 160(1): 83-89, 2003.

Rajkowska G, Miguel-Hidalgo JJ, Wei J, Dilley G, Pittman SD, Meltzer HY, Overholser JC, Roth BL, Stockmeier CA. Morphometric evidence for neuronal and glial prefrontal cell pathology in major depression. *Biol Psychiatry* 45(9): 1085-1098, 1999.

Roger MA, Bradshaw JL, Pantelis C, Phillips JG. Frontostriatal deficits in unipolar major depression. *Brain Res Bull* 47(4): 297-310, 1998.

Rosenblatt A, Leroi I. Neuropsychiatry of Huntington's disease and other basal ganglia disorders. *Psychosomatics* 41(1): 24-30, 2000.

Sapolsky RM. Depression, antidepressants, and the shrinking hippocampus. *Proc Natl Acad Sci U S A* 98 (22): 12320-12322, 2001.

Sapolsky RM. Glucocorticoids and hippocampal atrophy in neuropsychiatric disorders. *Arch Gen Psychiatry* 57(10): 925-935, 2000.

Sapolsky RM. Glucocorticoids, stress, and their adverse neurological effects: relevance to aging. *Exp Gerontol.* 34(6): 721-732, 1999.

Scahill RI, Schott JM, Stevens JM, Rossor MN, Fox NC. Mapping the evolution of regional atrophy in Alzheimer's disease: Unbiased analysis of fluid-registered serial MRI. *Proc Natl Acad Sci U S A* 99 (7): 4703-4707, 2002.

Scheltens P, Barkhof F, Leys D, Wolters EC, Ravid R, Kamphorst W. Histopathologic correlates of white matter changes on MRI in Alzheimer's disease and normal aging. *Neurology* 45 (5): 883-888, 1995.

Schirmer M, Fels S. Severe deep white matter lesions and outcome in major depressive disorder: might vasculitis be cause of these lesions in elderly depressive patients? *BMJ* 318(7185): 737-738, 1999.

Scott SA, Dekosky ST, Sparks DL, Knox CA, Scheff SW. Amygdala cell loss and atrophy in Alzheimer's disease. *Ann Neurol* 32(4): 555-563, 1992.

Selkoe DJ. Translating cell biology into therapeutic advances in Alzheimer's disease. *Nature* 399(6738): A23-31, 1999.

Shah PJ, Ebmeier KP, Glabus MF, Goodwin GM. Cortical grey matter reductions associated with treatment-resistant chronic unipolar depression. Controlled magnetic resonance imaging study. *Br J Psychiatry* 172: 527-532, 1998.

Sheline YI, Gado MH, Kraemer HC. Untreated depression and hippocampal volume loss. *Am. J. Psychiatry* 160(8): 1516 – 1518, 2003.

Sheline YI, Gado MH, Price JL. Amygdala core nuclei volumes are decreased in recurrent major depression. *Neuroreport* 9(9): 2023-2028, 1998.

Sheline YI, Sanghavi M, Mintun MA, Gado MH. Depression duration but not age predicts hippocampal volume loss in medically healthy women with recurrent major depression. *J Neurosci* 19 (12): 5034-5043, 1999.

Sheline YI, Wang PW, Gado MH, Csernanskey JG, Vannier MW. Hippocampal atrophy in recurrent major depression. *Proc Natl Acad Sci USA* 93(9): 3908-3913, 1996.

Sheline YI. Neuroimaging studies of mood disorder effects on the brain. *Biol Psychiatry* 54(3): 338-352, 2003.

Smith AD, Jobst KA. Use of structural imaging to study the progression of Alzheimer's disease. *Br Med Bull* 52 (3): 575-586, 1996.

Soares J, Mann J. The anatomy of mood disorders- review of structural neuroimaging studies. *Biol psychiatry* 41(1): 86-106, 1997.

Sultzer DL, Chen ST, Brown CV, Mahler ME, Cummings JL, Hinkin CH, Mandelkern MA. Subcortical hyperintensities in alzheimer's disease; associated clinical and metabolic findings. *J Neuropsychiatry Clin Neurosci* 14(3): 262-269, 2002.

Thomas RM, Peterson DA. A neurogenic theory of depression gains momentum. *Mol Interv* 3(8): 441-444, 2003.

Thompson PM, Megal MS, Woods RP, Zoumalan CI, Lindshield CJ, Blanton RE, Moussail J, Holmes CJ, Cummings JL, Toga AW. Cortical change in Alzheimer's disease detected with a disease-specific population-based brain atlas. *Cereb Cortex* 11 (1): 1-16, 2001.

Wenk GL. Neuropathlogic changes in Alzheimer's disease. *J Clin Psychiat* 64(9): 7-10, 2003.

In: Cognition and Mood Interactions
Editor: Miao-Kun Sun, pp. 137-148

ISBN 1-59454-229-5
2005 © Nova Science Publishers, Inc.

Chapter VIII

Possible Link between Cholesterol and Dementia, Depression

*Katsuhiko Yanagisawa**
National Institute for Longevity Sciences

The brain is an organ rich in cholesterol; however, it remains to be elucidated how cholesterol metabolism in the brain is regulated and how cholesterol is involved in the neuronal functions. Recently, evidence has been accumulating to indicate that alteration in the plasma cholesterol level is associated with the development of neurological and neuropsychological disorders, including Alzheimer's disease and depression.

1. Cholesterol in the Brain

1.1. General Aspects

Cholesterol is one of the major lipids in cellular membranes and is essential for many cellular functions. The brain is highly rich in cholesterol. It is of note that the brain accounts for only 2% of the whole body mass but contains almost one-quarter of the unesterified cholesterol in the whole body (Dietschy and Turley, 2001). Thus, it is likely that cholesterol plays a critical role in neuronal functions. However, little is known about cholesterol metabolism in the brain. This is partly due to the difficulty of performing lipid-chemical studies using cultured neurons. It is considered that cholesterol turnover is restricted to a very low rate only inside the brain. Only 0.02% of the cholesterol pool in the brain undergoes a turnover each day (Dietschy and Turley, 2001). This is less than 1% of the cholesterol turnover in the whole body (Dietschy and Turley, 2001). Although a recent study indicated the possibility of cholesterol transport across the blood-brain barrier (Refolo *et al.*, 2000), most cholesterol in the brain is likely produced by *in situ* synthesis. Interestingly, the rate of *in situ* cholesterol synthesis in many organs, including the nervous system, depends on age (Cenedella and Shi, 1994; Stahlberg *et al.*, 1991; Goodrum, 1990; Popplewell and Azhar, 1987). The rate of cholesterol synthesis decreases with age. Moreover, cholesterol is the only major lipid in the brain that cannot be synthesized at the end of neurites (Vance *et al.*, 1994), suggesting that cholesterol level at the ends of neurites depends on two inputs, such as axonal flow from the soma and uptake from the extracellular space through apolipoprotein receptors. Thus, it seems likely that the functions of neurons in the elderly depend on exogenous cholesterol levels to a higher degree than those in young individuals. In regard to the development of Alzheimer's disease (AD), aging is the strongest risk factor. Thus, it may be possible to assume that the pathological significance of aging for AD development is closely associated with the aging associated alteration of the synthesis and transport of cholesterol.

The shape of neuron is very unique and it has a large plasma membrane compared with any other cell type. Importantly, cholesterol accounts for more than 40 mol% of the total membrane lipids in synaptic plasma membranes (Schroeder *et al.*, 1991; Wood *et al.*, 1989). Thus, it is likely that cholesterol plays critical roles in maintaining the structure and functions of neurons. Wood and his colleagues and other groups previously performed quantitative analyses of synaptic plasma membranes and reported that cholesterol is not evenly distributed throughout neuronal membranes but is concentrated in different pools, including cholesterol lateral domains and transbilayer cholesterol domains Wood et al., 1999). Interestingly, they found that there seem to be two distinct pools of lateral domains: the cholesterol in one pool is not stable but rather easily exchangeable following biochemical treatment. Although the physiological significance of these two pools of lateral domains remains to be elucidated, a previous study revealed that the acetylcholine receptor is closely associated with the poorly exchangeable pool (Leibel *et al.*, 1987). Alternatively, in regard to transbilayer cholesterol domains, Igbavboa et al. previously reported that the exofacial leaflet of lipid bilayers of synaptic plasma membranes appears to contain substantially much less cholesterol than does the cytofacial leaflet (13 vs. 87%, respectively). The point which should be emphasized here is that the asymmetric distribution of cholesterol throughout the lipid bilayer of synaptic plasma membranes can be altered by biological factors, including risk factors for AD development; for example, aging (Igbavboa et al. 1996) and the expression of apolipoprotein E allele ε4 (Hayashi et al. 2002).

1.2. A novel Probe for Cholesterol Metabolism in the Brain

It remains to be elucidated how cholesterol homeostasis is maintained inside the brain despite continuous *de novo* cholesterol synthesis. Recently, novel information has been provided by a study on a cholesterol metabolite in serum. Bjorkhem et al. found that an endogenously oxidized metabolite of cholesterol, 24S-hydroxycholesterol (24S-OH- Chol) is almost exclusively synthesized in the brain (Bjorkhem et al., 1998). Indeed, the 24S-OH-Chol concentration in the brain is 30-1500-fold higher than those in any other organ. Thus, it is likely that 24S-OH-Chol has the ability to pass through the blood brain barrier and is involved in the cholesterol homeostasis in the brain. Moreover, 24SOH- Chol level in the plasma can be a useful peripheral marker to evaluate the levels of *de novo* cholesterol synthesis in the brain. Interestingly, plasma 24-OH-Chol level is age-dependent. The level is high before age 20 and then decreases with age. As discussed below, the determination of plasma 24S-OH-Chol levels in the individuals with AD and depression may provide information on the possibility of alterations in cholesterol metabolism in these psychoneurological disorders.

2. Cholesterol and Alzheimer's Disease

It is obvious that hypercholesterolemia is closely associated with the development of vascular dementia through the acceleration of atheroma formation; however, evidence is accumulating to indicate that alterations in cholesterol metabolism can be a risk factor for AD development. Previous studies revealed that a number of genetic polymorphisms are associated with the AD development. Importantly, they include various genes encoding proteins that are directly involved in the regulation of lipid metabolism.

2.1. Epidemiology

Alternatively, previous studies focused on serum cholesterol levels in association with AD development. Notkola et al. suggested on the basis of a longitudinal study that an increase in the serum total cholesterol (TC) level in midlife can be a risk factor for the development of late-life AD (Notkola et al., 1998). This relationship between AD development and serum cholesterol level was also suggested by the study of Kivipelto et al., who concluded that there was a correlation between midlife hypercholesterolemia and the prevalence of late-life mild cognitive impairment (MCI), a putative preclinical stage of AD (Kivipelto et al., 2001). These results suggest that hypercholesterolemia is a possible risk factor for AD development. This possibility has been further supported by recent studies of two groups. Jick et al. and Wolozin et al. have independently performed retrospective epidemiological studies and found that statin, an inhibitor of 3-hydroxy-3-methylglutaryl coenzyme A reductase, a key enzyme in cholesterol synthesis, may have an ability to suppress the development of AD (Jick et al., 2000; Wolozin et al., 2000).

2.2. Lipid analysis of human brain affected with AD. Direct lipid analysis of a brain affected with AD would be very informative. However, the results of previous studies to determine whether the net of cholesterol content is altered in the AD brain have been contradictory. Mason previously analyzed lipid membranes extracted from the cortices of AD brains by an X-ray diffraction method (Mason et al., 1992). They reported that the unesterified cholesterol: phospholipid molecular ratio significantly decreased by 30% in the AD brain compared with that in age-matched controls. Soderberg et al. performed a similar analysis using different brain regions of AD patients; however, they found increased levels of phosphatidylinositol but mostly unchanged cholesterol levels in the AD brains (Soderberg et al., 1992). This contradiction may arise from the different techniques employed to determine lipid levels.

It is also likely that the levels of lipids and proteins in autopsy samples may be modified during the postmortem stage and these levels may be different from those observed during the disease process.

2.3. Risk Factors for AD and Increase in Cholesterol Level: A Putative Biological Basis for Cholesterol-Dependent AD Development

2.3.1. Aging

The strongest risk factor for the development of AD is aging. Thus, scientists have focused on elucidating how aging plays a role in the development of AD. Igbavboa et al. previously performed lipid analysis of synaptic plasma membranes using aged mice (Igbavboa *et al.*, 1996). They attempted to determine the cholesterol distribution throughout lipid bilayers of the synaptic plasma membranes because there are two transbilayer cholesterol pools, such as the cholesterol pool in the exofacial and cytofacial leaflets; importantly, a cytofacial leaflet contains cholesterol sevenfold of that of an exofacial leaflet. Igbabvoa et al. examined the age-dependent alteration of membrane fluidity and cholesterol distribution. They isolated the synaptic plasma membranes (SPMs) from mice in three different age groups, namely, 3-4, 14-15, and 24-25 months old, and then they determined the fluidity and levels of cholesterol in the exofacial and cytofacial leaflets of the synaptic plasma membranes (SPMs). In this experiment, they found that the exofacial leaflet of SPMs from young mice was more fluid than the cytofacial leaflet. Interestingly, the difference in membrane fluidity between the exofacial and cytofacial leaflets was not significant in the SPM prepared from aged mice. In regard to the levels of cholesterol in these two leaflets, they found that there was an approximately twofold increase in the cholesterol level in the exofacial leaflet in the aged mice compared with that in the young mice. They also determined the level of total cholesterol in the synaptic plasma membrane; however, there was no difference among the three different-age groups. On the basis of these results, they concluded that the asymmetric distribution of cholesterol throughout the lipid bilayers of the SPMs changes with age.

2.3.2. Apolipoprotein E

Apolipoprotein E (apoE) is a major lipoprotein in the brain. Previous studies revealed that the genetic polymorphism of the *ApoE* gene is closely associated with the prevalence of AD (Corder et al., 1993; Poirier et al., 1993; Saunders et al., 1993; Strittmatter et al., 1993). To date, much effort has been exerted to elucidate the pathogenic role of one of the apoE isoforms, apoE4, a gene product of apoE allele e4, the presence of which is a strong risk factor for AD. It was suggested that apoE directly modulates the aggregation behavior of amyloid β-protein (Aβ) and tau protein, which are the proteinaceous components of senile plaques and neurofibrillary tangles in AD brains, respectively. However, the results of the studies are controversial and it still remains to be determined whether apoE4 directly accelerates the progression of AD pathology through direct binding to Aβ and tau protein. We have been attempting to elucidate the pathogenic role of apoE4 from the viewpoint of the physiological function of apoE, that is, the regulation of cholesterol metabolism in the brain (Michikawa and Yanagisawa, 1998). The results of our studies suggest that apoE regulates the turnover of lipids, including cholesterol, through the modulation of the influx and efflux of these lipids in an isoform-dependent manner (Gong et al., 2002; Michikawa et al., 2000). Moreover, we have also examined the possibility of whether apoE modulates cholesterol distribution throughout the lipid bilayers of synaptic plasma membranes in an isoform-dependent manner (Hayashi et al., 2002). In this experiment, we performed subcellular fractionation of human apoE3- and apoE4-knock-in mouse brains. We determined the levels of phospholipid and cholesterol (total and free) in fractions, including the plasma membrane fraction, endoplasmic fractions and also synaptosome fraction. Quantitative analyses revealed that there was no significant difference in lipid concentrations in these fractions among the wild-type, apoE3- and apoE4-knock-in mice. However, the asymmetric distribution of cholesterol in the SPMs prepared from apoE4-knock-in mice was markedly altered compared with that of apoE3-knock-in mice. The cholesterol level in the exofacial leaflet of apoE4-knock-in mice SPMs was approximately twofold that of wild-type and apoE3-knock-in mice. Interestingly, the total cholesterol level in the SPMs did not change. Thus, as in aged mice, the cholesterol distribution in the SPMs of apoE4-knock-in mice is likely to be altered so that the cholesterol level in the exofacial leaflet increases. The involvement of apoE in the regulation of cholesterol distribution throughout the lipid bilayers of the SPMs was also suggested by Wood and his colleagues. They previously performed experiments similar to those on aged mice using apoE- and LDL-receptor-deficient mice (Igbavboa et al., 1997). Importantly, the cholesterol level in the SPM exofacial leaflets of the apoE- and LDL-receptor-deficient mice showed a twofold increase compared with that of the wild-type mice.

2.3.3. Down Syndrome

Down syndrome (DS), caused by a trisomy of chromosome 21, is also a risk factor for the development of AD changes in the brain. The formation of senile plaques and neurofibrillary tangles is, without exception, observed in the brain of DS patients more than 45 years old. It is generally accepted that the development of AD changes in DS brains is due to the high expression level of the *APP* gene due to the trisomy of chromosome 21. However, an alternative possibility was also previously reported. Naeim and Walford reported that a membrane prepared from the mononuclear blood cells of DS patients showed an increased rigidity. This result indicated that the cholesterol level increases in the membrane of DS blood cells (Naeim and Walford, 1980). This possibility was supported by a study of Diomode et al. They found, in the trisomy 21 fetuses, an alteration of the activities of the sterol regulatory element binding proteins, SREBP-1 and SREBP-2, which are involved in the regulation of cholesterol synthesis (Diomede et al., 1999). Taken together, it is likely that cholesterol metabolism is altered in DS.

2.4. Cholesterol Metabolism in AD Brains

The most important and straightforward study may be to directly examine the lipid composition in the AD brain. However, as described above, it is difficult to obtain accurate information on alterations in lipid metabolism from autopsy brains. Lütjohann et al. examined the level of plasma 24S-OH-Chol in AD, non-AD demented and depressive patients and in healthy controls (Lütjohann et al., 1996). Interestingly, the plasma 24S-OH-Chol levels in the AD and non-AD demented patients was modestly but significantly elevated compared with those in the depressive patients and healthy controls. Although the plasma 24S-OH-Chol levels did not significantly differ between the AD and non-AD demented patients, importantly, plasma 24S-OH-Chol level negatively correlated with the severity of dementia. This intriguing finding was followed by the study of Papassotiropoulos et al.

(Papassotiropoulos et al., 2000), who found that the inheritance of the apoE4 allele is associated with a reduced plasma 24SOH-Chol level in a manner independent of the severity of dementia in the patients examined. In regard to the alteration in the plasma 24S-OH-Chol level in the early stage of AD, Papassotiropoulos et al. and Schonknecht et al. also reported that the plasma 24S-OH-Chol level increased in the cerebrospinal fluid (CSF) in patients with mild cognitive impairment (MCI) (Papassotiropoulos et al., 2002; Schonknecht et al., 2002).

These studies suggest that cholesterol turnover is accelerated in the brains of patients with AD, leading to a decrease in its turnover in the advanced stage of the disease. At present, we do not know how the plasma 24S-OH-Chol level is elevated in association with AD. One of the possible explanation was recently provided; polymorphism in the cholesterol *24S-hydroxylase (CYP46)* gene, which encodes the enzyme involved in the conversion of cholesterol to 24S-OH-Chol, is associated with AD (Papassotiropoulos et al., 2003; Kolsch et al., 2002). Interesting to note is that a genotype that is more prevalent in the AD group is associated with an increased 24S-OH-Chol/cholesterol ratio in CSF. Thus, it may be possible to assume that cholesterol metabolism or turnover is altered during the development of AD through the accelerated conversion of cholesterol to 24S-OH-Chol, which may or may not be associated with polymorphism of the *CYP46* gene.

2.5. Animal Models

The association between the prevalence of AD development and the serum cholesterol levels is supported by the results of previous studies using experimental animals. It was reported that a high-cholesterol diet may induce Aβ accumulation in the brain (Sparks et al. 1994). It is generally accepted that the blood-brain barrier prevents the transport of serum cholesterol to the brain. Thus, it remains to be determined whether oral excess intake of cholesterol can directly alter the metabolism of proteins and lipids in the brain so that Aβ deposits in brain parenchyma. Recently, Refolo et al. have also suggested a possible association with high-cholesterol diet and the facilitation of Aβ deposition using APP-transgenic mouse model of AD (Refolo et al., 2000). They extended their study using an inhibitor of cholesterol biosynthesis and concluded that hypocholesterolemia is associated with reduced Aβ deposition in the brain (Refolo et al., 2001). Again, it has been generally accepted that cholesterol turnover is only restricted inside the brain. These lines of evidence suggest that cholesterol is transportable across the blood-brain barrier.

2.6. Lessons from NPC

Nieman-Pick type C disease (NPC) is an autosomal recessive neurovisceral lipid storage disorder (Pentchev et al., 1995). The causative genes, including Niemann-Pick C1 (NPC1), have been identified and, to date, it is widely accepted that the abnormal trafficking of exogenous cholesterol is closely associated with the progression of this disease. Importantly, the formation of neurofibrillary tangles, which is indistinguishable from those formed in AD brains, was reported in the brain with NPC (Auer et al., 1995; Suzuki et al., 1995). Moreover, the deposition of Aβ has also recently been reported (Saito et al., 2002). This line of evidence strongly suggests that the alteration of cholesterol metabolism is a potent factor accelerating the pathological processes of AD. It was also suggested that we can obtain information regarding molecular pathophysiology from animal and cellular models of NPC. It seems likely that a mutation of *NPC* genes induces the alteration of trafficking and/or cholesterol accumulation in lysosomes. Thus, a question to answer is how Aβ deposition is accelerated under these conditions. Sugimoto et al. recently investigated the intracellular trafficking of lipids, including cholesterol and GM1 ganglioside, in NPC1-deficient cells and found that not only cholesterol but also GM1 ganglioside accumulates in different vesicular compartments of NPC1-deficient cells (Sugimoto et al., 2001). As described below, we and other groups have suggested that Aβ adopts an altered conformation through binding to GM1 ganglioside and that GM1-ganglioside-bound Aβ acts as a seed for Aβ fibrillogenesis (Yanagisawa et al., 1995; Mclaurin and Chakrabartty,, 1996; Choo-Smith et al, 1997). Furthermore, we also found that the binding of Aβ to GM1 ganglioside is facilitated in a cholesterol-rich environment due to the cluster formation of GM1 ganglioside (Kakio et al, 2001). Taken together, the accumulation of cholesterol and GM1 ganglioside due to the *NPC* mutation is a favorable condition for the initiation of Aβ aggregation. This possibility has been further supported by Yamazaki et al. They performed a culture study using NPC deficient cells (Yamazaki et al., 2001). They treated CHO cells with U18666A, which induces the NPC-mimicking accumulation of cholesterol in the cells. In this experiment, they quantified the amount of intracellular Aβ. Interestingly, Aβ accumulates in its aggregated form in the late endosomes of the cells in association with intracellular cholesterol accumulation.

2.7. Implications of Alterations in Cholesterol Distribution/Metabolism in the Brain for the AD Development

It remains to be elucidated how an increase in the cholesterol level in the brain accelerates the pathological processes of AD. Recently, evidence is growing to suggest that an increase in membrane cholesterol level enhances Aβ generation through the activation of β- and γ-cleavage of APP, which are proteolytic process of Aβ generation (Frears et al., 1999; Fassbender et al., 2001). Although further studies are required, it is suggested that these proteolytic cleavages of APP occur in the lipid raft (Wahrle et al., 2002; Ehehalt et al., 2003), which is a cholesterol-rich microdomain in the cells (Simons and Ikonen, 1997). An alternative possibility on the cholesterol-dependent acceleration of the amyloid cascade was suggested by our group and other groups. We previously performed the immunochemical analysis of AD brains to determine the Aβ species that initially deposits in the brain and found that a GM1-ganglioside-bound form of Aβ (GAβ) is selectively deposited in the brains that exhibit early pathological AD changes (Yanagisawa et al, 1995). On the basis of the molecular characteristics of GAβ, including its unique immunoreactivity and extremely high potential to form large aggregates of Aβ, we hypothesized that Aβ adopts an altered immunoreactivity via binding to GM1 ganglioside and then accelerates the aggregation of soluble Aβ by acting as a seed. Subsequently, we noticed that increase in the cholesterol level facilitates the binding of Aβ to GM1 ganglioside through the acceleration of GM1 clustering (Kakio et al., 2001). Thus, taken together, an increase in the membrane cholesterol level is likely to accelerate the amyloid cascade through the facilitation of both the generation and aggregation of Aβ.

At this point, it remains to be determined how the level of membrane cholesterol increases in AD. On the basis of recent epidemiological studies, hypercholesterolemia may be responsible. Alternatively, as discussed above, the distribution but not the total cholesterol level may be altered in association with risk factors for the development of AD, including aging and the expression of apoE4.

3. Cholesterol and Depression

Previous studies suggested that a low total cholesterol level is associated with an increased prevalence of psychiatric disorders, including depression and anxiety (Agargun, 2002). However, this is a controversial proposition as described below. We also cannot completely exclude the possibility that depression can cause a decrease in the serum cholesterol level through poor intake of food. In 1993, Morgan et al., reported that low plasma cholesterol level is associated with depressive symptoms in elderly men and suggested that a very low total cholesterol level may lead to suicide and violent death (Morgan et al., 1993). This possibility was supported by a recent study of Aijanseppa et al., suggesting that a low total serum cholesterol level is associated with a high amount of depressive symptoms (Aijanseppa et al., 2002). In contrast, Deisenhammer et al. reported that there was no positive association between the level of serum cholesterol and the course of depression and suicidal tendencies (Deisenhammer et al., 2004). Ledochowski et al., reported, in contrast to the widely accepted view, that a high cholesterol level is associated with signs of depressive mood (Ledochowski et al., 2003). It is difficult at this point to describe what these controversy stem from and how the serum cholesterol level is related to depression-associated neurochemical alteration in the brain. To date, no data have been reported to suggest that the depressive state directly or indirectly modulates the endogenous synthesis of cholesterol in the brain (Lutjohann et al., 2000). Further studies are required; however, it may be possible to assume that peripheral cholesterol modulates the cholesterol turnover in the brain, and subsequently, membrane-bound serotonergic structures (Papakostas et al., 2003).

References

Agargun MY. Serum cholesterol concentration, depression, and anxiety. *Acta Psychiatr Scand* **105**: 81-83, 2002.

Aijanseppa S, Kivinen P, Helkala EL, Kivela SL, Tuomilehto J, Nissinen A. Serum cholesterol and depressive symptoms in elderly Finnish men. *Int J Geriatr Psychiatry* **17**: 629-634, 2002.

Auer IA, Schmidt ML, Lee VM, Curry B, Suzuki K, Shin RW, Pentchev PG, Carstea 11 ED,Trojanowski JQ. Paired helical filament tau (PHFtau) in Niemann-Pick type C disease is similar to PHFtau in Alzheimer's disease. *Acta Neuropathol (Berl)* **90**: 547-551, 1995.

Bjorkhem I, Lutjohann D, Diczfalusy U, Stahle L, Ahlborg G,Wahren J. Cholesterol homeostasis in human brain: turnover of 24S-hydroxycholesterol and evidence for a cerebral origin of most of this oxysterol in the circulation. *J Lipid Res* **39**: 1594-1600, 1998.

Cenedella RJ, Shi H. Spatial distribution of 3-hydroxy-3-methylglutaryl coenzyme A reductase messenger RNA in the ocular lens: relationship to cholesterologenesis. *J Lipid Res* **35**: 2232-2240, 1994.

Choo-Smith LP, Garzon-Rodriguez W, Glabe CG, Surewicz WK. Acceleration of amyloid fibril formation by specific binding of Aβ-(1-40) peptide to gangliosidecontaining membrane vesicles. *J Biol Chem* **272**: 22987-22990, 1997.

Corder EH, Saunders AM, Strittmatter WJ, Schmechel DE, Gaskell PC, Small GW, Roses AD, Haines JL, Pericak-Vance MA. Gene dose of apolipoprotein E type 4 allele and the risk of Alzheimer's disease in late onset families. *Science* **261**: 921-923, 1993.

Deisenhammer EA, Kramer-Reinstadler K, Liensberger D, Kemmler G, Hinterhuber H,Wolfgang Fleischhacker W. No evidence for an association between serum cholesterol and the course of depression and suicidality. *Psychiatry Res* **121**: 253-261, 2004.

Dietschy JM, Turley SD. Cholesterol metabolism in the brain. *Curr Opin Lipidol* **12**: 105-112, 2001.

Diomede L, Salmona M, Albani D, Bianchi M, Bruno A, Salmona S, Nicolini U. Alteration of SREBP activation in liver of trisomy 21 fetuses. *Biochem Biophys Res Commun* **260**: 499-503, 1999.

Ehehalt R, Keller P, Haass C, Thiele C, Simons K. Amyloidogenic processing of the Alzheimer □-amyloid precursor protein depends on lipid rafts. *J Cell Biol* **160**: 113-123, 2003.

Fassbender K, Simons M, Bergmann C, Stroick M, Lutjohann D, Keller P, Runz H, Kuhl S, Bertsch T, von Bergmann K, Hennerici M, Beyreuther K, Hartmann T. Simvastatin strongly reduces levels of Alzheimer's disease β-amyloid peptides Aβ42 and Aβ40 in vitro and in vivo. *Proc Natl Acad Sci U S A* **98**: 5856-5861, 2001.

Frears ER, Stephens DJ, Walters CE, Davies H, Austen BM. The role of cholesterol in the biosynthesis of β-amyloid. *Neuroreport* **10**: 1699-1705, 1999.

Gong JS, Kobayashi M, Hayashi H, Zou K, Sawamura N, Fujita SC, Yanagisawa K, Michikawa M. Apolipoprotein E (ApoE) isoform-dependent lipid release from astrocytes prepared from human ApoE3 and ApoE4 knock-in mice. *J Biol Chem* **277**: 29919-29926, 2002.

Goodrum JF. Cholesterol synthesis is down-regulated during regeneration of peripheral nerve. *J Neurochem* **54**: 1709-1715, 1990.

Hayashi H, Igbavboa U, Hamanaka H, Kobayashi M, Fujita SC, Wood WG, Yanagisawa K. Cholesterol is increased in the exofacial leaflet of synaptic plasma membranes of human apolipoprotein E4 knock-in mice. *Neuroreport* **13**: 383-386, 2002.

Igbavboa U, Avdulov NA, Schroeder F, Wood WG. Increasing age alters transbilayer fluidity and cholesterol asymmetry in synaptic plasma membranes of mice. *J Neurochem* **66**: 1717-1725, 1996.

Igbavboa U, Avdulov NA, Chochina SV, Wood WG. Transbilayer distribution of cholesterol is modified in brain synaptic plasma membranes of knockout mice deficient in the low-density lipoprotein receptor, apolipoprotein E, or both proteins. *J Neurochem* **69**: 1661-1667, 1997.

Jick H, Zornberg GL, Jick SS, Seshadri S, Drachman DA. Statins and the risk of dementia. *Lancet* **356**: 1627-1631, 2000.

Kakio A, Nishimoto SI, Yanagisawa K, Kozutsumi Y, Matsuzaki K. Cholesteroldependent formation of GM1 ganglioside-bound amyloid β-protein, an endogenous seed for Alzheimer amyloid. *J Biol Chem* **276**: 24985-24990, 2001.

Kivipelto M, Helkala EL, Hanninen T, Laakso MP, Hallikainen M, Alhainen K, Soininen H, Tuomilehto J, Nissinen A. Midlife vascular risk factors and late-life mild cognitive impairment: A population-based study. *Neurology* **56**: 1683-1689, 2001.

Kolsch H, Lutjohann D, Ludwig M, Schulte A, Ptok U, Jessen F, von Bergmann K, Rao ML, Maier W, Heun R. Polymorphism in the cholesterol 24S-hydroxylase gene is associated with Alzheimer's disease. *Mol Psychiatry* **7**: 899-902, 2002.

Ledochowski M, Murr C, Sperner-Unterweger B, Neurauter G, Fuchs D. Association between increased serum cholesterol and signs of depressive mood. *Clin Chem Lab Med* **41**: 821-824, 2003.

Leibel WS, Firestone LL, Legler DC, Braswell LM, Miller KW. Two pools of cholesterol in acetylcholine receptor-rich membranes from Torpedo. *Biochim Biophys Acta* **897**: 249-260, 1987.

Lutjohann D, Breuer O, Ahlborg G, Nennesmo I, Siden A, Diczfalusy U, Bjorkhem I. Cholesterol homeostasis in human brain: evidence for an age-dependent flux of [24]S-hydroxycholesterol from the brain into the circulation. *Proc Natl Acad Sci U S A* **93**: 9799-9804, 1996.

Lutjohann D, Papassotiropoulos A, Bjorkhem I, Locatelli S, Bagli M, Oehring RD, Schlegel U, Jessen F, Rao ML, von Bergmann K, Heun R. Plasma 24Shydroxycholesterol (cerebrosterol) is increased in Alzheimer and vascular demented patients. *J Lipid Res* **41**: 195-198, 2000.

Mason RP, Shoemaker WJ, Shajenko L, Chambers TE, Herbette LG. Evidence for changes in the Alzheimer's disease brain cortical membrane structure mediated by cholesterol. *Neurobiol Aging* **13**: 413-419, 1992.

McLaurin J, Chakrabartty A. Membrane disruption by Alzheimer β-amyloid peptides mediated through specific binding to either phospholipids or gangliosides. Implications for neurotoxicity. *J Biol Chem* **271**: 26482-26489, 1996.

Michikawa M, Yanagisawa K. Apolipoprotein E4 induces neuronal cell death under conditions of suppressed de novo cholesterol synthesis. *J Neurosci Res* **54**: 58-67, 1998.

Michikawa M, Fan QW, Isobe I, Yanagisawa K. Apolipoprotein E exhibits isoform specific promotion of lipid efflux from astrocytes and neurons in culture. *J Neurochem* **74**: 1008-1016, 2000.

Morgan RE, Palinkas LA, Barrett-Connor EL, Wingard DL. Plasma cholesterol and depressive symptoms in older men. *Lancet* **341**: 75-79, 1993.

Naeim F, Walford RL. Disturbance of redistribution of surface membrane receptors on peripheral mononuclear cells of patients with Down's syndrome and of aged individuals. *J Gerontol* **35**: 650-655, 1980.

Notkola IL, Sulkava R, Pekkanen J, Erkinjuntti T, Ehnholm C, Kivinen P, Tuomilehto J, Nissinen A. Serum total cholesterol, apolipoprotein E epsilon 4 allele, and Alzheimer's disease. *Neuroepidemiology* **17**: 14-20, 1998.

Papakostas GI, Petersen T, Mischoulon D, Hughes ME, Alpert JE, Nierenberg AA, Rosenbaum JF, Fava M. Serum cholesterol and serotonergic function in major depressive disorder. *Psychiatry Res* **118**: 137-145, 2003.

Papassotiropoulos A, Lutjohann D, Bagli M, Locatelli S, Jessen F, Rao ML, Maier W, Bjorkhem I, von Bergmann K, Heun R. Plasma 24S-hydroxycholesterol: a peripheral indicator of neuronal degeneration and potential state marker for Alzheimer's disease. *Neuroreport* **11**: 1959-1962, 2000.

Papassotiropoulos A, Lutjohann D, Bagli M, Locatelli S, Jessen F, Buschfort R, Ptok U, Bjorkhem I, von Bergmann K, Heun R. 24S-hydroxycholesterol in cerebrospinal fluid is elevated in early stages of dementia. *J Psychiatr Res* **36**: 27-32, 2002.

Papassotiropoulos A, Streffer JR, Tsolaki M, Schmid S, Thal D, Nicosia F, Iakovidou V, Maddalena A, Lutjohann D, Ghebremedhin E, Hegi T, Pasch T, Traxler M, Bruhl A, Benussi L, Binetti G, Braak H, Nitsch RM, Hock C. Increased brain β-amyloid load, phosphorylated tau, and risk of Alzheimer disease associated with an intronic CYP46 polymorphism. *Arch Neurol* **60**: 29-35, 2003.

Pentchev PG. Vanier MT. Suzuki K. Patterson MC. Niemann-Pick disease, type C: a cellular cholesterol lipidosis, in: *The metabolic and Molecular Basis of Inherited Disease* (C. R Scriver, A. L. Beaudet, W.S. Sly, and D.Vall, eds), McGraw-Hill, New York. pp.2625-2640, 1995

Poirier J, Davignon J, Bouthillier D, Kogan S, Bertrand P, Gauthier S. Apolipoprotein E polymorphism and Alzheimer's disease. *Lancet* **342**: 697-699, 1993.

Popplewell PY, Azhar S. Effects of aging on cholesterol content and cholesterol metabolizing enzymes in the rat adrenal gland. *Endocrinology* **121**: 64-73, 1987.

Refolo LM, Malester B, LaFrancois J, Bryant-Thomas T, Wang R, Tint GS, Sambamurti K, Duff K, Pappolla MA. Hypercholesterolemia accelerates the Alzheimer's amyloid pathology in a transgenic mouse model. *Neurobiol Dis* **7**: 321-331, 2000.

Refolo LM, Pappolla MA, LaFrancois J, Malester B, Schmidt SD, Thomas-Bryant T, Tint GS, Wang R, Mercken M, Petanceska SS, Duff KE. A cholesterol-lowering drug reduces β-amyloid pathology in a transgenic mouse model of Alzheimer's disease. *Neurobiol Dis* **8**: 890-899, 2001.

Saito Y, Suzuki K, Nanba E, Yamamoto T, Ohno K, Murayama S. Niemann-Pick type C disease: accelerated neurofibrillary tangle formation and amyloid βdeposition associated with apolipoprotein E epsilon 4 homozygosity. *Ann Neurol* **52**: 351-355, 2002.

Saunders AM, Strittmatter WJ, Schmechel D, George-Hyslop PH, Pericak-Vance MA, Joo SH, Rosi BL, Gusella JF, Crapper-MacLachlan DR, Alberts MJ, et al. Association of apolipoprotein E allele epsilon 4 with late-onset familial and sporadic Alzheimer's disease. *Neurology* **43**: 1467-1472, 1993.

Schonknecht P, Lutjohann D, Pantel J, Bardenheuer H, Hartmann T, von Bergmann K, Beyreuther K, Schroder J. Cerebrospinal fluid 24S-hydroxycholesterol is increased in patients with Alzheimer's disease compared to healthy controls. *Neurosci Lett* **324**: 83-85, 2002.

Schroeder F, Nemecz G, Wood WG, Joiner C, Morrot G, Ayraut-Jarrier M, Devaux PF. Transmembrane distribution of sterol in the human erythrocyte. *Biochim Biophys Acta* **1066**: 183-192, 1991.

Simons K, Ikonen E. Functional rafts in cell membranes. *Nature* **387**: 569-572, 1997.

Soderberg M, Edlund C, Alafuzoff I, Kristensson K, Dallner G. Lipid composition in different regions of the brain in Alzheimer's disease/senile dementia of Alzheimer's type. *J Neurochem* **59**: 1646-1653, 1992.

Sparks DL, Scheff SW, Hunsaker JC, 3rd, Liu H, Landers T, Gross DR. Induction of Alzheimer-like β-amyloid immunoreactivity in the brains of rabbits with dietary cholesterol. *Exp Neurol* **126**: 88-94, 1994.

Stahlberg D, Angelin B, Einarsson K. Age-related changes in the metabolism of cholesterol in rat liver microsomes. *Lipids* **26**: 349-352, 1991.

Strittmatter WJ, Weisgraber KH, Huang DY, Dong LM, Salvesen GS, Pericak-Vance M, Schmechel D, Saunders AM, Goldgaber D, Roses AD. Binding of human apolipoprotein E to synthetic amyloid βpeptide: isoform-specific effects and implications for late-onset Alzheimer disease. *Proc Natl Acad Sci U S A* **90**: 8098-8102, 1993.

Steegmans PH, Fekkes D, Hoes AW, Bak AA, van der Does E, Grobbee DE. Low serum cholesterol concentration and serotonin metabolism in men. *B M J* **312**: 221, 1996.

Sugimoto Y, Ninomiya H, Ohsaki Y, Higaki K, Davies JP, Ioannou YA, Ohno K. Accumulation of cholera toxin and GM1 ganglioside in the early endosome of Niemann-Pick C1-deficient cells. *Proc Natl Acad Sci U S A* **98**: 12391-12396, 2001.

Suzuki K, Parker CC, Pentchev PG, Katz D, Ghetti B, D'Agostino AN, Carstea ED. Neurofibrillary tangles in Niemann-Pick disease type C. *Acta Neuropathol (Berl)* **89**: 227-238, 1995.

Vance JE, Pan D, Campenot RB, Bussiere M, Vance DE. Evidence that the major membrane lipids, except cholesterol, are made in axons of cultured rat sympathetic neurons. *J Neurochem* **62**: 329-337, 1994.

Wahrle S, Das P, Nyborg AC, McLendon C, Shoji M, Kawarabayashi T, Younkin LH, Younkin SG, Golde TE. Cholesterol-dependent γ-secretase activity in buoyant cholesterol-rich membrane microdomains. *Neurobiol Dis* **9**: 11-23, 2002.

Wolozin B, Kellman W, Ruosseau P, Celesia GG, Siegel G. Decreased prevalence of Alzheimer disease associated with 3-hydroxy-3-methyglutaryl coenzyme A reductase inhibitors. *Arch Neurol* **57**: 1439-1443, 2000.

Wood WG, Cornwell M, Williamson LS. High performance thin-layer chromatography and densitometry of synaptic plasma membrane lipids. *J Lipid Res* **30**: 775-779, 1989.

Wood WG, Schroeder F, Avdulov NA, Chochina SV, Igbavboa U. Recent advances in brain cholesterol dynamics: transport, domains, and Alzheimer's disease. *Lipids* **34**: 225-234, 1999.

Yamazaki T, Chang TY, Haass C, Ihara Y. Accumulation and aggregation of amyloid β-protein in late endosomes of Niemann-pick type C cells. *J Biol Chem* **276**: 4454-4460, 2001.

Yanagisawa K, Odaka A, Suzuki N, Ihara Y. GM1 ganglioside-bound amyloid β-protein (Aβ): a possible form of preamyloid in Alzheimer's disease. *Nat Med* **1**: 1062-1066, 1995.

In: Cognition and Mood Interactions
Editor: Miao-Kun Sun, pp. 149-160
ISBN 1-59454-229-5
2005 © Nova Science Publishers, Inc.

Chapter IX

Stress in Dementia and Depression

Noriyuki Kitayama and J. Douglas Bremner
Emory University School of Medicine

Animal models have been developed for the loss of memory function that occurs in some individuals with normal aging. One model posits that progressive increases in the stress hormone cortisol lead to progressive atrophy of the hippocampus, a brain area involved in memory, with progressive memory impairments and further increases in cortisol. Elevations in cortisol interfere with memory function in normal individuals, and dementia develops more commonly in a subgroup of elderly patients with recurrent depression, especially those who have reversible memory impairments during episodes of depression. This has led to the hypothesis that elevations in cortisol with depression lead to hippocampal atrophy and progressive memory impairments. Although some studies have shown relationships between cortisol, memory and hippocampal atrophy in the very elderly, it is not clear if elevations in cortisol cause the progressive memory impairment seen in some patients with recurrent depression. Future research in this area is needed.

1. Introduction

Stress plays a critical role in the development of depression, and stress has been proposed to play a role in the acceleration of memory loss with aging. Brain areas responsible for memory (e.g., hippocampus and amygdala) play an important role in the stress response. Hormones such as cortisol and adrenaline, which are released during stress, bathe these brain areas and modulate their function, bringing the organism back to a similar state as during prior times of danger, when there was a similar stress-induced outpouring of these stress hormones. In this way, the stress response mobilizes brain systems that are critical for survival.

With excessive or repetitive stress, the individual can develop long-term changes in these same brain systems that mediate memory and the stress response. Individuals exposed to repeated stress may develop dysfunction in their stress response systems, and can lose the capacity to properly adapt to new stressors. Stress responses that are useful for short-term survival can be at the expense of long-term function. For instance, excessive levels of cortisol result in a gastric ulcers, osteoporosis, cardiovascular disease, diabetes, and asthma. Stress also impairs the immune system, which increases the risk of developing infections and other medical disorders.

Stress has also been hypothesized to interact with aging to lead to a type of accelerated aging. For instance, in the "glucocorticoid cascade" model of aging, progressive increases in glucocorticoids (e.g., cortisol) lead to progressive hippocampal atrophy, which in turn results in a loss of inhibition on the hypothalamic-pituitary-adrenal (HPA) axis, leading to even higher glucocorticoid levels, hippocampal atrophy, and memory impairments, in a progressively accelerating cascade. Although more applicable to the rat than humans, this type of model provides a way to start thinking about the relationship between stress, dementia and depression. In this chapter, we review the interaction between stress, depression and dementia, with a focus on neurobiological models that link stress to both depression and dementia.

2. Effects of Stress on Memory and the Hippocampus

In 1990, Robert Sapolsky, Bruce McEwen, and colleagues at Stanford and Rockefeller Universities made the startling observation that stress may damage the brain. These scientists found that high levels of glucocorticoids seen in stress result in damage to the hippocampus, a brain area involved in learning and memory (McEwen et al., 1992; Sapolsky, 1996).

There are now a considerable numbers of studies in animals showing that stress is associated with structural changes in the hippocampus (McEwen et al., 1992; Sapolsky, 1996). When male and female vervet monkeys are caged together, the female monkeys attack the males, leading to extreme stress in the males, which is often fatal. Monkeys who were improperly caged and died spontaneously following exposure to severe stress were found to have damage to the CA3 subfield of the hippocampus (Uno et al., 1989). This hippocampal damage was reproducible when glucocorticoids were implanted directly into the hippocampus (Sapolsky et al., 1988, 1990). Psychosocial stress in monkeys (Uno et al., 1989) and tree shrews (Magarinos et al., 1996) resulted in decreased dendritic branching and /or neuronal loss in the CA3 region of the hippocampus. Studies in a variety of animal species showed that direct glucocorticoid exposure resulted in decreased dendritic branching (Packan and Sapolsky, 1990; Woolley et al., 1991), alterations in synaptic terminal structure (Magarinos and McEwen, 1995; Magarinos et al., 1997), a loss of neurons (Uno et al., 1989), and inhibition of neuronal regeneration (Gould et al., 1998) within the CA3 region of the hippocampus. These effects were felt to be mediated through disruption of cellular metabolism, leading to an increase in release of endogenously released excitatory amino acid, and an increase in vulnerability to their effects (Sapolsky, 1986; Sapolsky et al., 1988; Armanini et al., 1990; Lawrence and Sapolsky, 1994; Stein-Behrens et al., 1994; Magarinos and McEwen 1995). These findings are consistent with the hypothesis that glucocorticoids released during stress are associated with hippocampal damage and associated memory deficits. However, glucocorticoids have other actions besides a damaging a damage effect on hippocampal neurons. For instance, low levels of glucocorticoids following adrenalectomy result in damage to neurons of the dentate gyrus of the hippocampus (Vaher et al., 1994).

Stressors were also associated with deficits in memory functions that are mediated by the hippocampus. Stress was associated with both deficits in working memory tasks, as well as inhibition of long-term potentiation, which is dependent on the NMDA (excitatory amino acid) receptor (highly concentrated in the hippocampus, and felt to represent a model for memory at the molecular level (Diamond et al., 1995, 1996). High levels of glucocorticoids seen with stress were associated with deficits in new learning, in addition to damage to the hippocampus (Luine et al., 1994). Long-term subcutaneous implants of glucocorticoids which mimic chronic stress situation were shown to result in deficits in new learning and memory for maze escape behaviors. Moreover, the magnitude of deficits was correlated with the number of damaged cells in the CA3 region the hippocampus (Arbel et al., 1994). Physiologic levels of glucocorticoids can impair memory, even without the loss of hippocampal neurons (Bodnoff et al., 1995), an effect that may be mediated by modulation of hippocampal-based long-term potentiation (Pavlides et al., 1995).

3. Stress and Depression

Major depression is a common psychiatric disorder affecting 15% of the population at some time in their lives that is associated with considerable morbidity and loss of economic productivity (Bremner et al 2002). Stress exposure is an important factor in both the development of depression as well as vulnerability to relapse. Elevations in the stress hormone cortisol are seen in about a third of depressed patients.

Several pieces of evidence are consistent with elevations in cortisol in a subgroup of depressed patients. Depressive episodes were shown to be associated with high levels of urinary free cortisol (UFC) in subgroups of depressed patients. Over 40% of the depressed patients had UFC excretions in the range seen in Cushing's disease (Carroll et al., 1976). As reviewed above, elevated levels of glucocorticoids seen in stress have been associated with damage to hippocampal neurons. In addition, patients with a history of exposure to extreme stress and the diagnosis of posttraumatic stress disorder (PTSD) were found to have smaller hippocampal volume as measured with magnetic resonance imaging (MRI) and deficits in hippocampal based verbal declarative memory function (Bremner et al., 1995; Bremner, 1999). It has been hypothesized that elevated levels of glucocorticoids during depressive episodes could cause hippocampal damage, leading to a reduction in volume. In other words, chronic repeated episodes of depression may lead to progressive hippocampal atrophy over time, possibly increasing the risk for subsequent depressive relapse (Bremner et al., 2000). Hippocampal dysfunction may contribute to verbal declarative memory deficits in depression (Sass et al., 1990, Burt et al., 1995). Until recently there have been few studies of hippocampal volume in patients with depression (Sheline et al., 1996; Bremner et al., 2000).

Studies have highlighted the physical abnormalities seen in depressed patients that may be related to excessive levels of cortisol. The physical manifestations of depression, include deficits in hippocampal based memory function, association with cardiovascular disease, hypertension, osteoporosis, and diabetes, to name a few. These facts suggest that hypothalamic-pituitary-adrenal (HPA) axis abnormalities may have a direct effect on the physical health of patients with depression (Brown et al., 2004).

4. The Interaction of Stress and Aging in Producing Memory Impairments

Aging and stress may interact to promote hippocampal toxicity with related memory dysfunction. Sapolsky, Krey, and McEwen (1985) outlined a "glucocorticoid cascade" model for age-related memory deficits. They found that in rodents there is a progressive increase (due to a loss of hippocampal inhibition of glucocorticoid release) in peripheral glucocorticoid levels, and progressive memory deterioration. These rats also showed a delay in return of glucocorticoid levels to baseline after stress, possibly secondary to a down regulation of glucocorticoid receptors in the hippocampus with aging (Sapolsky et al., 1983a, 1983b). Aging was associated with a loss of the normal plasticity of these receptors (Eldridge et al., 1989a, 1989b).

Studies in elderly human subjects on the relationship between glucocorticoids, memory, and the hippocampus have been few and have had mixed findings (Stein-Behrens et al., 1992; Urban, 1992). Some studies support the idea that elevations in cortisol (Armanini et al., 1993; Lupien et al., 1994; Swaab et al., 1994; Van Cauter et al., 1996) and an impairment in feedback sensitivity to cortisol (O'Brien et al., 1994) occur with normal aging. Aging individuals had decreased numbers of glucocorticoid receptors measured on leukocytes (Armanini et al., 1992, 1993) and altered cortisol responsiveness to stressors (Gotthardt et al., 1995; Raskind et al., 1995; Seeman et al., 1995). Increases in cortisol (Lupien et al., 1994) and decreased sensitivity to the feedback inhibition of cortisol (O'Brien et al., 1994) with aging were correlated with progressive memory impairment. Acute administration of glucocorticoids resulted in greater memory impairment in young individuals compared to elderly, interpreted as secondary to decreased hippocampal glucocorticoid receptor sensitivity (Newcomer et al., 1994). Increased cortisol levels over time were correlated in one study of elderly subjects with declarative memory deficits and hippocampal atrophy on MRI (Lupien et al., 1998). In one study that looked at the relationship between stress and cortisol in the elderly, Seeman et al. (1995) measured cortisol and ACTH response to the stress of a driving simulation challenge test in 16 healthy men and women between 70 and 79 years of age. They found significant elevations in ACTH and Cortisol with stress in the elderly subjects. Furthermore, those subjects with a low self esteem exhibited a nearly six-fold greater Cortisol response to the driving challenge compared to those reporting a high self esteem. Another study in elderly normal subjects showed that subjects with increased cortisol reactivity to a social stressor had impaired verbal declarative memory function before the test. These subjects also had increased cortisol at baseline in anticipation of the stressor. This study suggested that an increase in anticipation of a stressful event with increased cortisol results in an impairment in verbal declarative memory function in the elderly (Lupien et al., 1997)

Posttraumatic stress disorder (PTSD) is a condition that has a high comorbidity with depression and, like depression, is linked to stress. There is a paucity of research on the relationship between aging and PTSD (reviewed in Ruskin & Talbot, 1996) and most of these studies have been epidemiological. Kato et al. (1996) measured the frequency of short-term PTSD symptoms amongst evacuees of the Hanshin-Awaji earthquake. Fifty subjects under the age of 60 years and 73 subjects over the age of 60 years were interviewed at 3 and 8 weeks after the earthquake. At the 3-week time point, all subjects from both age groups experienced sleep disturbances, depression, hypersensitivity, and irritability. At the 8-week time point, elderly subjects showed a significant decrease in 8 of 10 symptoms, while there was no change in the younger subjects. Goenjian et al. (1994) evaluated 179 subjects 1.5 years after the 1988 earthquake. Although the total mean score on the PTSD reaction index was not significantly different between elderly and younger adults, there was a significant difference in the symptom profile, with the elderly scoring higher on arousal symptoms and lower on intrusive symptoms than younger subjects. Even fewer biological studies were performed on aging and PTSD. One study found decreased cortisol levels in 24-hr urine samples in elderly Holocaust survivors with PTSD (Yehuda et al., 1995) and in middle aged Vietnam combat veterans with PTSD, while younger individuals with abuse-related PTSD actually had elevated cortisol levels (Lemieux and Coe, 1995). It may be that PTSD in younger individuals is associated with hypercortisolemia, while with aging there is hypocortisolemia, possibly secondary to long-term dysregulation of the HPA axis.

The findings reviewed up to this point raise the question, can stress-related disorders like depression and PTSD be considered to represent a form of accelerated aging? In animal studies both stress and aging are associated with declarative memory dysfunction and hippocampal atrophy. These findings hold based on human research in populations of stress and probably aging as well. Stress and aging may also interact to increase the vulnerability of the hippocampus to glucocorticoid mediated toxicity. For example, continuous administration of slow-release corticosterone to simulate mild stress in young (3 months old) and middle aged (12 months old) rats resulted in greater cognitive deficits in the middle aged rats (Levy et al., 1994). Findings related to the HPA axis may also be relevant to understanding the relationship between stress and aging. In animal studies, both chronic stress (Ladd et al., 1996) and aging (Sapolsky et al., 1983a, 1983b) are associated with down-regulation of glucocorticoid receptors and impaired return of baseline of glucocorticoids after reintroduction of stress. These findings also support the hypothesis that chronic stress can be thought of as a type of "accelerated aging." Clinical studies in PTSD patients, however, showed an increase in glucocorticoid receptors on peripheral lymphocytes. A clue about these apparent discrepancies may come from the results of studies looking at the effect of dexamethasone on memory function. Dexamethasone-induced impairments in memory function in normal younger subjects, but not in normal older subjects, is consistent with a loss of hippocampal glucocorticoid receptors with normal aging (Newcomer et al., 1994). A current study in our laboratory is looking at the effects of dexamethasone on memory function in depression and PTSD. If there is a loss of hippocampal glucocorticoid receptors, as is seen in normal aging, then there should be no effect of dexamethasone on memory in depression and PTSD (making it like a form of "accelerated aging"). In fact, preliminary data shows that both depression and PTSD show a lack of effect of dexamethasone on memory, making them look like normal elderly subjects, and corroborating the idea of stress-related disorders depression and PTSD as representing a form of "accelerated aging."

5. Age-Related Morphological Changes in the Brain in Normal Elderly Subjects

Studies using MRI have examined the examined changes in the brain with normal aging. Some studies (Convit et al., 1995), but not others (Sullivan et al., 1994), found a decrease in volume of the hippocampus measured with MRI in elderly subjects. Studies in individuals with age-associated memory impairment (AAMI) demonstrated alterations in hippocampal structure (Soininen et al., 1994; Parnetti et al., 1996) which were correlated with memory impairment (Soininen et al., 1994). It is clear that hippocampal atrophy, hypercortisolemia, and memory impairment do not progress as rapidly in humans as in rodents, although there is evidence to suggest that a similar process is taking place at a slower rate in at least a subgroup of the elderly. Future studies should focus on populations of "super elderly" individuals (e.g., subjects who are 75 or greater, rather than using conventional definitions of the elderly, such as greater than age 65).

There are a few studies which estimated age-related changes in white and gray matter volume. A study which reported the age-related reduction of cerebral volume demonstrated that a highly nonlinear increase in the volume of signal hyperintensities are observed in cortical and subcortical regions (Jernigan TL et al., 1990). In another study, significant decreases in the grey matter of both cortices and subcortices were reported (Jernigan TL et al., 1991). Additionally, another study found no correlation between aging and white matter volume but suggested decreased grey matter volume of the temporal lobe with normal aging (Sullivan et al., 1994). These findings are consistent with a loss of cortical grey matter volume, especially in the temporal lobe, with normal aging.

Functional brain imaging studies are consistent with decreased hippocampal function with aging. For instance, one study measuring functional brain changes (regional cerebral blood flow) using Positron Emission Tomography (PET) found a relative failure in hippocampal activation during a memory encoding task. The authors concluded that memory impairments with normal aging may be due to a failure to encode the stimuli adequately (Grady et al., 1995).

6. Geriatric Depression and Cognitive Disorders

Elderly patients with depression show essentially a similar symptom profile as younger patients with depression (Brodaty et al 1991). Patients with late-life depression, however, tend to have more severe psychomotor changes, and are more likely to have psychotic features associated with their depression (Alexopoulos 1990; Brodaty 1996). Patients with late-life depression also have more cognitive impairments, including deficits in memory and executive functions (Cummings, J.L. 1993). Furthermore, depression with an onset in late life is associated with increased rates of cerebrovascular disease and other neurodegenerative disorders (Krishnan et al 1994; Hickie et al 1995). Many patients with late-onset depressive disorders have extensive white matter hyperintensities on MRI that are felt to be secondary to micro-infarction, and that predispose patients to the development of chronic depression and progressive cognitive decline, probably through a disruption in neural circuits mediating mood and cognition (Hickie et al 1996; Greenwald et al 1998). PET studies demonstrated bilateral activation deficits in the anterior cingulate gyrus and hippocampus that were correlated with memory impairments depressed geriatric patients relative to comparison subjects (de Asis et al., 2001). The results suggested that hippocampal dysfunction was related to the memory dysfunction characteristic of late-life depression.

Some studies have examined the relationship between late-life depression and the development of dementia. Patients who developed cognitive impairment during depressive episodes were found to have irreversible dementia at later follow-up in 43% of cases, while those without cognitive impairments during depression developed dementia in only 12% of cases. The authors suggested that geriatric depression with reversible dementia is a clinical entity that includes a group of patients with early-stage dementing disorders (Alexopoulos et al 1993). Another study compared patients with late-onset major depression, Alzheimer's disease (AD), and age-matched healthy subjects. The AD subjects showed a significantly lower whole brain volume and a significantly higher CSF volume in comparision to the controls and depressed patients. Depressed patients exhibited a higher ventricle-brain ratio suggesting a higher degree of atrophy compared to healthy individuals. In contrast, Alzheimer patients showed significantly lower volumes than depressed patients and controls with respect to all volumetric parameters. These results suggested a marked difference in pattern of atrophy between geriatric depression and primary degenerative dementia (Pantel et al 1997).

7. Increased Cortisol Levels and Alzheimer's Disease

Elevations in cortisol have been associated with both late-life depression and dementia. As described above, stress is associated with an increase in cortisol activity, and a sub group of patients with late life depression show increased cortisol levels. Some studies found increased cortisol levels in patients with Alzheimer's disease (AD). Swaab et al. (1994) investigated cortisol levels in cerebrospinal fluid (CSF) of patients with Alzheimer's disease and healthy controls. Mean CSF total cortisol level was 83% higher in AD than in the controls. Additionally, Pomara et al. (2002) examined the effects of mifepristone (a central glucocorticoid receptor antagonist) on cognition in AD, and suggested the possibility that glucocorticoid receptor antagonist may be effective for the cognitive impairment in the patients with AD.

8. Conclusion

Studies in animals have outlined an interesting model by which increased cortisol levels with normal aging lead to progressive hippocampal atrophy, memory deficits, and further increases in cortisol. The fact that a subgroup of depressed patients show increased cortisol has led to the idea that cortisol could lead to hippocampal atrophy with cognitive deficits in depression. This may explain the progressive loss of memory seen in a subgroup of elderly patients with depression. There is some evidence to support such a relationship in normal aging. Not enough research has been performed in patients with depression that addresses this specific area. Future studies are needed to examine the relationship between depression and dementia in patients with depression.

References

Alexopoulos, G.S. (1990): Clinical and biological findings in late-onset depression. In Tassman, A., Goldfinger, S.M., Kaufman, C.A. (eds), *Review of Psychiatry,* vol 9. Washington, DC: American Psychiatric Press, pp 249-262.

Alexopoulos, G.S., Meyers, B.S., et al. (1993). The course of geriatric depression with "reversible ddementia": a control study. *Am J Psychiatry* **150** (11): 1693-1699.

Arbel, I., T. Kadar, et al. (1994). The effects of long-term corticosterone administration on hippocampal morphology and cognitive performance of middle-aged rats. *Brain Res* **657**(1-2): 227-35.

Armanini, D., I. Karbowiak, et al. (1992). Corticosteroid receptors and lymphocyte subsets in mononuclear leukocytes in aging. *Am J Physiol* **262**(4 Pt 1): E464-6.

Armanini, D., M. Scali, et al. (1993). Corticosteroid receptors and aging. *J Steroid Biochem Mol Biol* **45**(1-3): 191-4.

Armanini, M. P., C. Hutchins, et al. (1990). Glucocorticoid endangerment of hippocampal neurons is NMDA-receptor dependent. *Brain Res* **532**(1-2): 7-12.

Bodnoff, S. R., A. G. Humphreys, et al. (1995). Enduring effects of chronic corticosterone treatment on spatial learning, synaptic plasticity, and hippocampal neuropathology in young and mid-aged rats. *J Neurosci* **15**(1 Pt 1): 61-9.

Bremner, J. D. (1999). Does stress damage the brain? *Biol Psychiatry* **45**(7): 797-805.

Bremner, J. D. and M. Narayan (1998). The effects of stress on memory and the hippocampus throughout the life cycle: implications for childhood development and aging. *Dev Psychopathol* **10**(4): 871-85.

Bremner, J. D., M. Narayan, et al. (2000). Hippocampal volume reduction in major depression. *Am J Psychiatry* **157**(1): 115-8.

Bremner, J. D., P. Randall, et al. (1995). MRI-based measurement of hippocampal volume in patients with combat-related posttraumatic stress disorder. *Am J Psychiatry* **152**(7): 973-81.

Bremner, J. D., M. Vythilingam, et al. (2002). Reduced volume of orbitofrontal cortex in major depression. *Biol Psychiatry* **51**(4): 273-9.

Brodaty, H., Peters K., et al. (1991): Age and depression. *J Affect Disord* 23:137-149.

Brodatry, H. (1996): Melancholia and the aging brain. In Parker G, Hadzi-Pavlovic, D (eds), *Melancholia: A Disorder of Movement and Mood.* New York: Cambridge University Press, pp 237-251.

Brown, E. S., F. P. Varghese, et al. (2004). Association of depression with medical illness: does cortisol play a role? *Biol Psychiatry* **55**(1): 1-9.

Burt, D. B., M. J. Zembar, et al. (1995). Depression and memory impairment: a meta-analysis of the association, its pattern, and specificity. *Psychol Bull* **117**(2): 285-305.

Carroll, B. J., G. C. Curtis, et al. (1976). Urinary free cortisol excretion in depression. *Psychol Med* **6**(1): 43-50.

Cicchetti, D., Rogosch, F. A., et al. (1998). Maternal depressive disorder and contextual risk: contributions to the development of attachment insecurity and behavior problems in toddlerhood. *Dev Psychopathol* **10**(2): 283-300.

Convit, A., M. J. de Leon, et al. (1995). Age-related changes in brain: I. Magnetic resonance imaging measures of temporal lobe volumes in normal subjects. *Psychiatr Q* **66**(4): 343-55.

Cummings, J.L. (1993). The neuroanatomy of depression. *J Clin Psychiatry* **54** (suppl): 14-20.

de Asis, J. M., *et al.* 2001. Hippocampal and anterior cingulate activation deficits in patients with geriatric depression. *American Journal of Psychiatry* **158**: 1321-1323.

Diamond, D. M., B. J. Branch, et al. (1995). Effects of dehydroepiandrosterone sulfate and stress on hippocampal electrophysiological plasticity. *Ann N Y Acad i* **774**: 304-7.

Diamond, D. M., M. Fleshner, et al. (1996). Psychological stress impairs spatial working memory: relevance to electrophysiological studies of hippocampal function. *Behav Neurosci* **110**(4): 661-72.

Goenjian, A. K., L. M. Najarian, et al. (1994). Posttraumatic stress disorder in elderly and younger adults after the 1988 earthquake in Armenia. *Am J Psychiatry* **151**(6): 895-901.

Gotthardt, U., U. Schweiger, et al. (1995). Cortisol, ACTH, and cardiovascular response to a cognitive challenge paradigm in aging and depression. *Am J Physiol* **268**(4 Pt 2): R865-73.

Gould, E., Tanapat, P., et al. (1998) Proliferation of granule cell precursors in the dentate gyrus of adult monkeys is diminished by stress. *Proc Natl Acad Sci USA* **95**: 3168-3171.

Grady, C.L., McIntosh, A.R., et al. (1995). Age-related reductions in Human Recognition Memory Due to Impaired Encoding *Science* **269** (14): 218-221.

Hickie, I., Scott, E., et al. (1995): Subcortical hyperintensities on magnetic resonance imaging: Clinical correlates and prognostic significance in patients with severe depression. *Biol Psychiatry* **37**: 151-161.

Hickie, I., Scott, E., et al. (1997): Subcortical hyperintensities on magnetic resonance imaging in patients with severe depression – a longitudinal evaluation. *Biol Psychiatry* **42 (5)**: 367-374.

Jernigan, T.L., Press, G.A., Hesselink, J.R. (1990) Methods for measuring brain morphologic features on magnetic resonance images. *Arch Neuro* **47**: 27-32.

Jernigan, T.L., Archibald, S.L., Berhow M.T., et al. (1991) Cerebral structure on MRI, Part I: Localization of age-related changes *Biol Psychiatry* **29**: 55-67.

Kato, H., N. Asukai, et al. (1996). Post-traumatic symptoms among younger and elderly evacuees in the early stages following the 1995 Hanshin-Awaji earthquake in Japan. *Acta Psychiatr Scand* **93**(6): 477-81.

Kendler, K. S. (1998). Anna-Monika-Prize paper. Major depression and the environment: a psychiatric genetic perspective. *Pharmacopsychiatry* **31**(1): 5-9.

Kessler, R. C. (2000). Posttraumatic stress disorder: the burden to the individual and to society. *J Clin Psychiatry* **61 Suppl 5**: 4-12; discussion 13-4.

Kessler, R. C., K. A. McGonagle, et al. (1994). Lifetime and 12-month prevalence of DSM-III-R psychiatric disorders in the United States. Results from the National Comorbidity Survey. *Arch Gen Psychiatry* **51**(1): 8-19.

Krishnan, K.R.R., Ritchie, J.C., et al. (1994). Apolipoprotein E-4: Reply [correspondence]. *Neurology* **44**: 2420-2421.

Ladd, C. O., M. J. Owens, et al. (1996). Persistent changes in corticotropin-releasing factor neuronal systems induced by maternal deprivation. *Endocrinology* **137**(4): 1212-8.

Lawrence, M. S. and R. M. Sapolsky (1994). Glucocorticoids accelerate ATP loss following metabolic insults in cultured hippocampal neurons. *Brain Res* **646**(2): 303-6.

Lemieux, A. M. and C. L. Coe (1995). Abuse-related posttraumatic stress disorder: evidence for chronic neuroendocrine activation in women. *Psychosom Med* **57**(2): 105-15.

Levy, A., S. Dachir, et al. (1994). Aging, stress, and cognitive function. *Ann N Y Acad Sci* **717**: 79-88.

Luine, V., M. Villegas, et al. (1994). Repeated stress causes reversible impairments of spatial memory performance. *Brain Res* **639**(1): 167-70.

Lupien, S.J., S. Gaudreau, et al. (1997). Stress-induced declarative memory impairment in healthy elderly subjects: Relationship to cortisol reactivity. *J Clin End Metab*_82:2070-2075.

Lupien, S., A. R. Lecours, et al. (1994). Basal cortisol levels and cognitive deficits in human aging. *J Neurosci* **14**(5 Pt 1): 2893-903.

Lupien, S. J., M. de Leon, et al. (1998). Cortisol levels during human aging predict hippocampal atrophy and memory deficits. *Nat Neurosci* **1**(1): 69-73.

Lupien, S. J., N. P. Nair, et al. (1999). Increased cortisol levels and impaired cognition in human aging: implication for depression and dementia in later life. *Rev Neurosci* **10**(2): 117-39.

Magarinos, A. M. and B. S. McEwen (1995). Stress-induced atrophy of apical dendrites of hippocampal CA3c neurons: involvement of glucocorticoid secretion and excitatory amino acid receptors. *Neuroscience* **69**(1): 89-98.

Magarinos, A. M., B. S. McEwen, et al. (1996). Chronic psychosocial stress causes apical dendritic atrophy of hippocampal CA3 pyramidal neurons in subordinate tree shrews. *J Neurosci* **16**(10): 3534-40.

Magarinos, A.M., Verdugo, J.M., et al. (1997). Chronic stress alters synaptic terminal structure in hippocampus. *Proc Natl Acad Sci USA* **94**:14002-14008.

McEwen, B. S., J. Angulo, et al. (1992). Paradoxical effects of adrenal steroids on the brain: protection versus degeneration. *Biol Psychiatry* **31**(2): 177-99.

Newcomer, J. W., S. Craft, et al. (1994). Glucocorticoid-induced impairment in declarative memory performance in adult humans. *J Neurosci* **14**(4): 2047-53.

O'Brien, J. T., I. Schweitzer, et al. (1994). Cortisol suppression by dexamethasone in the healthy elderly: effects of age, dexamethasone levels, and cognitive function. *Biol Psychiatry* **36**(6): 389-94.

Packan, D. R. and R. M. Sapolsky (1990). Glucocorticoid endangerment of the hippocampus: tissue, steroid and receptor specificity. *Neuroendocrinology* **51**(6): 613-8.

Pantel, J., Schroder, J., et al. (1997). Quantitative magnetic resonance imaging in geriatric depression and primary degenerative dementia. *J Affect Disord* **42**: 69-83.

Parnetti, L., D. T. Lowenthal, et al. (1996). 1H-MRS, MRI-based hippocampal volumetry, and 99mTc-HMPAO-SPECT in normal aging, age-associated memory impairment, and probable Alzheimer's disease. *J Am Geriatr Soc* **44**(2): 133-8.

Pavlides, C., A. Kimura, et al. (1995). Hippocampal homosynaptic long-term depression/depotentiation induced by adrenal steroids. *Neuroscience* **68**(2): 379-85.

Pomara, N., P. M. Doraiswamy, et al. (2002). Mifepristone (RU 486) for Alzheimer's disease. *Neurology* **58**(9): 1436.

Raskind, M. A., E. R. Peskind, et al. (1995). The effects of normal aging on cortisol and adrenocorticotropin responses to hypertonic saline infusion. *Psychoneuroendocrinology* **20**(6): 637-44.

Sapolsky, R. M. (1986). Glucocorticoid toxicity in the hippocampus. Temporal aspects of synergy with kainic acid. *Neuroendocrinology* **43**(3): 440-4.

Sapolsky, R. M. (1996). Why stress is bad for your brain. *Science* **273**(5276): 749-50.

Sapolsky, R. M., L. C. Krey, et al. (1983a). The adrenocortical stress-response in the aged male rat: impairment of recovery from stress. *Exp Gerontol* **18**(1): 55-64.

Sapolsky, R. M., L. C. Krey, et al. (1983b). Corticosterone receptors decline in a site-specific manner in the aged rat brain. *Brain Res* **289**(1-2): 235-40.

Sapolsky, R. M., L. C. Krey, et al. (1985). Prolonged glucocorticoid exposure reduces hippocampal neuron number: implications for aging. *J Neurosci* **5**(5): 1222-7.

Sapolsky, R. M., L. C. Krey, et al. (1986). The neuroendocrinology of stress and aging: the glucocorticoid cascade hypothesis. *Endocr Rev* **7**(3): 284-301.

Sapolsky, R. M., D. R. Packan, et al. (1988). Glucocorticoid toxicity in the hippocampus: in vitro demonstration. *Brain Res* **453**(1-2): 367-71.

Sapolsky, R. M., H. Uno, et al. (1990). Hippocampal damage associated with prolonged glucocorticoid exposure in primates. *J Neurosci* **10**(9): 2897-902.

Sass, K. J., D. D. Spencer, et al. (1990). Verbal memory impairment correlates with hippocampal pyramidal cell density. *Neurology* **40**(11): 1694-7.

Seeman, T. E., L. F. Berkman, et al. (1995). Self-esteem and neuroendocrine response to challenge: MacArthur studies of successful aging. *J Psychosom Res* **39**(1): 69-84.

Sheline, Y. I., P. Wang, et al. (1996). Hippocampal atrophy in major depression. *Proc Nat Acad Sci USA* **93**: 3908-3913.

Soininen, H. S., K. Partanen, et al. (1994). Volumetric MRI analysis of the amygdala and the hippocampus in subjects with age-associated memory impairment: correlation to visual and verbal memory. *Neurology* **44**(9): 1660-8.

Stein-Behrens, B. A., W. J. Lin, et al. (1994). Physiological elevations of glucocorticoids potentiate glutamate accumulation in the hippocampus. *J Neurochem* **63**(2): 596-602.

Stein-Behrens, B. A. and R. M. Sapolsky (1992). Stress, glucocorticoids, and aging. *Aging (Milano)* **4**(3): 197-210.

Sullivan, E. V., L. Marsh, et al. (1994). Age-related decline in MRI volumes of temporal lobe gray matter but not hippocampus. *Neurobiol Aging* **16**(4): 591-606.

Swaab, D. F., F. C. Raadsheer, et al. (1994). Increased cortisol levels in aging and Alzheimer's disease in postmortem cerebrospinal fluid. *J Neuroendocrinol* **6**(6): 681-7.

Uno, H., R. Tarara, et al. (1989). Hippocampal damage associated with prolonged and fatal stress in primates. *J Neurosci* **9**(5): 1705-11.

Urban, R. J. (1992). Neuroendocrinology of aging in the male and female. *Endocrinol Metab Clin North Am* **21**(4): 921-31.

Vaher, P. R., V. N. Luine, et al. (1994). Effects of adrenalectomy on spatial memory performance and dentate gyrus morphology. *Brain Res* **656**(1): 71-8.

Van Cauter, E., R. Leproult, et al. (1996). Effects of gender and age on the levels and circadian rhythmicity of plasma cortisol. *J Clin Endocrinol Metab* **81**(7): 2468-73.

Virgin, C. E., Jr., T. P. Ha, et al. (1991). Glucocorticoids inhibit glucose transport and glutamate uptake in hippocampal astrocytes: implications for glucocorticoid neurotoxicity. *J Neurochem* **57**(4): 1422-8.

Woolley, C.S., Gould, E., et al. (1990).Exposure to excess glucocorticois alters dendritic morphology of adult hippocampal pyramidal neurons. *Brain Res* **531**: 225-231.

Yehuda, R., B. Kahana, et al. (1995). Low urinary cortisol excretion in Holocaust survivors with posttraumatic stress disorder. *Am J Psychiatry* **152**(7): 982-6.

Zola-Morgan, S. M. and L. R. Squire (1990). The primate hippocampal formation: evidence for a time-limited role in memory storage. *Science* **250**(4978): 288-90.

In: Cognition and Mood Interactions
Editor: Miao-Kun Sun, pp. 161-183
ISBN 1-59454-229-5
2005 © Nova Science Publishers, Inc.

Chapter X

Age-Related Changes in Memory and Mood

Elizabeth M. Zelinski* and Robert F. Kennison

Leonard Davis School of Gerontology, Andrus Gerontology Center
University of Southern California, Los Angeles, CA, USA

This chapter reviews the literature on population changes in memory and depression with age. Recent work shows the importance of going beyond cross-sectional comparisons to longitudinal follow up studies. However, selection bias affects outcomes in studies of change in memory and depression. Health, education, and other individual differences are also important to consider as covariates of both memory and mood change. Recent work on biological mechanisms of memory suggest that stress due to depression may be an important factor in memory decline in depressed individuals, but these studies are correlational and causality has not yet been clearly established. Similarly, research on memory complaints and their association with memory performance and depression has also been correlational, and despite limited evidence, all may need to be considered in predicting cognitive decline.

1. Introduction

Memory and mood in older adults are interrelated in complex ways, and they involve a broad array of issues ranging from effects of depression on performance in laboratory tasks to diagnosis of dementia. In this chapter, we briefly review recent issues in the evaluation of age associated memory change, specifically the role of depression, health, socioeconomic status, and other factors. Next, we discuss research issues in depression and mood, and review the literature on the relationship between memory and depression. We focus on linkages between memory and depression in both normal older adult population studies and in demented sample and population studies. We also briefly review biological and neurological changes that predict memory, depression, and their interaction, with emphasis on the recent allostatic load literature. Finally, we evaluate the relationship between self-reported memory complaints and their relationship to memory performance, depression, and dementia. We conclude with recommendations for new directions in research in these areas. Our focus will be on population studies, where possible, because they provide the best evidence of generalizable relationships between the measures of interest (as discussed below).

There are extensive reviews in the literature on the role of various cognitive mechanisms, including memory, that change "normally" with age (e.g., Zacks, Hasher, & Li, 2000). Many of these studies involve comparisons between college-aged individuals and people in their 60s and 70s, who are matched in education. Thus, although these studies can elucidate changes or differences in "the cream of the crop" older adults, they are silent as to changes that occur in older adults who are not college educated. Relatively few of these studies, in the experimental literature, address changes in the fastest growing segment of the older population, the oldest-old. As a result, we will review studies, where possible, that focus on populations of older adults with the full range of age and education, or those studies that examine age change longitudinally. We report that there are important covariates of memory performance, which are also correlated with one another, and that it is critical to identify both independent and shared variance in these predictors of memory in older adults. When this is done, there remain declines in memory performance that are associated with age.

As in the experimental psychology literature, the clinical literature on depression is subject to interpretive difficulties that are due, in part, to extensive use of convenience samples often with small numbers of people tested. For example, participants in convenience samples may vary greatly in mental health and depression history, medication use and compliance, and inpatient status. In such studies generalizability is limited, and results between studies are often found to be contradictory.

Another major concern that has yet to be resolved surrounds the complexity of classifying mental disorders. Depression is difficult to characterize in older adults (Lavretsky & Kumar, 2002). Reasons for this include (1) overlap between different characteristics such as anxiety and low mood, and issues related to cognitive aspects of mood, (2) instability of subtypes of depression over time, and (3) the finding that significant nonclinical depression that does not meet diagnostic criteria for a major depressive disorder still has major functional effects. In older adults, subclinical symptoms are more common than major depressive disorders (Judd et al., 1998). Blazer and colleagues have argued that adults over 60 have a unique symptom cluster profile relative to younger individuals that does not neatly fit DSM criteria. This includes depressed mood, psychomotor retardation, poor concentration, constipation, and poor self-perception of health (Blazer, Woodbury, Hughes, & George, 1989). Thus, in this chapter, we aim to characterize normative changes in mood, and we focus our review on age differences in response to depression scales in population surveys (as opposed to studies that focus on diagnosis of major depression with DSM criteria), only discussing the clinical literature in order to validate points made from the normative literature. That is, we evaluate both cross-sectional and longitudinal population studies in symptom reports.

2. "Normal" Memory Change with Age—Recent Studies

Age differences in episodic memory have consistently been observed between college aged and older participants (Zacks et al., 2000). There are also age differences between young-old and old-old participants, that is, people in their 60s vs. those in their 80s and up (e.g., Colsher & Wallace, 1991; Giambra, Arenberg, Zonderman, Kawas, & Costa, 1995; Small, Dixon, Hultsch, & Hertzog, 1999). To some extent these differences may be attributed to cohort effects, including generational differences in education and familiarity with cognitive testing. However, the few comparisons of individuals at the same age but of different generational cohorts suggest that these differences are less due to cohort and more due to age (e.g., Hultsch, Hertzog, Dixon, & Small, 1998; Zelinski & Burnight, 1997). This suggests that age difference comparisons do reflect age changes in memory.

However, the often mixed and contradictory results of longitudinal studies suggest that identification of age changes is complex. Age decrements in memory are consistent only when performance is assessed over either a minimum of five years or in a large sample (see Zelinski & Burnight, 1997, for a review) suggesting that average decline is slow to accumulate and low in statistical power. In contrast, studies with more frequent testings tend to report few age changes in those who do not progress to dementia (e.g., Haan, Shemanski, Jagust, Manolio, & Kuller, 1999; Rubin et al., 1998; Sliwinski, Hofer, Hall, Buschke, & Lipton, 2003; Wilson et al., 2002). This may occur because individuals who participate in frequent retestings are inherently higher performers or that they remain stable or improve in performance because of familiarity with the tests or because of practice (see Zelinski & Burnight, 1997). Longitudinal studies of memory disagree on when declines begin, the rate of decline, and whether declines are nonmonotonic (e.g., Colsher & Wallace, 1991; Giambra et al., 1995, Schaie, 1996, Singer, Verhaeghen, Ghisletta, Lindenberger, & Baltes, 2003). The lack of consistency in results may be due to selection issues, including those associated with the age range of participants.

Attrition in aging studies is associated with risk factors for mortality. Poor memory performance is associated with subsequent death (Bosworth & Schaie, 1999; Botwinick, West, & Storandt, 1978; Deeg, Hofman, & van Zonneveld, 1990; Rabbitt et al., 2002; Siegler, McCarty, & Logue, 1982; Small and Bäckman, 1997) and accelerated rates of decline prior to death have been reported (Hassing, Small, von Strauss, Fratiglioni, & Bäckman, 2002; Kennison & Zelinski, 2004, submitted; Sliwinski et al., 2003). However, dropout has been recently shown to be a better indicator of rapid memory decline than death in longitudinal research (Kennison & Zelinski, 2004, submitted; Sliwinski et al., 2003). Sliwinski et al. (2003) suggested that time to death may represent effects of illness and medical interventions, whereas time to dropout involves a wider series of attrition related phenomena and will therefore capture more variability in performance. Some of these effects are health related declines, perceived declines in self-appraisal of performance, and depression. The net effect of attrition is an increase in selectivity of samples in longitudinal research that tends to bias observed change.

Kennison and Zelinski (2004, submitted) found that there were substantial differences in memory performance in a population sample of Americans aged 70 and up depending on whether they remained in the study. Those who dropped out of the study had poorer performance at the average age of entry into the study and declined more quickly. However, the rate of decline varied with age—it increased into the 80s, then slowed during and after the mid-90s. This suggests that dropout status increased the rate of age declines whereas survival into very old age reduced them. However, there were declines with age in memory not accounted for by dropout status, suggesting that age still accounted for some of the variance in the observed declines.

Survival effects in very old age are the mirror image of death or dropout effects, whereby participants who may typically perform more poorly at baseline, such as nonwhites, compared to whites, and males, compared to females, may exhibit less age-related decline than their counterparts at the upper reaches of the lifespan (Bosworth & Schaie, 1999; Stewart, Zelinski, & Wallace, 2000). Survival may also moderate effects observed in earlier periods of old age. For example, Zelinski, Crimmins, Reynolds, and Seeman (1998) found that low health ratings, diabetes, or high blood pressure had negative effects on cognition for individuals in their 70s, but null or positive effects for individuals in their 80s and beyond.

3. Demographic and Health Effects on Memory Performance

Most theories of cognitive aging assume that similar mechanisms predict performance across individuals, at all points of the life span. But support for these theories is often based on findings comparing young adults with people in their 60s and 70s (Bäckman, Small, Wahlin, & Larsson, 2000). Recently however, the increase in the number of individuals living into their eighties and beyond, has led to inquiries about whether broad theories of cognition apply across the entire span of adulthood. Although the possibility that developmental discontinuities emerge in later life, that is, the predictors of cognition change as people age has some support (Baltes, 1987), several large population surveys in the US suggest that there is considerable continuity.

For example, education is a strong correlate of memory performance across the full range of old age (e.g., Colsher & Wallace, 1991; Zelinski et al., 1998; Zelinski & Gilewski, 2003). White race is also associated with an advantage in recall ability, as the effect of race is clearly associated with socioeconomic status variables, which are associated strongly with cognition (Neisser et al., 1996), into old age (Herzog & Wallace, 1997). Women have a slight advantage over men on recall tasks (Zelinski & Stewart, 1998). Direct evaluation of interactions of education, race, and gender with age has revealed few changes in the relative effects of education and race. Several surveys suggest that gender effects do not interact with age (e.g., Herlitz, Nilsson, & Bäckman, 1997; Stewart et al., 2000, Study 1), but one indicates that the female advantage reduces with very old age (Zelinski & Gilewski, 2003). It is likely that such effects, where found, reflect effects of mortality and poor health in the disadvantaged group (e.g., men), resulting in unbalanced attrition and survivor effects, and not the effects of age per se.

The role of health in memory ability is an important consideration in understanding age related memory change. Recently, Bäckman et al. (2000) predicted that individuals over the age of 75 would show small effects of demographic characteristics but large effects of health on performance, while those younger than 75 would have the opposite relationship. Increases in the prevalence of chronic medical conditions that may affect cognition such as hypertension, heart disease, diabetes, lung disease, and stroke, are associated with age (e.g., Elias, Elias, & Elias, 1990; Siegler & Costa, 1985), and so it is possible that the role of health in memory performance increases with age. Zelinski and Gilewski (2003) tested this hypothesis using data from Asset and Health Dynamics of the Oldest-Old, a representative survey of Americans over the age of 70, but found that the demographic variables had larger effects than health on recall. They suggested that those who live into very old age are hardier than those who do not (survival effects), that demographic variables are preeminent as predictors of cognition because of selection factors, and that interactions with age such as the one with gender may therefore reflect sampling differences between cross-sectional populations.

Although demographic predictors such as education are important in memory performance, the complication is that education is strongly related to the probability of experiencing specific medical conditions or reporting poorer health ratings (Feinstein, 1993) and will suppress effects of health on memory performance in correlational studies. In older adults, health ratings correlate with objective indicators such as physician ratings (La Rue, Bank, Jarvik, & Hetland, 1979; Linn & Linn, 1980; Maddox & Douglass, 1973), but they include not only a "health" component, but also subjective "psychological" components (e.g., Costa & McCrae, 1987; Liang, 1986). Some portion of this psychological component is manifested as depression, or negative affectivity (Watson & Pennebaker, 1989), which is associated with more negative health appraisals. Because depression is also associated with memory performance (Burt, Zembar, & Niederehe, 1995), as will be discussed in a subsequent section, associations of health ratings with memory may be related to the psychological component of health ratings rather than to actual disease-related impairments. Blazer and colleagues have suggested that low health ratings themselves are a manifestation of a specific geriatric depression symptom cluster (Blazer et al., 1989). Thus, education, health ratings, and depression scores are interrelated, leading to the possibility of suppression effects in analyses that attempt to partial out variance associated with each. These may, in turn, lead to faulty or misleading conclusions.

Studies examining aging and memory therefore should evaluate whether education, self-rated health, and depression predict variance independently. The few studies that have evaluated these covariates do report that there are independent effects of each source of variability. Thus, health, independent of education and depression, is a predictor of memory in large-sample studies that evaluate the full range of old age and of health experience (see Zelinski et al., 1998).

4. Measurement of Depression: Symptoms vs. Diagnosis in Old Age

One of the issues in evaluating memory and depression as covariates is that there are age differences in self-reports of depressive symptoms as well as in diagnosis of major depressive disorder. The direction of these differences is paradoxical: older adults report more symptoms but are less likely to be diagnosed as depressed (Kessler, Foster, Webster, & House, 1992). Diagnosis of depression is difficult for a number of reasons, especially in older adults (e.g., Lavretsky & Kumar, 2002). One of the major issues in an elderly population is the possible confounding of symptoms of depression with symptoms due to the disease. For example, Parkinson patients may show symptoms of psychomotor retardation but may not be depressed. In addition, it is not clear whether specific diseases affect neurological or endocrine systems that affect mood, whether these diseases cause physical or cognitive disabilities that lead to depression, or whether depression exacerbates the disabilities (see Krishnan et al., 2002). Thus, to avoid some of these difficulties and gain a clearer view, it may be wise take as preeminent, research on depression scales rather than on diagnosis of major depression or other affective disorders.

There are several major factors to consider in evaluating elevated depression scores in surveys. First, older adults are more at risk for health problems than younger ones, and people with medical conditions are more likely to have depressive symptoms than those without (e.g., Katon & Ciechanowski, 2002; Krishnan et al., 2002). Second, individuals with disabilities are more likely to be depressed, and risk for disability increases with age (see Lavretsky & Kumar, 2002). Third, women are more likely to score as depressed than men and the proportional increase in the number of women in the older population increases symptom reports when averaged (Dent et al., 1999). Fourth, many depression scales include somatic symptoms such as sleep and eating disturbances that increase in risk with age, but may not directly reflect depression (e.g., Lewinsohn, Seeley, Roberts, & Allen, 1997). Fifth, education is negatively related to depressive symptom reports, and because older adults have less education than younger ones, risk of such reports is greater. Studies attempting to tease out these multifarious effects report that after controlling for disability and health problems, as well as for vegetative symptom risk, older adults remain more at risk for symptoms of depression (Lewinsohn et al., 1997). There is also evidence from population surveys that depressive symptoms follow a parabolic course, with higher levels of symptoms in early and in late adulthood, and that these trends are found both for women and for men (e.g., Kessler et al., 1992). Thus, older adults are more likely to report all types of depressive symptoms even when confounding factors have been controlled.

As in the memory change literature, the best evidence for an increase with age in depressive symptoms should come from longitudinal research. Few changes are reported for the majority of subjects in these studies. Depression scores did not increase over a two year period for participants in the Australian Longitudinal Study of Ageing (ALSA: Anstey & Luszcz, 2002), with 77% of the sample with low and stable scores, 10% transitioning to depressed, 6% remitting, and 6% depressed at both occasions. Results from a 10-year prospective study in Helsinki indicated that on average, depression scores were stable, but that most of those scoring within a clinically significant range had remitted. However, some individuals did increase in depression score and they were more likely to have increased in cognitive impairment as well (Pitkälä, Kähönen-Väre, Valvanne, Strandberg, & Tilvis, 2003). The Longitudinal Aging Study of Amsterdam reported that the percentage of individuals with cutoff scores representing clinically significant depression increased over six years from 14 to

20% (van Gool et al., 2003). Thus, a minority of those who remain in depression studies show some increase in depression.

The validity of these longitudinal studies, however, is compromised by selection factors. In the ALSA study, those who dropped out had higher baseline depression scores and were also more likely to have died. This suggests that increases in depression may be underestimated because those who remain in the study have less baseline risk of depression. Survival effects may also be operative here, with those less depressed also more vigorous. In ALSA, eight year mortality was also associated with baseline depression score in men. Another concern is whether two points are sufficient to characterize patterns of depression change.

The Amsterdam Study on the Elderly (AMSTEL) study followed a group of 277 elderly individuals with high baseline depression scores over 6 years with a total of 14 repeated measurements. Only 14% remitted, and 44% fluctuated in depression score over the six-year period (Beekman et al., 2002). Those who remitted over time had relatively lower baseline scores. This suggests that repeated measurement reveals differential patterns of depression, and that the prognosis for permanent remission is poor in those with very high scores. Thus, two point longitudinal evaluations do little to reveal fluctuations in patterns of depression in older adults. Unfortunately, the depression score pattern of the majority of participants in AMSTEL has not yet been reported, so the study is agnostic as to the progression of depression scores in those who were not depressed at baseline.

These studies, taken together, suggest that selection bias is an issue in evaluating longitudinal change in depression, as those who drop out are more likely to have died, and those who remain alive were more depressed at baseline. It is not clear whether the general stability in depression scores reported in longitudinal research is an underestimate of incident depression, and whether the longitudinal course of depression scores parallels the age difference patterns observed in cross-sectional studies. Yet it appears that age related increases in depression are associated most strongly with poor health, the development of dementia, and mortality. Additional work is needed to characterize the course and correlates of depressive symptomatology in elderly populations.

A few studies have evaluated concurrent longitudinal change in depression and memory, but thus far, no association between depression change and memory decline has been observed (Comijs, Jonker, Beekman, & Deeg, 2001; Lavretsky, Ercoli, Siddarth, Bookheimer, Miller, & Small, 2003). These null effects may be attributed to practice effects as well as issues of selection and retention; depressed individuals are more likely to drop out of longitudinal studies, reducing the likelihood of identifying changes (see Kennison & Zelinski, 2004). Nevertheless, the use of sophisticated analytical techniques to examine longitudinal changes has not yet been incorporated into the study of depression in memory, and so we conclude that the evidence is very limited at this time.

5. The Relationship between Depression and Memory Performance in Nondemented Elderly Adults

Depression scores are negatively associated with recall (Cavanaugh & Murphy, 1986; Cipolli et al., 1995; La Rue, Swan, Carmelli, 1995; Luszcz, Bryan, & Kent, 1997; Zelinski et al., 1998). The association between depression and recall is stronger than that of depression and recognition (Bäckman & Forsell, 1994; Burt et al., 1995). Studies of recognition performance have suggested that people with higher depression scores are more cautious about responding when not certain about the correctness of answers (Dunbar & Lishman, 1984; Niederehe & Camp, 1985). Nevertheless, it appears that some portion of the memory deficit associated with depression involves memory processes and not just response bias.

Depression effects have been shown to affect attentional and working memory performance; systems that aid episodic memory performance. Effects of depression have been reported in both encoding and retrieval operations of episodic memory (Bäckman & Forsell, 1994), both of which involve strategy use. Depression related deficits have been reported for executive functions (Lyness, Eaton, & Schneider, 1994; McBride & Abeles, 2000), which impact the use of memory strategies in recall tasks. Similar results have been reported in working memory tasks that involve executive function or storage (Hayslip, Kennelly, & Maloy, 1990). Increased study times, and greater organizability of stimuli, improves performance in older adults with low depression scores, but not those with high scores (Bäckman & Forsell, 1994). Colby and Gotlib (1988) have suggested that depressed individuals show storage deficits that may be related to impaired rehearsal in depression. These results, taken together, indicate that some portion of the episodic memory deficit associated with depression involves strategy use or the lack there of in individuals with low mood. Strategy use involves cognitive effort, which may be decreased in depressed individuals. That is, strategy use may be affected by motivation problems due to apathy in individuals with higher depression scores.

In support of this assertion is the finding that measures of motivation are often more strongly predictive of cognitive performance than depression (Forsell, Jorm, Fratiglioni, Grut, & Winblad, 1993) and have been more strongly implicated in elderly men than women (Forsell, Jorm, & Winblad, 1994). Bäckman, Hill, and Forsell (1996) found that motivation related symptoms were related to performance decrements in memory whereas mood related symptoms were not, suggesting that motivational aspects of depression may have the strongest effects on memory performance. Both executive functioning and motivation reflect integrity of the frontal lobes, suggesting that frontal involvement may affect performance in depression.

6. Linking Depression and Memory Impairment

Biological theories of cognition suggest that memory impairment in depression may be linked not only to frontal or executive deficits, but to damage related to hippocampal function. A recent theory suggests that anatomical changes in hippocampus may be associated with stress. McEwen and colleagues, (1998; McEwen & Seeman, 1999) suggest that allostatic load may have major effects on a number of health outcomes, including hippocampal function. Adaptation to stress, allostasis, involves the recruitment of biological systems including the autonomic nervous system and the hypothalamic-pituitary-adrenal axis to promote adaptation. Allostatic load is a function of (1) the frequency of activation of the allostatic system, (2) the failure to reduce allostatic activity after stress, and (3) inadequate response of the allostatic system, which may elevate activity of counter-regulated allostatic systems (McEwen, 1998). The hippocampus has high levels of receptors for adrenal steroids, which are sensitive to allostatic load, and is involved in inhibition of hypothalamic-pituitary-adrenal axis activity. Destruction of hippocampal neurons occurs when stress levels are elevated over long periods such as months or years. In addition, short-term memory function is temporarily compromised when adrenal cortocoid levels are high.

Reductions in size and activation of the hippocampal formations, dorsal anterior cingulate, and frontal lobes have been noted in chronic depressives compared to normal controls and single episode depressives that parallel behavioral deficits in memory and executive functions (Bremner et al., 2000; Cummings, 1993; de Asis et al., 1999; Hickie et al., 1995; Shah, Klaus, Glabus, & Goodwin, 1998; Sheline, Sanghavi, Mintun, & Gado, 1999). The hippocampus, as well as the frontal lobes has been strongly associated with episodic memory performance, and individuals with high levels of allostatic load also show poorer memory performance. Hormones associated with high levels of stress, such as cortisol may be important in the atrophy of hippocampal tissue (McEdwen, recent), and higher cortisol levels are found in depression (Brown, Varghese, & McEwen, 2004). Thus, the link between depression and memory performance may be associated with allostatic load related reductions in brain structures associated with episodic memory performance.

However, the connection between glucocorticoids and memory performance is not as strong as might be expected. Higher basal cortisol is associated with decrements in performance on cognitive tests (e.g., Greendale, Kritz-Silverstein, Seeman, & Barrett-Connor, 2000). Decline in basal cortisol in successfully treated patients with Cushings' Disease (which causes high levels of endogenous cortisol for years) are associated with improvements in selective reminding recall and increase in hippocampal volume (Starkman, Giordani, Gebarski, & Schteingart, 2003). However, in all of these studies, multiple tests are administered with only some of the hypothesized to-be-affected tasks producing the expected results (e.g., Greendale, et al., 2000; Starkman et al., 2003). Cortisol level has no relationship to Mini Mental Status Exam performance (Greendale, 2000) but increasing cortisol levels or high levels at baseline are associated with poorer verbal and spatial delayed recall (Lupien et al., 1998). These effects may be low in statistical power, and it is very likely that structures other than hippocampus are involved during performance of different cognitive tasks, and that other variables such as education may affect performance. Thus, depression and stress appear to affect episodic memory performance but this relationship needs to be more clearly identified.

Another route to poorer memory functioning in depression is through cerebrovascular disorders. In MRI studies, deep white matter hyperintensities reported in patients with depression have been linked to impairments in memory and executive functioning (Hickie et al., 1995). Late-onset depression has also been linked to white matter hyperintensities and memory deficit (Lesser et al., 1995) suggesting that vascular effects of brain aging itself may be associated with both impaired cognition and depression.

7. Linking Depression and Memory Impairment in Dementia

Depression has been identified as a risk factor for dementia (Berger, Fratiglioni, Forsell, Winblad, & Bäckman, 1999; Tierney, Boyle, Lam, & Szalai, 1999). The prevalence of depression in dementia is considerably higher than in the normal population (Forsell & Winblad, 1998). In a population study, depression was associated with 3.2% of Alzheimer's disease cases and 21.2% of vascular dementia cases (odds ratio = 8.2), suggesting that it may distinguish between the two (Newman, 1999). Although prevalence of depression in Alzheimer's disease is fairly low, depression may be a predictor of development of Alzheimer's disease (Weiner, Edland, Luszczynska, 1994). Its association with memory and other cognitive impairments suggests that it is sensitive to pre-clinical cognitive difficulties, but see (O'Carroll, Conway, Ryman, & Prentice, 1997; Schmand, Jonker, Geerlings, & Lindeboom, 1997).

However, its utility as a diagnostic toll so far has been limited because the associations between cognitive functioning and dementias have generally been small (Jorm, 2000). Alexopoulos, Meyers, Young, Mattis, & Kakuma, (1993) in a small sample longitudinal study found that depressed patients with pseudo-dementia had an increased rate of dementia diagnosis approximately two years later and they concluded that "geriatric depression with reversible dementia is a clinical entity that includes a group of patients with early-stage dementing disorders...[and] is an indication that a thorough diagnostic workup and frequent follow-ups [are needed]" (p. 1693). In a recent meta-analysis, Jorm (2000) concluded that depression is a valid risk factor for dementia, although he cautioned that more research is needed to discriminate vascular dementia, cognitive decline, and perceived cognitive decline.

8. Memory Complaints, Depression, and Memory Performance

Low memory self-efficacy or the perception that memory function is poor is an important mental health construct in aging that is related to depression and to memory and may provide an important connection to understanding the development of dementia (see Hertzog & Hultsch, 2000). Negative self-efficacy ratings are related to increasing age (Gilewski, Zelinski, & Schaie, 1990; Herzog & Rodgers, 1989; Hultsch, Hertzog, & Dixon, 1987). Approximately 25% of Americans from a population sample over age 70 rate their memory ability as fair or poor (Soldo, Hurd, Rodgers, & Wallace, 1997). It may be assumed that concerns about memory abilities are based on concerns about developing cognitive impairment. However, low ratings are not veridical with respect to actual memory functioning.

Memory complaints have been associated with memory performance decrements in a number of studies (Bassett & Folstein, 1993; Cavanaugh & Poon, 1989; Bolla, Lindgren, Bonaccorsy, & Bleeker, 1991; Christensen, 1991; Erber, Szuchman, & Rothberg, 1992; Gagnon et al., 1994; Herzog & Rogers, 1989; Jonker, Launer, Hooijer, & Lindeboom, 1996; Lane & Zelinski, 2003; Levy-Cushman & Abeles, 1998; Niederehe & Yoder, 1989; Ponds & Jolles, 1996; Radziwillowicz & Radziwillowicz, 1998; Zelinski, Gilewski, & Anthony-Bergstone, 1990), but null or negative effects have also often been reported (Barker, Prior, & Jones, 1995; Bolla et al., 1991; Derouesne, Lacomblez, Thibault, & LePoncin, 1999; Jorm et al., 1997; Kahn, Zarit, Hilbert, & Niederehe, 1975; Niederehe & Camp, 1985; O'Connor, Pollitt, Roth, Brook, & Reiss , 1990; O'Hara, Hinrichs, Kohout, Wallace, & Lemke, 1986; Palsson, Johansson, Berg, & Skoog, 2000; Schofield et al.,1997).

Longitudinal studies too have had mixed results. Memory complaint has been associated with memory decline in some studies (Lane & Zelinski, 2003; Schofield et al., 1997; Taylor, Miller, & Tinklenberg, 1992) but not others (Flicker, Ferris, & Reisberg, 1993; Jorm et al., 1997; Zelinski, Gilewski, & Schiae, 1993). Lane and Zelinski (2003) reported that self assessed frequency of forgetting was negatively associated with text recall, while ratings of seriousness of forgetting and retrospective memory functioning were negatively associated with list recall. Paradoxically, nineteen-year declines in performance in list and text recall were associated with reports of more frequent mnemonic usage suggesting that accurate monitoring of memory functioning may result in appropriate increases in compensatory strategies to offset declines. Jorm, Christensen, Korten, Jacomb, & Henderson (2001) demonstrated that memory complaints predict future memory declines. The reverse was also found; memory complaints retroactively predicted memory declines. Wang et al. (2000) found that baseline memory complaint predicted memory performance after controlling for depression and other variables, however, memory complaint did not predict memory decline in longitudinal comparisons.

Studies that have used appropriate methodologies including longitudinal follow-ups, community and population sampling, and modeling with incomplete data, and which have controlled for the effects of depression have tended to lend support for a positive relationship between self reports and performance (Jonker, Greelings, & Schmand, 2000). With appropriate controls, memory complaints thus account independently for approximately 3-10% of the variance in performance (Zelinski, Lane, & Burnight, 2001; Lane & Zelinski, 2003).

Various explanations for the modest relationship between memory complaints and memory performance have been proposed. The implicit theory hypothesis (McFarland, Ross, & Giltrow, 1992) suggests that older adults are aware of general age related deficits in memory and cognition and expect these changes to occur in themselves (Hertzog & Hultsch, 2000). The belief that memory declines with age is widely held among people of differing ages (Kite & Johnson, 1988; Ryan, 1992). At least partial support of the implicit theory hypothesis has been obtained (Lane & Zelinski, 2003; McDonadl-Miszczak, Hertzog, & Hultsch, 1995), and it likely explains some of the inaccuracy found in reporting of memory performance.

Memory complaints as already indicated, are associated with depression scores (Cutler & Grams, 1988; Ponds, Commissaries, & Jolles, 1997). Older adults believe that they have less control over their memories than younger adults (Hultsch et al., 1987), and they fear that memory difficulties may lead to dementia (Commissaris, Verhey, Ponds, Jolles, & Kok, 1994).

Responses to memory self-efficacy questionnaires are more highly correlated with depression than with memory performance (e.g., Kahn, Zarit, Hilbert, & Niederehe, 1975; Levy-Cushman & Abeles, 1998; Niederehe & Yoder, 1989; Popkin, Gallagher, Thompson, & Moore, 1982; Schofield et al., 1997; West, Boatwright, & Schleser, 1984). Harwood, Barker, Ownby, Mullan, & Duara (1999; also see Harwood et al., 1999b) found in a large sample study of 3225 older adults that risk of depression was predicted by memory complaints and female gender, but not by age, education, presence of the APOE-4 allele, or marital status. Memory complaints have been shown to decrease as depressive symptoms subside (Plotkin, Mintz, & Jarvik, 1985), and following treatment of depression (Popkin et al., 1985). Niederehe and Yoder (1989) found that depressed people reported more generalized memory difficulties that were also more extensive than controls, and that age did not interact with reports.

Nevertheless, the relationship between memory self-efficacy and depression remains rather modest, with bivariate correlations ranging from -.30 to -.36 or with depression independently accounting for up to 16% of the variance in self-efficacy (e.g., Bolla et al., 1991; Johannson, Allen-Burge, & Zarit, 1997; West et al., 1984).

Recently it has been suggested that the relationship between memory self-efficacy and depression is more closely associated with personality-related depression rather than low mood. Memory self-efficacy is more pessimistic for people with high neuroticism than for people with low neuroticism. This has been confirmed in studies that have reported higher negative affectivity and lower memory self-efficacy (Barker, Carter, & Jones, 1994; Cavanaugh & Murphy, 1986; Cavanaugh & Poon, 1989; Christensen, 1991; Lane & Zelinski, 2003; Ponds & Jolles, 1996; Smith, Petersen, Ivnik, Malec, & Tangalos, 1996). A meta-analysis confirmed that neuroticism is an independent predictor of self-efficacy ratings on a wide range of cognitive tasks, including memory (Judge & Ilies, 2002). However, Zelinski and Gilewski (2003) found that depression scores suppressed effects of neuroticism in predicting memory self-efficacy. This may indicate that mood has effects over and above a major personality factor in predicting memory complaints. However, the direction of causality with respect to depression and neuroticism is controversial.

Individuals treated for major depression do decline in neuroticism (e.g., Griens, Jonker, Spinhove, & Blom, 2002) but other work suggests that neuroticism may represent a mood-dispositional trait that remains high in individuals prone to experience negative affect, even after treatment has reduced depression (e.g., Harkness, Bagby, Joffe, & Levitt, 2002). It is likely that variance associated with either state or trait depression, or both, is associated with memory complaints.

Besides age, memory performance declines, depressive affect or personality, other covariates of memory self-efficacy include education, with more educated people rating themselves higher in efficacy, and health ratings, with those reporting better health reporting better memory (Zelinski et al., 2001). Relationships between memory self-efficacy, age, education, depression, education, and health are similar for both convenience samples as well as the population sample of over 7000 American adults over age 70 in the Asset and Health

Dynamics of the Oldest-old (AHEAD) study (Zelinski et al., 2001). The consistency of identified covariates of memory self-efficacy across samples suggests that these individual differences predictors represent stable sources of variance in self reported memory (Zelinski & Gilewski, 2003). These are similar predictors for memory performance at the population level.

In sum, memory complaints should not be considered to be accurate descriptions of actual memory performance. They nevertheless have some predictive value when considered in the context of the reporting individual's tendency towards neuroticism and towards depression, and are tempered in the context of the belief held by most elders that memory declines with age (Lane & Zelinski, 2003). Memory complaints may indicate the presence of depression, and when they are voiced, should prompt clinicians to further evaluate whether depression exists.

9. Depression, Memory Complaints, and Dementia

Studies evaluating clinical populations report reliable associations between memory complaints and performance in the pre-clinical and early stages of Alzheimer's disease (Geerlings, Jonker, Bouter, Adèr, & Schmand, 1999) and other forms of dementia (Derouesné, Lacomblez, Thibault, & LePoncin, 1996), but the accuracy of self-reports drops as the disease progresses (Grut et al., 1993). For example, Geerlings et al. (1999) found that memory complaints predicted incidence of Alzheimer's disease, but only in patients that did not have associated memory impairment at baseline. Given difficulties associated with differentiating pre-clinical dementia from normal age associated memory impairments, and that denial and other factors may affect ratings of memory functioning in these populations, pre-clinical dementia is likely to cloud the accuracy of memory complaints.

Memory complaints have been assessed as a diagnostic indicator of Alzheimer's disease (c.f., Jonker et al., 2000), but the association is often weak (Schmand et al., 1997), and differentiating between pseudo-Alzheimer's symptoms in depression and the actual disease has been difficult (O'Carroll et al., 1997; O'Connor et al., 1990). The fact that memory deficits are found in patients with either Alzheimer's disease or depression has lead to difficulties in diagnosis and frequent misdiagnosis, particularly for Alzheimer's disease (Feinberg & Goodman, 1984). People with pre-clinical or early Alzheimer's disease often deny or mask symptoms by avoiding memory intense situations, and they frequently experience depression associated symptoms that may or may not rise to the level of diagnosis (see Jonker et al., 2000). In addition, memory and executive functioning complaints and deficits are common in depression. Some studies have reported that it was not possible to distinguish early dementia from depression based on standard diagnostic criteria, and on psychometric test batteries (Rubin, Kinscherf, Grant, & Storandt, 1991).

In a review of both cross-sectional and longitudinal studies, Jonker et al. (2000) concluded that memory complaints predict dementia when associated with mild cognitive impairment and the duration is greater than two-years. We agree with Grut et al's. conclusion that "the patient's own complaints should not be ignored, as subjects in the mild state of dementia often have some insight into their own memory deficit" (p. 1295). Yet complaints lack diagnostic specificity and should be evaluated in the context of a thorough diagnostic workup and corroborating reports from others.

10. Conclusions

Despite a number of methodological issues in the measurement of memory change and depression change, both memory declines and increases in depressive symptomatology are affected by aging. Because symptoms of depression occur at high levels in both young and old adults (Kessler et al., 1989) this suggests that memory deficits in older adults are not only due to depression. Meta-analysis confirms that depression-associated memory deficits are greater in young than in older adults (Burt et al., 1995). Nevertheless, the declines in memory performance and increase in depression and correlations between the two observed in most older adults, indicate that depression is one of a host of factors that may be contributing to poor memory performance, and that clinical memory decline may also contribute to depression, and that underlying brain changes may be responsible for both. Much remains to be done in identifying and clarifying causal relationships. Data emerging from ongoing longitudinal population studies of memory, depression, and health changes in aging will provide some answers and undoubtedly new questions to our understanding of memory and mood changes with age.

References

Alexopoulos, G. S., Meyers, B. S., Young, R. C., Mattis, S., & Kakuma, T. (1993). The course of geriatric depression with "reversible dementia": A controlled study. *American Journal of Psychiatry, 150,* 1693-1699.

Anstey, K. J., & Luszcz, M. A. (2002). Mortality risk varies according to gender and change in depressive status in very old adults. *Psychosomatic Medicine, 64,* 880-888.

Bäckman, L., & Forsell, Y. (1994). Episodic memory functioning in a community-based sample of old adults with major depression: Utilization of cognitive support. *Journal of Abnormal Psychology, 103,* 361-370.

Bäckman, L., Hill, R. D., & Forsell, Y. (1996). The influence of depressive symptomatology on episodic memory functioning among clinically nondepressed older adults. *Journal of Abnormal Psychology, 105,* 97-105.

Bäckman, L., Small, B. J., Wahlin, A. & Larsson, M. (2000). Cognitive functioning in very old age. In F. I. M. Craik & T. A. Salthouse (Eds.), *The handbook of aging and cognition* (2nd ed., pp. 499-558). Mahwah, NJ: Lawrence Erlbaum Associates.

Baltes, P. (1987) Theoretical propositions of life-span developmental psychology: On the dynamics between growth and decline. *Developmental Psychology, 23,* 611-626.

Barker, A., Carter, C., & Jones, R. (1994). Memory performance, self-reported memory loss and depressive symptoms in attenders at a GP-referral and a self-referral memory clinic. *International Journal of Geriatric Psychiatry, 9,* 305-311.

Barker, A., Prior, J., & Jones, R. (1995). Memory complaint in attenders at a self-referral memory clinic: The role of cognitive factors, affective symptoms and personality. *International Journal of Geriatric Psychiatry, 10,* 777-781.

Bassett, S. S., & Folstein, M. F. (1993). Memory complaint, memory performance, and psychiatric diagnosis: A community study. *Journal of Geriatric Psychiatry and Neurology, 6,* 105-111.

Beekman, A. T. F., Geerlings, S. W., Deeg, D. J. H., Smit, J. H., Schoevers, R. S., de Beurs, E., et al. (2002). The natural history of late-life depression. *Archives of General Psychiatry, 59,* 605-611.

Berger, A.K., Fratiglioni, L., Forsell, Y., Winblad, B., & Bäckman, L. (1999). The occurrence of depressive symptoms in the preclinical phase of AD: A population-based study. *Neurology, 53,* 1998-2002.

Blazer, D. G., Woodbury, M., Hughes, D. C., & George, L. K. (1989). A statistical analysis of the classification of depression in a mixed community and clinical sample. *Journal of Affective Disorders, 16,* 11-20.

Bolla, K. I., Lindgren, K. N., Bonaccorsy, C., & Bleecker, M. L. (1991). Memory complaints in older adults: Fact or fiction? *Archives of Neurology, 48,* 61-64.

Bosworth, H. B., & Schaie, K. W. (1999). Survival effects in cognitive function, cognitive style and sociodemographic variables in the Seattle longitudinal study. *Experimental Aging Research, 25,* 121-139.

Botwinick, J., West, R. L., & Storandt, M. (1978). Predicting death from behavioral test performance. *Journal of Gerontology, 33,* 755-762.

Bremner, J. D., Narayan, M., Anderson, E. R., Staib, L. H., Miller, H. L., & Charney, D. S. (2000). Hippocampal volume reduction in major depression. *American Journal of Psychiatry, 157,* 115-117.

Burt, D. B., Zembar, M. J., & Niederehe, G. (1995). Depression and memory impairment: A meta-analysis of the association, its pattern, and specificity. *Psychological Bulletin, 117,* 285-305.

Cavanaugh, J. C., & Murphy, N. Z. (1986). Personality and metamemory correlates of memory performance in younger and older adults. *Educational Gerontology, 12,* 385-394.

Cavanaugh, J. C., & Poon, L. W. (1989). Metamemorial predictors of memory performance in young and older adults. *Psychology and Aging, 4,* 365-368.

Christensen, H. (1991). The validity of memory complaints by elderly persons. *International Journal of Geriatric Psychiatry, 6,* 307-312.

Cipolli, C., Neri, M., De Vreese, L. P., Pinelli, M., Rubichi, S., & Lalla, M. (1995). The influence of depression on memory and metamemory in the elderly. *Archives of Gerontology and Geriatrics, 23,* 111-127.

Colby, C. A., & Gotlib, I. H. (1988). Memory deficits in depression. *Cognitive Therapy and Research, 12,* 611-627.

Colsher, P. L., & Wallace, R. B. (1991). Longitudinal application of cognitive function measures in a defined population of community-dwelling elders. *Annals of Epidemiology, 1,* 215-230.

Comijs, H. C., Jonker, C., Beekman, A. T. F., & Deeg, D. J. H. (2001). The association between depressive symptoms and cognitive decline in community-dwelling elderly persons. *International Journal of Geriatric Psychiatry, 16*, 361-367.

Commissaris, C. J. A. M., Verhey, F. R. J., Ponds, R. W. H. M., Jolles, J. & Kok, G. (1994). Public education about normal forgetfulness and dementia: Importance and effects. *Patient Education and Counseling, 24*, 109-115.

Costa, P. T., & McCrae, R. R. (1987). On the need for longitudinal evidence and multiple measures in behavioral-genetic studies of adult personality. *Behavioral and Brain Sciences, 10*, 22-23.

Cummings, J. L. (1993). Frontal-subcortical circuits and human behavior. *Archives of Neurology, 50*, 873-880.

Cutler, S. J., & Grams, A. E. (1988). Correlates of self-reported everyday memory problems. *Journal of Gerontology, 43*, S82-S90.

de Asis, J. M., Stern, E., Alexopoulos, G. S., Pan, H., Van Gorp, W., Blumberg, H., et al. (2001). Hippocampal and anterior cingulate activation deficits in patients with geriatric depression. *American Journal of Psychiatry, 158*, 1321-1323.

Deeg, D. J. H., Hofman, A., & van Zonneveld, R. J. (1990). The role of change in cognitive function in survival of Dutch elderly. In P. J. D. Drenth & J. A. Sergeant (Eds.), *European perspectives in psychology, Vol. 1: Theoretical, psychometrics, personality, development, educational, cognitive, gerontological* (pp. 451-467). Oxford, England: John Wiley & Sons.

Dent, O. F., Waite, L. M., Bennett, H. P., Casey, B. J., Grayson, D. A., Cullen, J. S., et al. (1999). A longitudinal study of chronic and depressive symptoms in a community sample of older people. *Aging and Mental Health, 3*, 351-357.

Derouesné, C., Lacomblez, L., Thibault, S., & LePoncin, M. (1999). Memory complaints in young and elderly subjects. *International Journal of Geriatric Psychiatry, 14*, 291-301.

Dunbar, G. C., & Lishman, W. A. (1984). Depression, recognition-memory and hedonic tone: A signal detection analysis. *British Journal of Psychiatry, 144*, 376-382.

Elias, M. F., Elias, J. W., & Elias, P. K. (1990). Biological and health influences on behavior. In J. E. Birren & K. W. Schaie (Eds.), *Handbook of the psychology of aging* (3rd ed., pp. 79-102). San Diego, CA: Academic Press, Inc.

Erber, J. T., Szuchman, L. T., & Rothberg, S. T. (1992). Dimensions of self-report about everyday memory in young and older adults. *International Journal of Aging and Human Development, 34*, 311-323.

Feinberg, T., & Goodman, B. (1984). Affective illness, dementia, and pseudodementia. *Journal of Clinical Psychiatry, 45*, 99-103.

Feinstein, J. S. (1993). The relationship between socioeconomic status and health: A review of the literature. *Milbank Quarterly, 71*, 279-322.

Flicker, C., Ferris, S. H., & Reisberg, B. (1993). A longitudinal study of cognitive function in elderly persons with subjective memory complaints. *Journal of the American Geriatric Society, 41*, 1029-1032.

Forsell, Y., Jorm, A. F., Fratiglioni, L., Grut, M., & Winblad, B. (1993). Application of DSM-III-R criteria for major depressive episode to elderly subjects with and without dementia. *American Journal of Psychiatry, 150*, 1199-1202.

Forsell, Y., Jorm, A. F., & Winblad, B. (1994). Association of age, sex, cognitive dysfunction, and disability with major depressive symptoms in an elderly sample. *American Journal of Psychiatry, 151*, 1600-1604.

Forsell, Y., & Winblad, B. (1998). Major depression in a population of demented and nondemented older people: Prevalence and correlates. *Journal of the American Geriatrics Society, 46*, 27-30.

Gagnon, M., Dartigues, J. F., Mazaux, J. M., Dequae, L., Letenneur, L., Giroire, J. M., et al. (1994). Self-reported memory complaints and memory performance in elderly French community residents: Results of the PAQUID research program. *Neuroepidemiology, 13*, 145-154.

Geerlings, M. I., Jonker, C., Bouter, L. M., Adèr, H. J., & Schmand, B. (1999). Associated between memory complaints and incident Alzheimer's disease in elderly people with normal baseline cognition. *American Journal of Psychiatry, 156*, 531-537.

Giambra, L. M., Arenberg, D., Zonderman, A. B., Kawas, C., & Costa, P. T. (1995). Adult life span changes in immediate visual memory and verbal intelligence. *Psychology and Aging, 10*, 123-139.

Gilewski, M. J., Zelinski, E. M., & Schaie, K. W. (1990). The Memory Functioning Questionnaire for assessment of memory complaints in adulthood and old age. *Psychology and Aging, 5*, 482-490.

Greendale, G. A., Kritz-Silverstein, D., Seeman, T., & Barrett-Connor, E. (2000). Higher basal cortisol predicts verbal memory loss in postmenopausal women: Rancho Bernardo Study. *Journal of the American Geriatrics Society, 48*, 1655-1658.

Griens, A. M. G. F., Jonker, K., Spinhove, P. & Blom, M. B. J. (2002). The influence of depressive state features on trait measurement. *Journal of Affective Disorders, 70*, 95-99.

Grut, M., Jorm, A. F., Fratiglioni, L., Forsell, Y., Viitanen, M., & Winblad, B. (1993). Memory complaints of elderly people in a population survey: Variation according to dementia stage and depression. *Journal of the American Geriatrics Society, 41*, 1295-1300.

Haan, M. N., Shemanski, L., Jagust, W. J., Manolio, T. A., & Kuller, L. (1999). The role of APOE epsilon4 in modulating effects of other risk factors for cognitive decline in elderly persons. *Journal of the American Medical Association, 282*, 40-46.

Harkness, K. L., Bagby, R. M., Joffe, R. T., & Levitt, A. (2002). Major depression, chronic minor depression, and the Five-Factor Model of Personality. *European Journal of Personality, 16*, 271-281.

Harwood, D. G., Barker, W. W., Ownby, R. L., Mullan, M., & Duara, R. (1999). Factors associated with depressive symptoms in non-demented community-dwelling elderly. *International Journal of Geriatric Psychiatry, 14*, 331-337.

Hassing, L. B., Small, B. J., von Strauss, E., Fratiglioni, L., & Bäckman, L. (2002). Mortality-related differences and changes in episodic memory among the oldest old: Evidence from a population-based sample of nonagenarians. *Aging, Neuropsychology, and Cognition, 9*, 11-20.

Hayslip, B. J., Kennelly, K. J., & Maloy, R. M. (1990). Fatigue, depression, and cognitive performance among aged persons. *Experimental Aging Research, 16*, 111-115.

Herlitz, A., Nilsson, L.G., & Bäckman, L. (1997). Gender differences in episodic memory. *Memory and Cognition, 25*, 801-811.

Hertzog, C., & Hultsch, D. F. (2000). Metacognition in adulthood and old age. In F. I. M. Craik, & T. A. Salthouse (Eds), *The handbook of aging and cognition (2nd ed.)* (pp. 417-466). Mahwah, NJ: Lawrence Erlbaum Associates, Publishers.

Herzog, A. R., & Rodgers, W., L. (1989). Age differences in memory performance and memory ratings as measured in a sample survey. *Psychology and Aging, 4,*173-182.

Herzog A. R., & Wallace, R. B. (1997). Measures of cognitive functioning in the AHEAD study. *Journal of Gerontology: Psychological and Social Sciences, 52B (special issue),* 37-48.

Hickie, I., Scott, E., Mitchell, P., Wilhelm, K., Austin, M.-P., & Bennett, B. (1995). Subcortical hyperintensities on magnetic resonance imaging: Clinical correlates and prognostic significance in patients with severe depression. *Biological Psychiatry, 37,* 151-160.

Hultsch, D. F., Hertzog, C., & Dixon, R. A. (1987). Age differences in metamemory: Resolving the inconsistencies. *Canadian Journal of Psychology. Special Issue: Aging and cognition, 41,* 193-208.

Hultsch, D. F., Hertzog, C., Dixon, R. A., & Small, B. J. (1998). *Memory change in the aged.* New York: Cambridge University Press.

Johannson, B., Allen-Burge, R., & Zarit, S. H. (1997). Self-reports on memory functioning in a longitudinal study of the oldest-old: Relation to current, prospective, and retrospective performance. *Psychological Sciences, 52B*, P139-P146.

Jonker, C., Geerlings, M. I., & Schmand, B. (2000). Are memory complaints predictive for dementia? A review of clinical and population-based studies. *International Journal of Geriatric Psychiatry, 15*, 983-991.

Jonker, C., Launer, L. J., Hooijer, C., & Lindeboom, J. (1996). Memory complaints and memory impairment in older individuals. *Journal of the American Geriatrics Society, 44,* 44-49.

Jorm, A. F. (2000). Is depression a risk factor for dementia or cognitive decline? *Gerontology, 46*, 219-227.

Jorm, A. F., Christensen, H., Korten, A. E., Henderson, A. S., Jacomb, P. A., & Mackinnon, A. (1997). Do cognitive complaints either predict future cognitive decline or reflect past cognitive decline? A longitudinal study of an elderly community sample. *Psychological Medicine, 27*, 91-98.

Jorm, A. F., Christensen, H., Korten, A. E., Jacomb, P. A., & Henderson, A. S. (2001). Memory complaints as a precursor of memory impairment in older people: A longitudinal analysis over 7-8 years. *Psychological Medicine, 31*, 441-449.

Judd, L. L., Akiskal, H. S., Maser, J. D., Zeller, P. J., Endicott, J., Coryell, W., et al. (1998). Major depressive disorder: A prospective study of residual subthreshold depressive symptoms as predictor of rapid relapse. *Journal of Affective Disorders. Special Issue: George Winokur, 50*, 97-108.

Judge, T. A., & Ilies, R. (2002). Relationship of personality to performance motivation: A meta-analytic review. *Journal of Applied Psychology, 87*, 797-807.

Kahn, R. L., Zarit, S. H., Hilbert, N. M., & Niederehe, G. (1975). Memory complaint and impairment in the aged: The effect of depression and altered brain function. *Archives of General Psychiatry, 32,* 1569-1573.

Katon, W., & Ciechanowski, P. (2002). Impact of major depression on chronic medical illness. *Journal of Psychosomatic Research, 53,* 859-863.

Kennison, R. F., & Zelinski, E. M. (2004). *Estimating age change in 7-year list recall in AHEAD: The effects of independent predictors of missingness and dropout.* Manuscript submitted for publication.

Kessler, R. C., Foster, C., Webster, P. S., & House, S. (1992). The relationship between age and depressive symptoms in two national surveys. *Psychology and Aging, 7,* 119-126.

Kite, M. J. & Johnson, B. T. (1988). Attitudes toward older and younger adults: A meta-analysis. *Psychology and Aging, 3,* 233-244.

Krishnan, K. R. R., Delong, M., Kraemer, H., Carney, R., Spiegel, D., Gordon, C., et al. (2002). Comorbidity of depression with other medical diseases in the elderly. *Biological Psychiatry,* 52, 559-588.

Lane, C. J., & Zelinski, E. M. (2003). Longitudinal hierarchical linear models of the Memory Functioning Questionnaire. *Psychology and Aging, 18,* 38-53.

La Rue, A., Bank, L., Jarvik, L., & Hetland, M. (1979). Health in old age: How do physicians' ratings and self-ratings compare? *Journal of Gerontology, 34,* 687-691.

La Rue, A., Swan, G. E., & Carmelli, D. (1995). Cognition and depression in a cohort of aging men: Results from the Western Collaborative Group study. *Psychology and Aging, 10,* 30-33.

Lavretsky, H., Ercoli, L., Siddarth, P., Bookheimer, S., Miller, K., & Small, G. (2003). Apolipoprotein epsilon-4 allele status, depressive symptoms, and cognitive decline in middle-aged and elderly persons without dementia. *American Journal of Psychiatry, 11,* 667-673.

Lavretsky, H., & Kumar, A. (2002). Clinically significant non-major depression. *American Journal of Geriatric Psychiatry, 10,* 239-255.

Lesser, I. M., Boone, K. B., Mehringer, C. M., Wohl, M. A., Miller, B. L., & Berman, N. G. (1996). Cognition and white matter hyperintensities in older depressed patients. *American Journal of Psychiatry, 153,* 1280-1287.

Levy-Cushman, J., Abeles, N. (1998). Memory complaints in the able elderly. Clinical *Gerontologist, 19,* 3-24.

Lewinsohn, P. M., Seeley, J. R., Roberts, R. E., & Allen, N. B. (1997). Center for Epidemiologic Studies Depression Scale (CES-D) as a screening instrument for depression among community-residing older adults. *Psychology and Aging, 12,* 277-287.

Liang, J. (1986). Self-reported physical health among aged adults. *Journal of Gerontology, 41,* 248-260.

Linn, M. W., & Linn, B., S. (1980). Qualities of institutional care that affect outcome. *Aged Care and Services Review, 2,* 1, 3-14.

Lupien, S. J., de Leon, M., de Santi, S., Convit, A., Tarshish, C., Nair, N. P. V., et al. (1998). Cortisol levels during human aging predict hippocampal atrophy and memory deficits. *Nature Neuroscience, 1,* 69-73.

Luszcz, M. A., Bryan, J., & Kent, P. (1997). Predicting episodic memory performance of very old men and women: Contributions from age, depression, activity, cognitive ability, and speed. *Psychology and Aging, 12*, 340-351.

Lyness, S. A., Eaton, E. M., & Schneider, L. S. (1994). Cognitive performance in older and middle-aged depressed outpatients and controls. *Journal of Gerontology: Psychological Sciences, 49*, P129-P136.

Maddox, G. L., & Douglass, E. B. (1973). Aging and individual differences: A longitudinal analysis of social, psychological, and physiological indicators. *Journal of Gerontology, 29*, 555-563.

McBride, A. M., & Abeles, N. (2000). Depressive symptoms and cognitive performance in older adults. *Clinical Gerontologist, 21*, 27-47.

McEwen, B. S. (1998). Stress, adaptation, and disease: Allostasis and allostatic load. In S. M. McCann & J. M. Lipton (Eds.), *Annals of the New York Academy of Sciences, Vol. 840: Neuroimmunomodulation: Molecular aspects, integrative systems, and clinical advances* (pp. 33-44). New York: New York Academy of Sciences.

McEwen, B. S., & Seeman, T. (1999). Protective and damaging effects of mediators of stress: Elaborating and testing the concepts of allostasis and allostatic load. In N. E. Adler & M. Marmot (Eds.), *Socioeconomic status and health in industrial nations: Social, psychological, and biological pathways. Annals of the New York Academy of Sciences, Vol. 896* (pp. 30-47). New York: New York Academy of Sciences.

McFarland, C., Ross, M., & Giltrow, M. (1992). Biased recollections in older adults: The role of implicit theories of aging. *Journal of Personality and Social Psychology, 62*, 837-850.

Neisser, U., Boodoo, G,. Bouchard, T. J., Jr., Boykin, A. W., Brody, N., Ceci, S., J., et al. (1996). Intelligence: Knowns and unknowns. *American Psychologist, 51*, 77-101.

Newman, S. C. (1999). The prevalence of depression in Alzheimer's disease and vascular dementia in a population sample. *Journal of Affective Disorders, 52*, 169-176.

Niederehe, G., & Camp, C. J. (1985). Signal detection analysis of recognition memory in depressed elderly. *Experimental Aging Research, 11*, 207-213.

Niederehe, G., & Yoder, C. (1989). Metamemory perceptions in depressions of young and older adults. *Journal of Nervous and Mental Disease, 177*, 4-14.

O'Carroll, R. E., Conway, S., Ryman, A., & Prentice, N. (1997). Performance on the delayed word recall test (DWR) fails to differentiate clearly between depression and Alzheimer's disease in the elderly. *Psychological Medicine, 27*, 967-971.

O'Connor, D. W., Pollitt, P. A., Roth, M., Brook, P. B., & Reiss, B. B. (1990). Memory complaints and impairment in normal, depressed, and demented elderly persons identified in a community survey. *Archives of General Psychiatry, 47*, 224-227.

O'Hara, M. W., Hinrichs, J. V., Kohout, F. J., Wallace, R. B., & Lemke, J. H. (1986). Memory complaint and memory performance in the depressed elderly. *Psychology and Aging, 1*, 208-214.

Palsson, S., Johansson, B., Berg, S., & Skoog, I. (2000). A population study on the influence of depression on neuropsychological functioning in 85-year-olds. *Acta Psychiatrica Scandinavica, 101*, 185-193.

Pitkälä, K., Kähönen-Väre, M., Valvanne, J., Strandberg, T. E., Tilvis, R. S. (2003). Long-term changes in mood of an aged population: Repeated Zung-tests during a 10-year follow up. *Archives of Gerontology and Geriatrics, 36*, 185-195.

Plotkin, D. A., Mintz, J., & Jarvik, L. F. (1985). Subjective memory complaints in geriatric depression. *American Journal of Psychiatry, 142*, 1103-1105.

Ponds, R. W. H. M., & Jolles, J. (1996). Memory complaints in elderly people: The role of memory abilities, metamemory, depression, and personality. *Educational Gerontology, 22*, 341-357.

Ponds, R. W. H. M., Commissaris, K. J. A. M., & Jolles, J. (1997). Prevalence and covariates of subjective forgetfulness in a normal population in the Netherlands. *International Journal of Aging and Human Development, 45*, 207-221.

Popkin, S. J., Gallagher, D., Thompson, L. W., & Moore, M. (1982). Memory complaint and performance in normal and depressed older adults. *Experimental Aging Research, 8*, 141-145.

Rabbitt, P., Watson, P., Donlan, C., McInnes, L., Horan, M., Pendleton, N., et al. (2002). Effects of death within 11 years on cognitive performance in old age. *Psychology and Aging, 17*, 468-481.

Radziwillowicz, W., & Radziwillowicz, P. (1998). Memory functions in endogenous depression. *Psychiatria Polska, 32*, 187-197.

Ryan, E. B. (1992) Beliefs about memory changes across the adult life span. *Journals of Gerontology, 47*, P41-P46.

Rubin, E. H., Kinscherf, D. A., Grant, E. A., & Storandt, M. (1991). The influence of major depression on clinical and psychometric assessment of senile dementia of the Alzheimer type. *American Journal Psychiatry, 148*, 1164-1171.

Rubin, E. H., Storandt, M., Miller, P., Kinscherf, D. A., Grant, E. A., Morris, J. C., et al. (1998). A prospective study of cognitive function and onset of dementia in cognitively healthy elders. *Archives of Neurology, 55*, 395-401.

Schaie, K. W. (1996). Intellectual development in adulthood. In J. E. Birren & K. W. Schaie (Eds.), *Handbook of the psychology of aging* (4th ed., pp. 266-286). San Diego, CA: Academic Press, Inc.

Schofield, P. W., Marder, K., Dooneief, G., Jacobs, D. M., Sano, M., & Stern, Y. (1997). Association of subjective memory complaints with subsequent cognitive decline in community-dwelling elderly individuals with baseline cognitive impairment. *American Journal of Psychiatry, 154*, 609-615.

Schmand, B., Jonker, C., Geerlings, M. I., & Lindeboom, J. (1997). Subjective memory complaints in the elderly: Depressive symptoms and future dementia. *British Journal of Psychiatry, 171*, 373-376.

Shah, P. J., Ebmeier, K. P., Glabus, M. F., & Goodwin, G., M. (1998). Cortical grey matter reductions associated with treatment-resistant chronic unipolar depression: Controlled magnetic resonance imaging study. *British Journal of Psychiatry, 172*, 527-532.

Sheline, Y. I., Sanghavi, M., Mintun, M. A., & Gado, M. H. (1999). Depression duration but not age predicts hippocampal volume loss in medically healthy women with recurrent major depression. *Journal of Neuroscience, 19*, 5034-5043.

Siegler, I. C., & Costa, P. T. (1985). Health behavior relationships. In J. E. Birren & K. W. Schaie (Eds.), *Handbooks of the psychology of aging* (2ⁿᵈ ed., pp. 144-166). New York: Van Nostrand Reinhold Co., Inc.

Siegler, I. C., McCarty, S. M., & Logue, P. E. (1982). Wechsler Memory Scale scores, selective attrition, and distance from death. *Journal of Gerontology, 37*, 176-181.

Singer, T., Verhaeghen, P., Ghisletta, P., Lindenberger, U., & Baltes, P. B. (2003). The fate of cognition in very old age: Six-year longitudinal findings in the Berlin Aging Study (BASE). *Psychology and Aging, 18,* 318-331.

Sliwinski, M. J., Hofer, S. M., Hall, C., Buschke, H., & Lipton, R. B. (2003). Modeling memory decline in older adults: The importance of preclinical dementia, attrition, and chronological age. *Psychology and Aging, 18,* 658-671.

Small, B. J., & Bäckman, L. (1997). Cognitive correlates of mortality: Evidence from a population-based sample of very old adults. *Psychology and Aging, 12,* 309-313.

Small, B. J., Dixon, R. A., Hultsch, D. F., & Hertzog, C. (1999). Longitudinal changes in quantitative and qualitative indicators of word and story recall in young-old and old-old adults. *Journals of Gerontology: Series B: Biological Sciences and Medical Sciences, 54B*, P107-P115.

Smith, G. E., Petersen, R. C., Ivnik, R. J., Malec, J. F., & Tangalos, E. G. (1996). Subjective memory complaints, psychological distress, and longitudinal change in objective memory performance. *Psychology and Aging, 11*, 272-279.

Soldo, B. J., Hurd, M. D., Rodgers, W. L., & Wallace, R. B. (1997). Asset and Health Dynamics Among the Oldest-old: An overview of the AHEAD study. *Journal of Gerontology: Psychological and Social Sciences, 52B,* (special Issue), 1-20.

Starkman, M. N., Giordani, B., Gebarski, S. S., & Schteingart, D. E. (2003). Improvement in learning associated with increase in hippocampal formation volume. *Biological Psychiatry, 53*, 233-238.

Stewart, S. T., Zelinski, E. M., & Wallace, R. B. (2000). Age, medical conditions, and gender as interactive predictors of cognitive performance: The effects of selective survival. *Journals of Gerontology: Series B: Psychological Sciences and Social Sciences, 55B*, P381-P383.

Taylor, J. L., Miller, T. P., & Tinklenberg, J. R. (1992). Correlates of memory decline: A 4-year longitudinal study of older adults with memory complaints. *Psychology and Aging, 7*, 185-193.

Tierney, M. C., Boyle, E., Lam, R. E., & Szalai, J. P. (1999). Do depressive symptoms in memory-impaired elders predict probable Alzheimer's disease? *Aging and Mental Health, 3*, 88-93.

van Gool, C. H., Kempen, G. I. J. M., Penninx, B. W. J. H., Deeg., D. J. H., Beekman, A. T. F., & van Eijk, J. T. M. (2003). Relationship between changes in depressive symptoms and unhealthy lifestyles in late middle aged and older persons: Results from the Longitudinal Aging Study Amsterdam. *Age and Ageing, 32*, 81-87.

Wang, P. N., Wang, S. J., Fuh, J. L., Teng, E. L., Liu, C. Y., Lin, C. H., et al. (2000). Subjective memory complaint in relation to cognitive performance and depression: A longitudinal study of a rural Chinese population. *Journal of the American Geriatrics Society, 48*, 295-299.

Watson, D., & Pennebaker, J. W. (1989). Health complaints, stress, and distress: Exploring the central role of negative affectivity. *Psychological Review*, *96*, 234-254.

Weiner, M. F., Edland, S. D., Luszczynska, H. (1994). Prevalence and incidence of major depression in Alzheimer's disease. *American Journal of Psychiatry*, *151*, 1006-1009.

West, R., Boatwright, L. K., Schleser, R. (1984). The link between memory performance, self-assessment, and affective status. *Experimental Aging Research*, *10*, 197-200.

Wilson, R. S., Schneider, J. A., Barnes, L. L., Beckett, L. A., Aggarwal, N. T., Cochran, E. J., et al. (2002). The apolipoprotein E epsilon4 allele and decline in different cognitive systems during a 6-year period. *Archives of Neurology*, *59*, 1154-1160.

Zacks, R. T., Hasher, L., & Li, K. Z. H. (2000). Human memory. In F. I. M. Craik & T. A. Salthouse (Eds.), *The handbook of aging and cognition* (2nd ed., pp. 293-357). Mahwah, NJ: Lawrence Erlbaum Associates.

Zelinski, E. M., & Burnight, K. P. (1997). Sixteen-year longitudinal and time lag changes in memory and cognition in older adults. *Psychology and Aging*, *12*, 503-513.

Zelinski, E. M., Burnight, K. P., & Lane, C. J. (2001). The relationship between subjective and objective memory in the oldest old: Comparisons of findings from a representative and a convenience sample. *Journal of Aging and Health*, *13*, 248-266.

Zelinski, E. M., Crimmins, E., Reynolds, S., & Seeman, T. (1998). Do medical conditions affect cognition in older adults? *Health Psychology*, *17*, 504-512.

Zelinski, E. M., & Gilewski, M. J. (2003). Effects of demographic and health variables on Rasch scaled cognitive sores. *Journal of Aging and Health, 15,* 435-464.

Zelinski, E. M., Gilewski, M. J., & Anthony-Bergstone (1990). Memory Functioning Questionnaire: Concurrent validity with memory performance and self-reported memory failures. *Psychology and Aging*, 5, 388-399.

Zelinski, E. M., Gilewski, M. J., & Schaie, K. W. (1993). Individual differences in cross-sectional and 3-year longitudinal memory performance across the adult life span. *Psychology and Aging*, *8*, 176-186.

Zelinski, E. M., & Stewart, S. T. (1998). Individual differences in 16-year memory changes.*Psychology and Aging*, *13*, 622-630.

In: Cognition and Mood Interactions

Editor: Miao-Kun Sun, pp. 185-224

ISBN 1-59454-229-5

2005 © Nova Science Publishers, Inc.

Chapter XI

Convergence of Antidementia and Antidepressant Pharmacology

*Marta Weinstock**

Department of Pharmacology, School of Pharmacy

Hebrew University Hadassah Medical Center, Israel

Depression and mild cognitive impairment (MCI) in elderly subjects are risk factors for dementia. Reductions in hippocampal size and dendritic branching are seen in both conditions, accompanied by decreases in rCBF and glucose utilization. In Alzheimer's disease (AD), progressive neurodegeneration occurs with loss of cholinergic synapses and aminergic transmitters. Feedback regulation of the hypothalamic-pituitary-adrenal axis (HPA) axis through hippocampal glucocorticoid receptor (GR) is impaired in depression and dementia and affects 5-HT receptor signaling. Some of the behavioral changes seen in depression including hyperanxiety, learned helplessness, anhedonia and MCI can be induced in rodents by chronic inescapable stress. These are probably caused by increased activity of corticotropin-releasing hormone (CRH) and corticosterone and excessive release of glutamate, noradrenaline and dopamine in the prefrontal cortex (PFC) and hippocampus. Chronic stress decreases the release of 5-HT and of 5-HT_{1A} receptors in the PFC and hippocampus respectively, and dopamine in the nucleus accumbens. Alterations in the activity of glutamate, NA and 5-HT may be responsible for the depression of long-term potentiation (LTP), reduction in cAMP response-element binding protein (CREB) and brain-derived neurotrophic factor (BDNF) and impaired neurogenesis. As in depressed humans, chronic treatment of stressed rats with different classes of antidepressants normalizes mood and alterations in transmitter release and partially restores LTP, BDNF and neurogenesis. However, the majority of drugs are unable to reverse the cognitive impairment that occurs in some elderly depressed patients, probably because they do not increase cholinergic transmission or affect neurodegenerative processes resulting from vascular disease. This may be achieved by combinations of acetylcholinesterase (AChE) inhibitors and antidepressants, or by a novel drug TV3326, which has neuroprotective, monoamine oxidase (MAO) and AChE-inhibiting activity.

1. Introduction

The greater longevity of modern society has resulted in a marked increase in age-dependent diseases, including dementia, Parkinson's disease (PD), type II diabetes and osteoporosis. Late onset depression occurs in about 15% of older subjects in the community (Blazer, 1989), and may affect a much higher proportion of those in residential care (Evers et al., 2002). It is difficult to diagnose in elderly people because it may be masked by somatic complaints and because it is mistakenly considered by some patients and physicians to be part of the aging process (Gareri et al., 2002).

Cognitive impairment occurs in a significant proportion of elderly patients with depression. Many of them develop irreversible dementia within 3 years of the initial diagnosis, and several studies indicate that depression may be a risk factor for Alzheimer's disease (AD) (Kral and Emery, 1989; Alexopoulos et al., 1993; Stoudemire et al., 1993; Green et al., 2003). Although the mood disorder can be successfully treated with antidepressant drugs there is little evidence that cognitive deficits also improve with such treatment (Devanand et al., 2003). Failure to do so may be due to the choice of antidepressant drug, (some of which, like amitriptyline, actually impair memory, Van-Laar et al., 2002), the time at which treatment is commenced and its duration. It is more likely that neurodegeneration, vascular lesions or a combination of these are already present when the patients come to seek treatment for their depression (Geerlings et al., 2000). These are not always detected at diagnosis and are usually insensitive to antidepressant treatment. Imaging and *post mortem* studies in depressed subjects with cognitive impairment show signs of hippocampal (Bremner et al., 2000; Vakili et al., 2000) and/or cortical atrophy, ventricular enlargement and white matter degenerative changes, particularly in the frontal lobes (Mitchell and Dening, 1996; Murata et al., 2001). White matter lesions may be present due to vascular disease and cause cognitive slowing by interruption of fronto-subcortical connections (Greenwald et al., 1998).

In younger patients with major depression there are relatively few structural abnormalities. A decrease has been reported in the number or density of glia and in neuronal size in the prefrontal cortex (PFC), as well as in the amount of dendritic branching in the hippocampus. There also appears to be a decrease in the expression of reelin, a gene involved in neuronal migration and synaptogenesis (Harrison, 2002). Although there is little evidence for overt neurodegeneration in subjects with major depression without vascular complications, in contrast to those with dementia, a constellation of abnormalities in cerebral blood flow and glucose metabolism has been detected in the PFC and limbic system by neuro-imaging techniques. While some of these abnormalities are restored to normal during symptom remission, others persist and could reflect underlying genetic differences from control subjects or signs of impaired neuronal function (Drevets, 2000).

Depression is a heritable disorder with a risk of 50% among close family members, but no consistent genetic abnormality has yet been identified (Merikangas et al., 2002). Most likely, it results from a combination of genetic and environmental factors, which begin to have an influence on the developing fetus and continue throughout life. Major depression has been separated into two distinct types according to its presentation, termed "melancholic" and "atypical" (Gold and Chrousos, 1999). These may have a different etiology and genetic basis, which could determine the response to drug treatment. Patients with the melancholic type are hyper-aroused, overanxious, have poor appetite, suffer from insomnia, impaired concentration, feelings of guilt, are unable to feel pleasure and are poorly responsive to the environment. Those with atypical depression are lethargic and fatigue easily, have hypersomnia and hyperphagia but are reactive to the environment. There is evidence that the melancholic type may be associated with periods of chronic stress and shares many of its features (Wong et al., 2000a; Gold and Chrousos, 2002).

AD is the commonest form of primary progressive dementia among the elderly and is familial in about 2-5% of subjects showing an autosomal dominant inheritance. The incidence of AD is estimated to be around 2% in persons in the 7th decade and increases to more than 30% at the age of 90 or more (Hafner, 1990). In about 15-20% of the total number of subjects with dementia, vascular disease is the underlying cause. The characteristic symptoms of both types of dementia are cognitive impairment and abnormalities in behavior that result from damage to selective neuronal circuits in the neocortex, hippocampus and basal forebrain cholinergic systems (Mesulam, 1996). As in depression, glucose metabolism is reduced by 30-50% in the posterior cingulate, parietal and temporal regions of the cortex, even at an early stage of mild cognitive impairment (Salmon et al., 1996; Small et al., 2000; Arnaiz et al., 2001). This leads to neuronal dysfunction and a loss of specific neuronal populations. In AD there is a loss of synapses, which may be preceded by widening of the synaptic cleft, resulting in reduced efficiency of communication between neurons (Waggie et al., 1999).

Although the underlying cause of AD is not yet known, *post mortem* brain histopathology has revealed either or both dystrophic neurites and intracellular neurofibrillatory tangles, composed of tau protein (Goedert et al., 1996) and extracellular senile plaques containing β-amyloid peptide (Aβ), a proteolytic product of amyloid precursor protein (APP). Aβ is neurotoxic and can decrease the synthesis and release of acetylcholine (ACh) from cortical and hippocampal neurons (Vaucher et al., 2001). Like some of those with depression, AD subjects have a smaller hippocampal volume (Cardenas et al., 2003) and fewer apical dendrites in hippocampal and cortical areas than aged matched healthy subjects (Ohm et al., 2002). They have deficits in noradrenaline (NA) in the locus coeruleus (LC) and in the frontal, parietal and temporal lobes of the cortex (Matthews et al., 2002) and of serotonin (5-HT) in the frontal and temporal cortices (Lai et al., 2003). These neurotransmitter changes probably contribute to the cognitive impairment and behavioral abnormalities, which commonly include paranoia, apathy or disinhibition, hallucinosis, aggressiveness and depressive symptoms (Levy et al., 1996). Thus, although AD and depression have different etiologies, there is an overlap of functional abnormality associated with neurotransmitter deficits. This may explain why a significant proportion of subjects with AD show depressive symptoms while many with depression develop dementia.

1.1. Mal-Adaptation to Chronic Stress in the Etiology of Depression and Generalized Anxiety Disorder

1.1.1. Neurotransmitter Changes in Response to Acute Stress

In response to acute stress, corticotropin-releasing hormone (CRH) is released from the paraventricular nucleus (PVN) and activates a number of systems that strongly affect attention, mood and motor performance (Cole and Robbins, 1992; Makino et al., 2002). These include the hypothalamic-pituitary-adrenal (HPA) axis and the LC (Butler et al., 1990; Van Bockstaele et al., 1996) and result in increased circulating levels of adrenocorticotropic hormone (ACTH) and cortisol, and of NA in the hippocampus and prefrontal cortex (PFC) (Mangiavacchi et al., 2001). CRH also activates a gamma amino butyric acid (GABA) inhibitory input to the dorsal raphé region (Roche et al., 2003) thereby reducing 5-HT release in the hippocampus, PFC and amygdaloid nuclei. Both acute stress (Bagley et al., 1997) and CRH stimulate the release of glutamate and dopamine (DA) in the PFC, which are involved in anticipatory phenomena and regulation of cognitive function. On the other hand, stress decreases DA release in the nucleus accumbens, which regulates pleasure and reward.

The effect of stress and CRH on neurotransmitter release in the PFC is mimicked by a benzodiazepine inverse agonist (Tam and Roth, 1985) and prevented by diazepam and zolpidem (Claustre et al., 1986; Kaneyuki et al., 1991; Bagley et al., 1997). These drugs enhance GABA-ergic transmission from inter-neurons in the piriform cortex, which in turn, inhibit cortical glutamate release. Since the GABA neurons are normally activated by 5-HT via 5-HT$_{2A}$ receptors (Van Oekelen et al., 2003), the reduction by stress of the release of PFC 5-HT provides an additional explanation for the higher glutamate output in response to increased neuronal activity. In a healthy individual, the activation of these systems is short-lived and homeostasis is rapidly restored at the completion of the response.

1.1.2. Effect of Chronic Stress on Behavior, Regulation of HPA Axis and Neurotransmitter Function in Experimental Animals

Behavioral alterations reminiscent of those seen in depressed human subjects can be induced in experimental animals by a various forms of chronic stress. The latter include inescapable electric footshock, chronic mild stress of a variable nature or alteration of social heirarchies. Among the behavioral changes seen in rats are hyperanxiety, (Weiss et al., 1981) an escape deficit when faced with a noxious stimulus (Gambarana et al., 1995a, 1995b), learned helplessness (Neumaier et al., 1997) anhedonia (Willner et al., 1992; Di Chiara and Tanda, 1997) and mild cognitive impairment. Similar behavioral changes are seen in adult rats that had been subjected to prenatal (Weinstock, 1997; 2001) or early life stress of maternal deprivation (Plotsky and Meaney, 1993; Vazquez, 1998).

Prolonged activation of the HPA axis and exaggerated activity of CRH in the LC and raphé nuclei is seen in adult animals subjected to chronic stress (Chrousos, 1998) and in those exposed to early life stress (Weinstock, 1997). This occurs because NA acts as part of a positive feedback loop on the HPA axis, promoting further release of CRH (Plotsky et al., 1989) and cortisol (Leibowitz et al., 1989). The result is a greater increase in the synthesis and release of NA in response to an acute stress than in naïve rats (Nisenbaum et al., 1991; Finlay et al., 1995) and disruption of the normal pattern of release of 5-HT and DA. The disturbance in neurotransmitter function is responsible for the impairment in cognition, mood regulation and the ability to feel joy or pleasure (McEwen, 1999; Duman et al., 2000). Anxiogenic behavior results from a direct action of both CRH and NA in the amygdala (Davis et al., 1994; Wong et al., 2000a), since it can be prevented by intracerebroventricular (icv) injection of CRH antagonists (Ward et al., 2000).

The effect of excess release of NA in the PFC on cognition may depend on the balance of its activity at α_1 and α_2 post-synaptic receptors. Thus, stimulation of α_2 receptors has been shown to enhance cognitive function (Arnsten et al., 1988), while it is impaired by activation of α_1 receptors (Arnsten et al., 1999). Overstimulation of NA systems by persistent stress also results in down–regulation of β-adrenergic receptors, together with a decrease in the sensitivity of adenyl cyclase to catecholamines (Stone and Platt 1982; Stone et al., 1985). It is not known what happens to α_1 and α_2 post-receptor signaling as a result of chronic stress. However, if the stressful situation is unrelieved, the alterations in the noradrenergic system become maladaptive to the organism, resulting in the precipitation of a generalized anxiety or depressive disorder.

Adult rats subjected to repeated inescapable stress (Adell et al., 1988; Finlay et al; 1995), or prenatal stress during the last week of gestation (Fride and Weinstock, 1989), have a higher release of DA in the PFC. It has been suggested that cortical DA regulates the emotional and behavioral sequelae of exposure to unavoidable aversive events, and may be responsible for learned helplessness and the escape deficit (Cuadra et al., 2001). Both inescapable stress in adult rats and prenatal stress also depressed the release in the nucleus accumbens more than after acute stress (Di Chiara and Tanda, 1997; Gambarana et al., 1999; Fride and Weinstock, 1989; Alonso et al., 1994), resulting in the anhedonia. The release of 5-HT in the PFC (Mangiavacchi et al., 2001) was also decreased more after chronic than after acute stress in rats and monkeys. In the latter, 5-HT release was still lower than in the basal condition 14 months after termination of exposure to chronic social stress (Fontenot et al., 1995). Although not measured in the monkeys, an increase in 5-HT_2 receptor binding was found in the cortex of depressed humans and is consistent with decreased 5-HT release. Thus, it appears that certain types of chronic stress can cause long-term alterations in serotoninergic transmission that could contribute to the hyperanxiety and depressive symptoms.

A reduction of 5-HT release in the PFC can diminish even more the inhibitory effect of GABA on cortical and hippocampal glutamate neurons. The resulting excess activity of glutamate on N-methyl D-aspartate (NMDA) receptors could explain the hippocampal and cortical cell loss found in chronically stressed rats or tree shrews (McEwen, 1999) since it was prevented by NMDA receptor antagonists and by benzodiazepines and phenytoin, which reduce glutamate release (McEwen, 1999).

In addition to its effects on neurotransmitter release, chronic stress attenuates the negative feedback by corticosterone via glucocorticoid receptors (GR) in the PFC (Mizoguchi et al., 2003), hippocampus, hypothalamus, anterior pituitary and brain stem nuclei (Makino et al., 2002), resulting in higher circulating levels of the glucocorticoid. Excess corticosterone acting on GR (Wissink et al., 2000) further alters serotoninergic transmission by reducing the expression of 5-HT_{1A} receptors in the granule layer of the dentate gyrus in rats (Meijer et al., 1997), through suppression of transcription induced by NF-κB. The sensitivity of the dentate gyrus can be explained by the fact that it contains the highest densities in the brain of GR and mineralocorticoid receptors (MR) for glucocorticoids (Fujita et al., 2000).

1.1.3. Alterations in the Regulation of the HPA Axis and of Neurotransmitter Activity in Human Subjects with Depression

Dysregulation of the HPA axis has been reported in women that had been subjected to severe childhood abuse (Heim et al., 2000) and also occurs, together with pronounced activation of central noradrenergic systems, in a significant proportion of human subjects with melancholic depression (Wong et al., 2000a). These data support the suggestion that early adverse events may predispose to depressive illness in later life.

Patients with depressive illness were found to have higher urinary and plasma levels of cortisol and did not decrease the latter in response to dexamethasone or dexamethasone plus CRH, indicating a loss of feedback regulation of the HPA axis via GR receptors (Holsboer-Trachsler et al., 1991). Higher concentrations of CRH (Nemeroff et al., 1984) and lower levels of neuropeptide Y (NPY), which has anxiolytic activity (Heilig and Thorsell, 2002), were found in the cerebrospinal fluid (CSF) of depressed patients (Westrin et al., 1999). The number of neurons in the PVN expressing CRH (Raadsheer et al., 1994) and levels of its mRNA were reported to be higher in patients with depression and in those with AD than in normal age-matched controls (Raadsheer et al., 1995). Thus, melancholic depression is associated with excess activity of CRH and decreased activity of NPY.

Dysregulation of aminergic transmission in discrete brain regions is much more difficult to demonstrate in humans, but those with melancholic depression had higher 24 hr levels of NA in the CSF than normal subjects (Wong et al., 2000a) suggesting a greater release, as was found in chronically stressed rats. The finding of lower levels of 5-hydroxy-indoleacetic acid (5HIAA) a major metabolite of 5-HT, in the CSF suggests that 5-HT release is reduced in depression (Maes and Meltzer, 1995), and could explain the greater number of $5-HT_2$ receptors in the frontal cortex in suicide victims (Mann et al., 1986). More recently, neuroimaging studies with positron emission tomography (PET) and [*carbonyl*-^{11}C] WAY-100635 have shown that brain $5-HT_{1A}$ receptor binding is also decreased (Drevets, 2000), as reported after repeated stress in rats. Excess glutamate release may occur in humans as in stressed rats and could explain hippocampal cell loss and dorsolateral prefrontal deficits in subjects with recurrent major depression (Sheline, 1996; Rogers et al., 1998; Rajkowska et al., 1999). The effects of chronic stress on CRH activity, biogenic amine transmission and behavior are summarized in Table 11.1.

Role of Hippocampus and Cortex in Learning and Memory

The hippocampus is a key brain area implicated in arousal, attention and motivation and plays a crucial role in the regulation of the response of the HPA axis to stress, because it has the highest concentration of GR in the brain. It also has an important function in the organization of learning, memory and attention, as well as memory consolidation and retrieval (Dubrovsky, 1991). One of the mechanisms by which the hippocampus is able to regulate the storage of information is known as long-term potentiation (LTP) (Bliss and Collingridge, 1993). This is an activity-dependent form of synaptic plasticity that occurs via glutamatergic collaterals synapsing onto dendritic spines in CA1 cells in the hippocampus.

LTP is also seen in cortical pyramidal neurons and may last for days or weeks (Stewart and Reid, 2002). LTP is induced by the entry of calcium into the cell through activation of NMDA receptors (Martin et al., 2000). Ca^{2+} ions activate Ca^{2+}/calmodulin-dependent protein kinase II, which is present in postsynaptic spines and is the molecular effector for the expression of the early phase of LTP. A later phase requires new protein synthesis (Popoli et al., 2002) as it is inhibited by actinomycin.

Table 11.1. Effects of chronic stress in rats on CRH activity and aminergic transmission

Neuro-transmitter	Alteration in release and/or activity	Consequence
CRH	↑ activity in LC ↑ activity in GABA interneurons to dorsal raphé nucleus	↑ NA release in PFC and hippocampus ↓ 5-HT release in PFC and hippocampus, ↑ 5-HT$_{2A}$ receptors in PFC
NA	↑ release in PFC	Altered attention and cognition, ↓ β receptors
5-HT	↓ release in PFC and hippocampus	Hyperanxiety, memory impairment
DA	↑ release in PFC ↓ release in n. accumbens shell	Hyperanxiety, behavioral suppression, cognitive impairment Anhedonia, behavioral suppression
Glutamate	↑ release in PFC, hippocampus	Neuronal atrophy, cognitive impairment

LC = locus coeruleus; PFC = prefrontal cortex

NMDA receptor activation promotes signaling to the nucleus in response to elevation of cytoplasmic cAMP or Ca^{2+} that culminates in the phosphorylation of cyclic AMP (cAMP) response-element binding protein (CREB), activation of multiple genes and long-term synaptic plasticity. CREB controls many genes including that of brain-derived neurotrophic factor (BDNF), which is directly involved in the regulation of protein machinery at postsynaptic nerve terminals. BDNF is directly involved in the regulation of protein machinery at postsynaptic nerve terminals, which could account for its ability to modulate synaptic transmission (Popoli et al., 2002). CREB activates BDNF by attaching to cAMP response-element binding elements in its promoter region (Nibuya et al., 1996), while the addition of BDNF to neurons stimulates phosphorylation of CREB and activation via kinase-regulated pathways (Walton and Dragunow, 2000), suggesting the presence of a positive feedback between BDNF and CREB. Chronic infusion of BDNF into the brain of adult rats can promote differentiation and survival of neurons. Furthermore, similar to environmental enrichment and hippocampal-dependent learning, BDNF can induce neurogenesis, indicated by a robust sprouting of 5-HT nerve terminals in the dentate gyrus and neocortex of the adult rat (Altar, 1999; Gould et al., 2000). Neurogenesis also occurs to a lesser extent in the brain of non-human primates and humans (Gould et al., 1999).

Long-term depression (LTD) is a long-lasting, activity-dependent decrease in synaptic efficacy, which was first observed in the hippocampus, but is also seen in the amygdala and cortex. Like LTP, it appears be dependent on glutamate activation of NMDA receptors but may also be glutamate-independent (Martin et al., 2000). The processing of this information via LTP and LTD can be modulated by noradrenergic and serotoninergic inputs from the LC and raphé nuclei, respectively (Mongeau et al., 1997). Thus, alterations in LTP, LTD and cognitive processes could be influenced by alterations in NA and 5-HT transmission that occur in prolonged stress and after antidepressant treatment.

2.1. Effect of Chronic Stress or Aging on Hippocampal Neurogenesis, Neural Plasticity and Memory in Rats

Chronic inescapable foot-shocks or psychosocial stress in rats that caused hyperanxiety, anhedonia, and hypophagia, depressed LTP (Foy et al., 1987; Shors et al., 1989) and facilitated LTD (Xu et al., 1997; Von Frijtag et al., 2002). Depression of LTP and the subsequent excitotoxicity occurs through excess glutamate stimulation of NMDA receptors. High concentrations of glucocorticoids also depressed LTP and increased LTD in the dentate gyrus (Xu et al., 1998), which may explain impaired memory in patients with Cushing's disease (Dubrowsky, 1991). Chronic stress in rats (McEwen, 1999), tree shrews (Van der Hart et al., 2002) or nonhuman primates (Gould et al., 1998) resulted in a reduction in the rate of proliferation of granule precursor cells in the dentate gyrus, suggesting suppression of adult neurogenesis, and a decrease in the number of branch points and total dendritic length in the apical dendritic trees of CA3 pyramidal neurons (McKittrick et al., 2000).

Others have shown that chronic stress produced cognitive deficits in spatial learning and memory (McEwen, 1999) that were associated with a reduction in the expression of BDNF in the hippocampus (Smith et al., 1995; Butterweck et al., 2001). This, in turn, may have resulted from a decrease serotoninergic signaling via 5-HT$_{1A}$ receptors (Fujita et al., 2000). Stimulation of such receptors releases the neurotrophic factor S100β from glial cells and protects neurons from the damaging effects of excess glutamate (Azmitia, 1999). The chain of events leading to decreased neurogenesis and memory impairment by persistent stress is summarized in Fig. 11.1.

Indirect evidence of excess glutamatergic activity in the PFC of depressed human subjects that could contribute to their frontostriatal deficits and cognitive impairment (Rogers et al., 1998) was seen in suicide victims who showed a down-regulation of NMDA receptors (Nowak et al., 1995). Extracellular concentrations of glutamate may be further increased by a reduction in the number of glial cells (Harrison, 2002), into which glutamate is transported from the synaptic gap (Drevets, 2000).

Impaired cognitive function in aging rats was associated with a decrease in GR and MR in the hippocampus and GR in the PVN (Hassan et al., 1999). Aged rats also showed a loss of cholinergic synapses and fewer dendritic branches in layer V pyramidal neurons of the parietal cortex, and alterations in cortical LTP (Wong et al., 2000b). About 30% of aged humans have high circulating levels of cortisol, and those with depression and cognitive impairment show similar changes to those in elderly rats in the cingulate and prefrontal cortices (Harrison, 2002). Thus, both aging and chronic stress can cause deficits in spatial learning and memory through adverse influences on neural plasticity and structure. The presence of excess amounts of glucocorticoid through impaired feedback regulation could ultimately cause irreversible neuronal damage by increasing the deleterious effects of environmental toxins and oxidative free radicals (Saplosky, 2000). This scenario provides a common link between the etiologies of depression and dementia and indicates potential avenues of treatment.

Convergence of Antidementia and Antidepressant Pharmacology

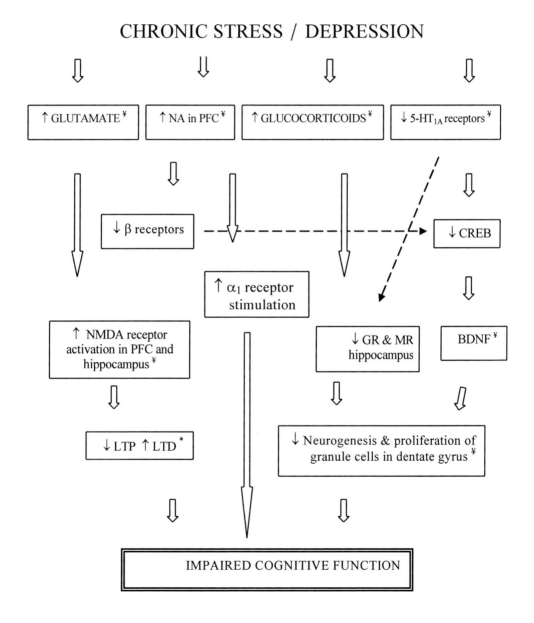

Fig 11.1. Effect of depression and chronic stress on cognitive function through alteration of HPA axis regulation, neurotransmitter function and transcription factors. ¥ reversed by chronic treatment with all groups of antidepressants; * to date, reversed by chronic treatment only with tianeptine & imipramine.

3. Therapeutic Agents Currently Used to Treat Depression

At the present time several different classes of drugs are in clinical use for the treatment of depression. These were originally classified on the basis of their pharmacological actions *in vitro* or after acute treatment in experimental animals. The early ones like isoniazid, a monoamine oxidase (MAO) inhibitor, or imipramine, a tricyclic tertiary amine were discovered by chance in the 1950s. This led to an alteration in the perception of depression and to the belief that it may be due abnormalities in the function of brain biogenic amines (Schildkraut, 1965). With the discovery of the action of tricyclic antidepressants (TCA)s imipramine and amitriptyline on the NA and 5-HT transporters, many second-generation drugs were developed, like desipramine and protriptyline, which were more selective reuptake inhibitors of NA. In the 1980s, different structures were prepared which only prevented 5-HT re-uptake (selective serotonin reuptake inhibitors, SSRIs) like fluvoxamine and fluoxetine, or were selective inhibitors of the NA transporter (NRIs), like reboxitine.

Irreversible MAO inhibitors, more potent than isoniazid, like tranylcypromine and pargyline had been synthesized and found to be very effective antidepressants. However, their use was severely limited because of the potential danger of producing hypertensive crises when tyramine-containing food and beverages were ingested. This was due to their inhibition of MAO-A in the gastro-intestinal tract (Blackwell et al., 1967). The problem of tyramine potentiation was considerably reduced with the introduction of reversible selective MAO-A inhibitors, like moclobemide (Da Prada et al., 1988). The realization that MAO inhibitors and TCAs increase synaptic levels of mononoamines led to the preparation of other drugs like mianserine and mirtazepine that also increase amine levels by blocking presynaptic NA and/or 5-HT autoreceptors.

After several decades of therapeutic experience with the different classes of drugs, it has become increasingly clear that their antidepressant effect does not result simply from the ability to increase amine levels in the synapse. This is based on three major findings.

1. There was no correlation between the clinically effective dose of drug and its affinity for the amine transporter. The latter can differ over a 1000-fold between drugs with similar clinical efficacy at a dose range of 75-150 mg a day.
2. Tianeptine, an effective antidepressant, was found to increase 5-HT re-uptake in contrast to SSRIs (Datla et al., 1993).
3. Improvement in depressive symptoms only appeared 2 or more weeks after the beginning of daily administration with all classes of these drugs (Mongeau et al., 1997), whereas the increase of 5-HT and NA in the synapse occurred immediately. The last finding prompted a large volume of pre-clinical research in which the different types of antidepressants were given for periods of 2-4 weeks to normal rats in an attempt to elucidate their mode of action. Several of them highlighted the differences in the effects of the classes of drugs on amine transporters, and receptors. Thus, chronic treatment with TCAs but not SSRIs caused down-regulation of the β adrenoceptors in the amygdala (Ordway et al., 1991) and also had different effects on pre- and post-synaptic 5-HT receptors and amine transporters (Herbert et al., 2001).

These alterations in normal animals almost certainly reflect a mechanism to prevent overstimulation of the respective aminergic system resulting from increased synaptic concentrations, and may be quite different from the mode of action of the drugs in depression.

More relevant differences between the actions of SSRIs and NRIs emerged from a comparison of their effects in patients. Administration of α-methyl p-tyrosine, an inhibitor of tyrosine hydroxylase, induced a relapse of depressive symptoms in those treated successfully with NRIs but not SSRIs (Miller et al., 1996). On the other hand, tryptophan depletion abolished the antidepressant effect of fluvoxamine, imipramine, phenelzine and tranycypromine, but not of desipramine (Delgado et al., 1990), a more selective inhibitor of the NA transporter. While a few weeks of antidepressant administration can often alleviate the behavioral symptoms of depression, treatment needs to be continued for several months to prevent their recurrence, a fact that is not always recognized by physicians. This suggests that the clinical features of depression may be eliminated by short-term neuro-adaptations caused by antidepressants, but long-term cellular alterations are critical for maintaining their clinical efficacy.

4. Novel Drugs with Potential Anxiolytic and Antidepressant Activity

4.1. CRH$_1$ Receptor Antagonists

In view of the experimental data implicating excess activity of CRH in hyperanxiety and behavioral suppression, and the demonstration that CRH$_1$ receptor-knockout mice display reduced anxiety and greater activity in intimidating situations, it was hypothesized that CRH$_1$ antagonists may provide a novel class of drugs with anxiolytic and antidepressant activity (Owens and Nemeroff, 1999). This was supported by the demonstration that an icv injection of peptide CRH antagonists and CRH antisense oligonucleotides induce anxiolytic activity in rodents. Three non-peptide CRH$_1$ antagonists, CP-154-526, its analog, antalarmin and R121919 were shown to have anxiolytic and antidepressant activity in a variety of experimental situations in rodents after parenteral administration. Moreover, the drugs did not prevent the normal release of ACTH and corticosterone in response to stress, indicating that they are unlikely to cause adrenal insufficiency (Deak et al., 1999; Arborelius et al., 2000). Antalarmin also inhibited behaviors associated with hyperanxiety in chronically-stressed monkeys and reduced the elevation in plasma NA, adrenaline, ACTH and cortisol produced by exposure to unfamiliar subjects in an adjacent cage (Habib et al., 2000). A preliminary open-label study was conducted with R121919 on 23 patients with depression who had Hamilton rating scores above 18 on a 21-item Depression Rating Scale. The drug significantly reduced patient and clinician-rated depression and anxiety scores in the majority of subjects within 30 days of treatment, but did not prevent the rise in plasma ACTH and cortisol induced by administration of CRH (Zobel et al., 2000). No untoward adverse effects were reported. In view of the strong placebo effect in patients with depression, a placebo-controlled trial of the drug given for longer period of time is awaited.

4.2. Neurokinin Antagonists

Neurokinins are a family of peptides related to substance P (SP) located in peripheral and central nervous system neurons and include SP, neurokinins A (NKA) and B (NKB). While all peptides can bind to three 3 NK receptors, SP shows preferential binding to NK_1 receptor and NKA and NKB show preference for NK_2 and NK_3 receptors, respectively. High concentrations of SP are found in the medial and central nuclei of the amygdala (Emson et al., 1978) LC, hypothalamus, substantia nigra and is expressed in cell bodies and dendrites (Ljungdhal et al., 1978). SP is released with NKA in response to chronic stress (Duggan and Furmidge, 1994) and may contribute to the exacerbation of the stress response and its consequences by activating NK_1 receptors in the amygdala and its projections to the hypothalamus, periaqueductal gray, and reticulopontine nucleus (Santarelli et al., 2001).

Inactivation of the NK_1 receptor of SP by cytotoxin saporin conjugates or by deletion, as in NK_1 receptor knockout mice induced antidepressant and anxiolytic effects and the appropriate alterations in 5-HT and NA transmission (Mantyh, 2002). NK1 knockout mice also showed raised levels of BDNF and neurogenesis in the hippocampus, similar to that seen in rodents that have been subjected to chronic stress and treated with conventional antidepressants (Morcuende et al., 2003). These findings led to the synthesis and pharmacological evaluation of a specific NK_1 antagonist, MK-0869. In several animal species MK-0869 prevented stress-induced anxiogenic and depressive behavior and activation of NA neurons by acute stress without inducing sedation (Rupniak, 2002). In preliminary clinical testing, MK-0869 also showed anxiolytic and antidepressant activity similar to that of SSRIs and greater than that of placebo (Ranga and Krishnan, 2002). It is not known whether MK-0869 has a more rapid onset of action than conventional antidepressants or whether it affects cognitive function in depressed subjects.

Recent studies have provided evidence that NKA promotes an increase in NA release in the PFC by activating NK_2 receptors in the LC (Steinberg et al., 2001). Selective NK_2 antagonists were synthesized, one of which, SR48968, was shown to suppress activation of the LC by CRH and to reduce NA release in the medial PFC induced by tail pinch (Steinberg et al., 2001). This suggested that NK_2 receptor activation by NKA mediates the stress-induced stimulation of the locus coeruleus by CRH. SR48968 also showed anxiolytic activity and a similar pattern of antidepressant-like properties to those of imipramine and fluoxetine in the forced swim test in mice and rats (Griebel et al., 2001). Clinical studies have not yet been performed with NK_2 antagonists.

4.3. NMDA Antagonists

Several studies have reported that chronic treatment with TCAs, MAO inhibitors and SSRIs led to a decrease in NMDA receptor functioning, probably via phosphorylation of CREB. NMDA antagonists were found to have antidepressant-like activity in the forced swim and chronic mild stress anhedonia models, and intravenous administration of ketamine, a use-dependent NMDA Na^+ channel blocker, produced rapid improvement of mood in depressed patients (Skolnick 1999). These observations provided support for a role of decreased NMDA-mediated transmission in the action of antidepressants. Furthermore, the implication that excess glutamate activity in the PFC is involved in disruption of cognitive function has led to further investigation of the molecular biology of the NMDA receptor complex. It was hoped that selective antagonists could be produced that would modify excess glutamate activity, without causing hallucinations, hypertension, catatonia and anesthesia by suppressing normal neuronal transmission. Four subunits of the NMDA receptor have been identified of which the NR_{2B} subtype is restricted to the forebrain. It is possible that selective antagonists of this subunit may have both antidepressant and antidementia activity of a more rapid onset than conventional drugs. As yet there are no reports of experimental data with such drugs.

In spite of the variety of medications currently available for the treatment of depression we do not yet have the means to enable us to decide which of these would be most effective for a given individual. We also cannot yet predict which depressed patient will develop dementia. Moreover, little attention has been paid to the gender differences in depressive disorders, which could well affect the response to different treatments (Kornstein et al., 2000; Frankiewicz et al., 2000). This may become possible with the identification of genes that increase the risk for the different types of depression, and with a greater understanding of the changes in the brain that underlie its diverse symptoms.

5. Preclinical Studies on the Action of Antidepressants on the HPA Axis, Behavior, Aminergic Transmission and Hippocampal Plasticity

5.1. Effect of Chronic Treatment with Antidepressants on Stress-Induced Abnormalities in Behavior

Research into the mechanism of action of antidepressants has been hampered by the lack of suitable animal models that can adequately replicate the human condition. At best, as indicated in preceding sections, some models can reproduce a few of the features of depression. To cause these changes in behavior, rats must either be subjected chronically for 3-4 weeks to different types of relatively mild stress to avoid adaptation (Willner et al., 1992), or to a single more severe stress like disruption of social hierarchy, or persistent foot-shock from which they cannot escape or over which they have no control (Shors et al., 1989; Von Frijtag et al., 2000). Others have shown that hyperanxiety and depressive-like behavior can be detected at adulthood in the offspring of rats that had been subjected to uncontrollable stress during pregnancy (Weinstock, 1997; 2001) or were stressed by maternal deprivation during early life (Plotsky and Meaney, 1993; Vazquez, 1998). Prenatal stress was shown to induce a loss of hippocampal neurons (Hayashi et al., 1998) and memory deficits at adulthood (Jaiswal and Bhattacharya, 1993; Lemaire et al., 2000). This early disturbance during critical brain development may sensitize the appropriate neural systems to the effects of stressful situations in later life and result in poor coping behavior (Weinstock, 1997). The consequences of prenatal and early life stress may also explain why some individuals are more susceptible than others to develop depression and cognitive impairments (Weinstock, 2001).

Many studies have shown that anhedonia, hyperanxiety and suppression of general activity induced by chronic inescapable stress can be corrected by treatment for at least two weeks with all the known types of clinically effective antidepressants including TCAs, SSRIs, NRIs and MAO inhibitors (Gambarana et al., 1995a; 1995b; Grappi et al., 2003; Muscat et al., 1992; Von Frijtag et al., 2002). The beneficial effect of the various types of drugs appears to be mediated by different neurotransmitters as shown by its prevention by specific receptor antagonists. Thus, the pharmacological effect of TCAs depended on activation of dopamine D_1 receptors; that of SSRIs depended on 5-HT activity via 5-HT$_{1A}$ receptors, and that of NRIs on NA activity through β-adrenergic receptors. In other experiments, intact 5-HT transmission was shown to be necessary for the action of fluoxetine but not that of desipramine in the forced swim test, since only the effect of fluoxetine was abolished by 5-HT depletion with parachlorophenylalanine (Page et al., 1999). Differences in the neurotransmitters involved in the mode of action of NRIs and SSRIs were also seen in human subjects (Miller et al., 1996; Delgado et al., 1990).

5.2. Effect of Chronic Treatment with Antidepressants on Stress-Induced CRH Hyperactivity and Dysregulation of HPA Axis

In spite of the fact that most antidepressants do not cause any changes in mood or in the regulation of the HPA axis in normal individuals, the majority of studies has assessed their effects in naïve, unstressed rats. Under such conditions, no changes were found in the levels of CRH or its mRNA in the PVN, even though antidepressants of different types were given daily for 4 weeks (Stout, et al., 2002). However, the elevation of CRH mRNA by 15 min of swim stress was significantly reduced by venlafaxine (an inhibitor of NA and 5-HT re-uptake) and tranylcypromine, but not by reboxetine or fluoxetine, administered for 26 days prior to the stress (Stout et al., 2002). There have also been a large number of investigations into the effect of different classes of antidepressants and electroconvulsive shock (ECS) on GR protein and mRNA in the hippocampus and hypothalamus of unstressed rats (Pariente and Miller, 2001). While the TCAs, ECS, MAO inhibitors and mirtazepine all up-regulated GR protein and its mRNA in the hippocampus, and occasionally also in the hypothalamus, the SSRIs were ineffective (Pariente and Miller, 2001). Nevertheless, both SSRIs and the other drugs reduced basal and stress-induced increases in plasma corticosterone, indicating that HPA axis regulation can be altered by all the antidepressants even in the absence of GR receptor upregulation.

Far fewer studies have been made in animals with evidence of HPA axis dysregulation, GR suppression and raised plasma corticosterone. Two weeks of daily stress induced a relatively small increase in CRH in the PVN mRNA, which was somewhat reduced towards normal levels by treatment with venlafaxine and tranylcypromine (Stout et al., 2002). It is possible that the increase in CRH and its suppression would have been greater had both the stress and antidepressants been given for longer time. Thus, eight, but not two weeks of daily treatment with imipramine was found to normalize mRNA of CRH in the PNV and of TH in the LC after its elevation in rats by recurring immobilization stress (Butterweck et al., 2001). In rats subjected to early life stress, chronic treatment with desipramine prevented the rise in brain CRH-2 receptor mRNA (Vaszuez et al., 2003). In a transgenic mouse model of reduced GR expression that showed several of the endocrine and behavioral abnormalities seen in depressed human subjects, chronic treatment with moclobemide or desipramine corrected the behavior and restored the elevated ACTH and corticosterone to normal levels (Pepin et al., 1992; Montkowski et al., 1995).

While amitriptyline administered for six weeks to prepubertal prenatally-stressed rats prevented the development of hyperanxiety, it actually increased anxiety in control rats exposed to an intimidating situation (Poltyrev et al., 2004). Both amitriptyline and a novel MAO-inhibitor, TV3326 also normalized the HPA axis response to acute stress in prenatally-stressed rats indicating a restoration of normal feedback control, whereas they caused an increase in basal levels of corticosterone in rats of unstressed mothers (Poltyrev et al., 2002). This serves to underscore the importance of using appropriate animal models in which both behavior and the regulation of the HPA axis have been altered by chronic or early-life stress, in order to investigate of the mode of action of anxiolytics and antidepressants.

5.3. Effect of Chronic Treatment with Antidepressants on Stress-Induced Alterations in Biogenic Amine Release and Transmission

Almost all the studies on the effects of chronic antidepressant treatment on 5-HT release and neurotransmission have also been performed in normal, unstressed rats (Mongeau et al., 1997). Thus, in naïve rats, SSRIs, TCAs and MAO inhibitors all increased 5-HT release by down-regulating $5-HT_{1A}$ autoreceptors. In other studies, TCAs, MAO inhibitors and mianserin caused a down-regulation of $5-HT_{2A}$ receptors, an action shared by some, but not all SSRIs (Van Oekelen et al., 2003). Since chronic stress brings about a reduction in 5-HT release in the cortex and hippocampus and thereby also increases $5-HT_{2A}$ receptors, it would have been much more relevant to see whether antidepressants could restore 5-HT transmission to control levels in chronically-stressed rats in association with the normalization of behavior. An indication of such a mode of action was obtained by neuroimaging techniques with labeled ligands in human subjects. These showed that four weeks of treatment with clomipramine and desipramine, which ameliorated their depressive symptoms, reduced cortical $5-HT_{2A}$ receptors to normal levels. This is compatible with a restoration of serotoninergic activity (Fujita et al., 2000).

Acute treatment with antidepressants in normal animals increased cortical NA release in the cortex (Dazzi et al., 2002a; 2002b). By contrast, both the excessive NA release and anxiogenic behavior induced by chronic stress were reduced to normal levels by two weeks daily administration of mirtazepine, venlafaxine or imipramine (Dazzi et al., 2002a; 2002b). In rats previously exposed to chronic variable stress or footshock, TCAs, MAO inhibitors, SSRIs and venaflaxine prevented the excessive DA release in the PFC induced by acute stress (Cuadra et al., 2001; Dazzi et al., 2001). Chronic administration of imipramine and reboxetine also raised DA release in the nucleus accumbens to control levels after it had been depressed by chronic stress (Gambarana et al., 1999; Grappi et al., 2003). The effect of chronic treatment with antidepressants on changes in transmitter release induced by chronic stress is shown in Table 11.2.

In summary, the data suggest that different classes of antidepressants can restore normal behavior in chronically-stressed rodents and depressed humans through their respective effects on the HPA axis, 5-HT, DA or NA transmission or a combination of these. However, the exact mechanism by which this is achieved varies according to the class of drug. Although this has not yet been fully elucidated, the reduction by antidepressants of abnormally high glucocorticoid levels probably contributes to the restoration of normal aminergic function. We do not yet know whether NK_1, NK_2 and CRH_1 antagonists also restore normal amine release and activity after their disruption by chronic stress, nor if they do so more rapidly than the older antidepressants.

Table 11.2. Restoration to normal values by chronic treatment with antidepressants of the alterations in neurotransmitter release induced by chronic stress.

Neuro-transmitter	Antidepressant	Duration of drug treatment	Consequence
NA	Imipramine, mirtazepine[1]	2 weeks	↓ in excess release in PFC
" "	Venaflaxine[2]	" "	↓ in excess release in PFC
DA	Imipramine[3], reboxetine[4]	3 weeks	↑release to normal levels in n. accumbens
" "	Imipramine, mirtazepine[5]	2 weeks	↓ in excess release in PFC
" "	Desipramine, fluoxetine phenelzine[7]	2 days	↓ in excess release in PFC
Glutamate	Imipramine, phenelzine[8*]	3 weeks	↓ in excess release in PFC

1. Dazzi et al., 2002a. 2. Dazzi et al., 2002b. 3. Gambarana et al., 1999; 4. Grappi et al., 2003. 5. Mangiavacchi et al., 2001. 6. Dazzi et al., 2001. 7. Cuadra et al., 2001. 8. Michael-Titus, et al., 2000. * acute stress. ↑ = increase; ↓ = decrease.

5.4. Effect of Antidepressants on Memory and Hippocampal Synaptic Plasticity

Changes in the actions of neurotransmitters in the PFC and hippocampus involved in the regulation of arousal, attention and motivation can influence the acquisition and retrieval of memory. The reduction by chronic stress of 5-HT and increase in NA activity in these brain areas could impair the normal processing of information, leading to an emphasis on unpleasant at the expense of pleasant memories, so characteristic of depression. By increasing 5-HT and NA activity on postsynaptic 5-HT1$_A$ and α_2 receptors respectively, and decreasing that of NA on β-adrenergic receptors, antidepressants may not only be able to restore normal mood, but also attention, memory acquisition, the normal number of dendritic spines and neurogenesis. However, as described above for the studies on the HPA axis and serotoninergic transmission, the effects of antidepressant on synaptic plasticity have almost all been carried out in normal rats. It was therefore not surprising that most of these found that the antidepressants suppressed LTP (O'Conner et al., 1993; Massicotte et al., 1993; Stewart and Reid, 2000), presumably because they disturbed intact aminergic transmission. By contrast, 3 months treatment with imipramine of rats that had been subjected to chronic social stress partially reversed both the decrease in LTP and increase in LTD (Von Frijtag et al., 2002). It is not known whether different classes of antidepressants share this activity, or can induce more robust increases in LTP within a shorter time than that shown by imipramine.

Tianeptine has several effects on synaptic plasticity and memory impairment that do not seem to be shared by other antidepressants. It reversed impaired memory consolidation induced by cholinergic and glutamatergic antagonists (Meneses, 2002) and when given daily for three weeks prevented the attenuation by chronic stress of NMDA-receptor-mediated excitatory postsynaptic currents (EPSCs) at hippocampal CA3 glutamate receptor ion channels (McKittrick et al., 2000). Tianeptine, but not desipramine or fluoxetine, also prevented atrophy of dendrites in CA3 pyramidal neurons and impairment of spatial memory induced by repeated restraint stress in rats (McEwen et al., 1997). Moreover, unlike other antidepressants, tianeptine strengthened the slope of the input-output relation of EPSCs both in control and stressed animals and in *in vitro* preparations. This may have occurred because unlike that of TCAs and SSRIs, acute administration of tianeptine does not increase synaptic levels of 5-HT above normal in control animals. The enhancement of EPSCs was blocked by the kinase inhibitor staurosporine suggesting that tianeptine targets the phosphorylation-state of glutamate receptors rather then presynaptic release mechanisms at CA3 synapses (Kole et al., 2002). The only other antidepressant that has been reported to counteract a memory deficit induced by prolonged stress is the reversible MAO-A inhibitor, moclobemide (Nowakowska et al., 2001), possibly because unlike tricyclic depressants, it does not block cholinergic transmission at muscarinic receptors. Although the authors claimed that this treatment decreased the turnover of DA, NA and 5-HT because it reduced the levels of dihydroxy- phenylalanine and 5HIAA in the hippocampus, these changes probably reflect MAO inhibition rather than a restoration of normal aminergic transmission. Moclobemide also improved performance of spatial navigation in GR-impaired transgenic mice and shifted the threshold for induction of hippocampal LTP at low stimulation frequencies (Steckler et al., 2001). It is not known whether SSRIs or other drugs that improve NA transmission and do not block muscarinic receptors can also improve cognitive function.

6. Effect of Antidepressants on Glutamate Transmission, BDNF and CREB

It was mentioned previously that the cognitive impairment induced by chronic stress could also be associated with an increase in glutamate release in the PFC. Chronic treatment with imipramine or phenelzine selectively decreased the excess glutamate output induced by stress in the PFC without affecting that in the striatum (Michael-Titus et al., 2000). However, the authors did not determine whether the stress caused an impairment of memory and whether this was prevented by antidepressants. The latter may have reduced glutamate release by restoring serotoninergic transmission, which acts to prevent excess glutamate release in the cerebral cortex (Maura et al., 1998).

Antidepressants of different types and NMDA antagonists can restore neurogenesis after its suppression by chronic stress, and promote hippocampal granule cell proliferation (Malberg et al., 2000; Manev et al., 2001). A TCA, clomipramine, tianeptine and the selective NK_1 antagonist L-760,735 all prevented the reductions in N-acetyl-aspartate (NAA), creatine and phosphocreatine and hippocampal volume induced in male tree shrews and in rats by repeated psychosocial stress (Czeh et al., 2001; Van der Hart et al., 2002). Since a decrease in NAA represents a reduction in neuroaxonal cellular density and /or dysfunction it suggests that the drugs were able to restore neurogenesis.

Chronic treatment for 21 days with tranylcypromine, sertraline, desipramine, mianserin, SSRIs or ECS restored the levels of BDNF mRNA and the expression of CREB in the hippocampus after these had previously been depressed by electroconvulsive shock in rats (Nibuya et al., 1995; 1996). However, daily treatment with imipramine for 8 weeks did not restore hippocampal levels of BDNF in rats that had been subjected to immobilization stress for one week, although it decreased the elevation of CRH mRNA in the PVN (Butterweck, 2001). Although not measured in this study, the failure by imipramine to increase BDNF could have occurred because it did not improve 5-HT_{1A} signaling and the expression of CREB. On the other hand, desipramine, but not fluoxetine, was able to increase BDNF in CREB-deficient mice (Conti et al., 2002). This suggests that some antidepressants raise BDNF in intact animals by increasing 5-HT1_A signaling and CREB while others can do so by another mechanism. Although the activation of CREB appears to be necessary for the restoration of BDNF and neurogenesis by antidepressants in chronically-stressed rats, it may not mediate their behavioral or neuroendocrine effects which are still seen in CREB-deficient mice. While the treatment of depression has usually focused on the relief of the behavioral symptoms, it is likely that transcriptional factors like CREB and BDNF must also be maintained in order to restore neural plasticity and neurogenesis, thereby preventing the development of cognitive deficits and the reappearance of symptoms on cessation of drug administration.

7. Effect of Antidepressants on Cognitive Impairment in Human Subjects

Depressive symptoms are commonly found in subjects with mild cognitive impairment (MCI) and dementias of the Alzheimer and vascular types (Levy et al., 1996). Moreover, it has been shown that MCI and associated depressive symptoms are risk factors or precursors of AD and vascular dementia (Li et al., 2001). Although all the different classes of antidepressants have been shown to improve mood in depressed elderly subjects with MCI or dementia and to increase to normal the concentrations of CREB in the temporal cortex (Dowlatshani et al., 1998), no consistent improvement in cognitive function has been reported. Even tianeptine, which produced the most consistent effects on impaired memory, synaptogenesis and hippocampal function in animal experiments (McEwen et al., 1997; Meneses, 2002; McKittrick et al., 2000), did not affect cognitive function, when given for 42 days, although it improved depressive symptomatology in a manner similar to paroxetine and normalized the hyperactivity of the HPA axis (Nickel et al., 2003). However, it is possible that drug treatment was not given for long enough to affect hippocampal plasticity in these subjects.

Some studies claimed an improvement in cognitive function with small doses of imipramine (Peselow et al., 1991) or with moclobemide (Pancheri et al., 1994) in elderly subjects without dementia. Others, performed in subjects with dementia, reported a worsening of cognitive function with TCAs that also block muscarinic receptors (Teri et al., 1991). Some improvement in memory occurred in a few studies but this could have been due to the fact that an appropriate control group of elderly subjects without depression were not included to account for an effect of familiarity with the testing procedures. In a study by Nebes et al. (2003) in which such controls were also tested, it was found that 12 weeks of treatment with nortriptyline or paroxetine failed to affect cognitive processes that are specifically impaired in geriatric depression: speed of information processing, working memory attention and episodic memory, although both drugs improved depressive symptoms. By contrast, another well-controlled study found that reboxetine, but not paroxetine, significantly improved the ability to sustain attention and the speed of cognitive processes in depressed AD subjects (Ferguson et al., 2003). There was no significant correlation between the improvement of depressed mood and measures of cognitive functioning. It is possible that the latter resulted from an alteration of the balance of activity NA in favor of α_2 rather than α_1 receptors in the PFC (Arnsten et al., 1988; 1999). Such an action is probably not be shared by the SSRI, paroxetine. However, the absence of any effect on cognitive function by another NRI nortriptyline, suggests that reboxetine may have additional actions not shared by other members of this group.

The lack of a clear improvement in cognitive function during chronic treatment with antidepressants in the majority of subjects with AD could also be due to the presence of deficits in cholinergic transmission (Coyle et al., 1983), irreversible neuronal damage, such as white matter hyperintensities (Murata et al., 2001) or right frontal lobe atrophy (Almeida et al., 2003), which are not affected by antidepressants. This agrees with the data in aged, cognitively impaired rats, in which 4 weeks of treatment with fluoxetine failed to improve memory in spite of the fact that it increased MR mRNA in the CA2 region of the hippocampus (Yau et al., 2002). Thus, the overall impression gained from these studies is that improvement in cognitive ability may only occur after chronic treatment of elderly subjects with depression with certain drugs and if this is not accompanied by irreversible brain damage or loss of cholinergic transmission.

8. Drugs Currently Used to Treat Impaired Cognitive Function and Slow Degeneration

8.1. Acetylcholinesterase Inhibitors

The finding that brain cholinergic neurons degenerate in AD, and that lesions of these systems in animals result in memory impairments, led to the administration of acetylcholinesterase (AChE) inhibitors, cholinergic agonists and precursors in an attempt to restore cholinergic transmission. Among these, the AChE inhibitors tacrine, donepezil, rivastigmine and galantamine have been the most successful in improving cognitive function. They increased attention and short-term memory for periods of up to two years in about 30% of patients with AD (Rösler et al., 1999a; Farlow et al., 2001, Feldman et al., 2001; Erkinjuntti et al., 2002) vascular dementia (Moretti et al., 2001) and dementia with Lewy bodies (Samuel et al., 2000; Wesnes et al., 2002). There are preliminary reports that AChE inhibitors may also improve memory in subjects with schizophrenia (Lenzi et al., 2003; Stryjer et al., 2003) and after this has been impaired by electroconvulsive therapy (Zink et al., 2002).

Central cholinergic systems play an important role in the coupling between neuronal activity and the accompanying increase in regional cerebral blood flow (rCBF) (Tsukada et al., 1997). Subjects with MCI and AD have reduced rCBF and glucose utilization probably because of a loss of cholinergic transmission to cortical areas (Arnaiz et al., 2001; Nobili et al., 2002). AChE inhibitors have been reported to increase rCBF (Ebmeier et al., 1992; Harkins et al., 1997) and brain activation in association with better working memory in AD patients (Rombouts et al., 2002). Moreover, the beneficial effect on cognitive performance induced by rivastigmine was accompanied by significant enhancement of frontal, parietal and temporal blood flow (Venneri et al., 2002). It is possible that the improvement in mood induced by AChE inhibitors in some subjects (Rösler et al., 1999b; Gauthier et al., 2002) could also have resulted from a restoration of rCBF in those brain areas in which a deficiency is associated with depressive symptoms.

AChE inhibitors may provide more than symptomatic relief of cognitive impairment since they also slow disease progression (Farlow et al., 2000; Mohs et al., 2001; Doraiswamy et al., 2002), which can even be detected after cessation of treatment (Farlow et al., 2003). Although the mechanism for this is not known, it has been suggested that it is related to their ability to slow down the formation of amyloidogenic compounds in the brain (Giacobini, 2001) and to improve mitochondrial function (Casademont et al., 2003), which is impaired in AD patients.

In spite of the undoubted beneficial effects of AChE inhibitors on attention, cognitive function and behavioral symptoms in subjects with dementia, there are still many in whom no significant improvement is seen. Moreover, there appear to be differences in the response of patients to the individual drugs. Thus, a considerable proportion of patients who failed to derive benefit from donepezil showed significant improvement in cognitive ability and activities of daily living when switched to rivastigmine (Auriacombe et al., 2002). It is not yet known whether this also applies to galantamine and whether patients who did not respond to rivastigmine can show improvement when switched to donepezil.

8.2. NMDA Antagonists

The NMDA receptor is a subtype of ionotropic glutamate receptors that is involved in synaptic mechanisms of LTP that are believed to play an important role in learning and memory (Martin et al., 2000). However, excess activation by glutamate can cause excitotoxic neuronal injury resulting in cognitive impairment (Greenamyre, 1986; McEwen, 1999). This could occur in the aging brain through a decrease in the astroglial glutamate transporter (Li et al., 1997), which has been shown to correlate with neuronal pathology in AD patients (Masliah et al., 1996). Continuous unco-ordinated stimulation of NMDA receptors by glutamate may also occur in AD because of an inability of Mg^{2+} to filter these stimuli. This leads to excess influx of Ca^{2+} and neurodegeneration.

Although experimental studies have shown that neurodegeneration and cell death can be prevented by direct blockade of glutamate NMDA type receptors (Meldrum and Garthwaite, 1990), competitive NMDA antagonists have detrimental effects on brain function. On the other hand, memantine has low affinity for the NMDA receptor but possesses some of the properties of Mg^{2+} showing strong voltage dependency (Danyz and Parsons, 2003). It is therefore less likely than competitve antagonists to impair brain function. In support of this, memantine was shown to restore LTP, which had been impaired in hippocampal slices by excess NMDA stimulation without interfering with normal LTP (Frankiewicz and Parsons, 1999). In a recent placebo-controlled trial in AD patients with moderate to severe dementia, memantine was found to reduce the rate of further decline in memory, behavior and basic activities of daily living (Reisberg et al., 2003). It is not known whether memantine has antidepressant activity like ketamine, another use dependent NMDA antagonist (Skolnick, 1999), or whether it can actually improve cognitive function in AD patients, if like AChE inhibitors it is given when memory is only mildly impaired. From a single study performed so far it appears that a combination of memantine with an AChE inhibitor is well tolerated (Hartmann and Mobius, 2003). It now needs to be determined whether this can confer additional benefits over each drug given alone.

8.3. Monoamine Oxidase B Inhibitors

MAO-B activity increases with age and may be partly responsible for the rise in oxidative free radicals during oxidative deamination of catecholamines (Saura et al., 1994). Selegiline a selective MAO-B inhibitor protected actions cultured neuronal cells against oxidative stress (Maruyama and Naoi, 1999), attenuated neuronal death and hastened functional recovery after ischemia (Knollema et al., 1995; Lahtinen et al., 1997). Selegiline also protected CA3-CA1 hippocampal connections against overactivation of NMDA receptors by acting downstream from these receptors (Niittykoski et al., 2003). The brains of patients with AD and PD show signs of oxidative stress (Yoritaka et al., 1996; Nunomura et al., 2001) which could be partially responsible for promoting the neurodegeneration. This prompted the use of the MAO-B selective inhibitor selegiline in PD in whom it slowed disease progression and delayed the time for the necessary introduction of L-DOPA (Shoulson, 1998). It was thought that selegiline could also slow disease progression in AD, in addition to improving cognitive function by preserving the levels of DA and NA. However, the general consensus from several placebo-controlled clinical trials is that selegiline does not significantly affect attention and memory in AD, unlike AChE inhibitors (Birks and Flicker, 2003). In one of the studies it did appear to slow dementia progression (Freedman et al., 1998). This effect may have been greater if selegiline had not been metabolized to methamphetamine, which has potential neurotoxic activity (Oh et al., 1994). At higher doses than those used in these studies, selegiline also blocks MAO-A and has some antidepressant effect (Mann et al., 1989), but like other irreversible MAO-A inhibitors, it potentiates the cardiovascular effects of tyramine found in cheese and other foods (Shulz et al., 1989).

A newer selective MAO-B inhibitor, rasagiline has all the neuroprotective effects of selegiline both *in vitro* and *in vivo* (Maruyama et al., 2000; Huang et al., 1999; Finberg et al., 1998), but lacks its neurotoxic activity as it is metabolized to aminoindan and not methamphetamine (Youdim and Weinstock, 2002). Rasagiline also delays the necessity for administration L-DOPA, indicating that it may have neuroprotective effects in human subjects (Rabey et al., 2000). It has not been tested in patients with AD.

9. Combination Therapies for the Treatment of Patients with Depression and Dementia

9.1. Dual Inhibitor of AChE and MAO, TV3326 (N-propargyl-3R-aminoindan-5yl)-ethyl methylcarbamate

Since most antidepressants do not appear to be able to improve cognitive function in depressed subjects with dementia, with the possible exception of moclobemide and reboxetine, attempts have been made to synthesize novel drugs, which have both antidepressant and AChE inhibitory activity. One of these, TV3326, is based on the rasagiline molecule but contains a carbamate moiety to confer AChE inhibitory activity (Weinstock et al., 2000b). TV3326 was found to be a more potent inhibitor of butyryl than of AChE but showed relatively weak inhibition of MAO-A and B *in vitro*. However, after chronic oral administration in mice, rats and monkeys it inhibited AChE, MAO-A and B in a similar dose range, because it is metabolized to more active inhibitors of both AChE and MAO than the parent drug (Weinstock et al., 2003).

TV3326 retained all the neuroprotective effects of rasagiline *in vivo* and *in vitro* (Youdim and Weinstock, 2002) and also speeded recovery of memory and motor function induced by closed head injury in mice. It corrected spatial memory deficits induced by icv injection of streptozotocin (Weinstock et al., 2001), which disrupted hippocampal cholinergic transmission by damaging the fornix (Shoham et al., 2004), and by parenteral administration of scopolamine in rats (Weinstock et al., 2000a). TV3326 also improved some measures of attention and cognitive function in old rhesus monkeys without inducing any adverse effects (Buccafusco et al., 2003). In cultured neuronal cells, TV3326 increased the formation of neuroprotective soluble APPα from APP, thereby reducing the likelihood of its conversion to toxic Aβ peptide (Yogev-Falach et al., 2002). It is not known whether MAO-A inhibition contributes to the cognitive effects of AChE inhibition with this drug, but the neuroprotective activities appear to depend on the propargylamine and not the carbamate moiety (Maruyama et al., 2003).

In the forced swim test in rats, TV3326 acted like conventional antidepressants, moclobemide and amitriptyline, in reducing immobility after chronic oral administration to rats indicating that it may have antidepressant potential (Weinstock et al., 2002b). This effect clearly resulted from MAO inhibition since it was not shared by the S-enantiomer, which inhibits AChE but not MAO. MAO inhibition by TV3326 was brain-selective with virtually no effect on the intestinal enzyme. Therefore, unlike other irreversible MAO inhibitors, TV3326 caused only minimal potentiation of the pressor response to oral tyramine in rabbits (Weinstock et al., 2002a), possibly because it was converted to an active MAO-A and B inhibitor in the brain. These unique properties, combined with its beneficial effects on memory in various animal models, suggest that TV3326 may be a safe and efficacious drug for the treatment of dementia co-morbid with depression. Its neuroprotective properties may help to slow the progression of neurodegeneration in AD patients, and represents a good example of convergence of antidepressant and antidementia pharmacology.

9.2. Dual Inhibitor of AChE and Serotonin Transporter RS-1259, (4-[1S)-methylamino-3-(4-nitrophenoxy)] proylphenyl N,N-dimethylcarbamate)

Another drug, RS-1259, with potential antidepressant and antidementia activity has recently been synthesized and its initial pharmacological activity described (Abe et al., 2003). This compound also contains a carbamate moiety to inhibit AChE but also acts as an SSRI, blocking the re-uptake of 5-HT. These actions enabled RS-1259 to increase extracellular levels of ACh and 5-HT in the hippocampus as measured by in vivo microdialysis in conscious rats. Acute administration of RS-1259 to aged rats reversed their impairment in short-term memory and increased duration of wakeful periods during daytime sleep. It is not known whether like other SSRIs, the drug has antidepressant-like activity in animal models or whether it can increase BDNF or promote neurogenesis. Further studies are awaited in order to determine whether this drug has any advantages over SSRIs or AChE inhibitors alone in the treatment of depression and dementia, respectively.

In this review, some of the pathophysiological and behavioral alterations in depression and dementia have been described. Similar alterations to those seen in depressed human subjects in the regulation of the HPA axis, aminergic transmission and transcription factors regulating neurogenesis, have been found in rats that had been subjected to chronic inescapable stress. In spite of this, the majority of studies on the mechanism of action of antidepressants have been performed in naive rats. In such animals, the drugs cause changes in neurotransmitter release and receptor activity, which are similar to those seen in response to acute stress, and usually in the opposite direction to those seen in depressed patients. Chronically stressed rats therefore present a more suitable model for the evaluation of the mechanism of action of different classes of antidepressants. In such animals, most classes of antidepressant drugs normalize behavior, dysregulation of the HPA axis and neurotransmitter function, but the aminergic receptors through which these effects are mediated, appear to differ among TCAs, NRIs and SSRIs. While, there is some overlap in the pathophysiological changes and neurotransmitter deficits in dementia and depression, the majority of antidepressants do not seem to be able to improve cognitive function in depressed elderly subjects with dementia, although they can ameliorate their depressive symptoms. It is hoped that novel drugs that have both anticholinesterase activity, to improve cortical cholineric transmission, and neuroprotective and antidepressant properties, will provide a therapeutic solution to this problem.

References

Abe Y, Aoyagi A, Hara T, Abe K, Yamazaki R, Kumagae Y, Naruto S, Koyama S, Tago K, Toda N, Takami K, Yamada N, Ori M, Kogen H, Kaneko T. Pharmacological characterization of RS122259, an orally active dual inhibitor of acetylcholinesterase and serotonin transporter, in rodents: Possible treatment of Alzheimer's disease. *J Pharmacol Sci* **93**: 95-105, 2003.

Adell A, Garcia-Marquez C, Armario A, Gelpi E. Chronic stress increases serotonin and noradrenaline in rat brain and sensitizes their responses to a further acute stress. *J Neurochem* **50**: 1678-1681, 1988.

Alexopoulos GS, Meyers BS, Young R C, Mattis S, Kakuma T. The course of geriatric depression with "reversible dementia": a controlled study. *Am J Psychiatry* **150**: 1693-1699, 1993.

Almeida OP, Burton EJ, Ferrier N, McKeith IG, O'Brien JT. Depression with late onset is associated with right frontal lobe atrophy. *Psycholog Med* **33**: 675-681, 2003.

Alonso SJ, Navarro E, Rodriguez M. Permanent dopaminergic alterations in the n. accumbens after prenatal stress. *Pharmacol Biochem Behav* **49**: 353-358, 1994.

Altar C. Neurotrophins and depression. *Trends Pharmacol Sci* **20**: 59-61, 1999.

Arborelius L, Skelton KH, Thrivikraman KV, Plotsky PM, Schulz DW, Owens MJ. Chronic administration of the selective corticotropin-releasing factor 1 receptor antagonist CP-154,526: behavioral, endocrine and neurochemical effects in the rat. *J Pharmacol Exptl Ther* **294**: 588-597, 2000.

Arnaiz E, Jelic V, Almkvist O, Wahlund LO, Winblad B, Valind S, Nordberg A. Impaired cerebral glucose metabolism and cognitive functioning predict deterioration in mild cognitive impairment. *Neuroreport* **12**: 851-855, 2001.

Arnsten AF, Cai JX, Goldman-Rakic PS. The alpha-2 adrenergic agonist guanfacine improves memory in aged monkeys without sedative or hypotensive side effects: evidence for alpha-2 receptor subtypes. *J Neurosci* **8**: 4287-4298, 1988.

Arnsten AF, Mathew R, Ubriani R, Taylor JR, Li BM. Alpha-1 noradrenergic receptor stimulation impairs prefrontal cortical cognitive function. *Biol Psychiatry* **45**: 26-31, 1999.

Auriacombe S, Pere J-J, Loria-Kanza Y, Vellas B. Efficacy and safety of rivastigmine in patients with Alzheimer's disease who failed to benefit from treatment with donepezil. *Curr Med Res* **18**: 129-138, 2002.

Azmitia EC. Serotonin neurons, neuroplasticity, and homeostasis of neural tissue. *Neuropsychopharmacology* **21(suppl 2)**: 33S-45S, 1999.

Bagley J, Moghaddam B. Temporal dynamics of glutamate efflux in the prefrontal cortex and in the hippocampus following repeated stress: effects of pretreatment with saline or diazepam. *Neuroscience* **77**: 65–73, 1997.

Birks J, Flicker L. Selegiline for Alzheimer's disease. *Cochrane Database Syst Rev* **2**: CD000442, 2003.

Blackwell B, Marley E, Price J, Taylor D. Hypertensive interactions between monoamine oxidase inhibitors and foodstuffs. *Br J Psychiatry* **113**: 349-365, 1967.

Blazer D. Depression in the elderly. *New Engl J Med* **320**: 164-166, 1989.

Bliss TVP, Collingridge GL. A synaptic model of memory: long-term potentiation in the hippocampus. *Nature* **361**: 31-39, 1993.

Bremner JD, Narayan M, Anderson ER, Staib LH, Miller HL, Charney DS. Hippocampal volume reduction in major depression. *Am J Psychiatry* **157**: 115-118, 2000.

Buccafusco JJ, Terry Jr AV, Goren T, Blaugrund E. Potential cognitive actions of (n-propargly-(3r)-aminoindan-5-yl)-ethyl, methyl carbamate (TV3326), a novel neuroprotective agent, as assessed in old rhesus monkeys in their performance of versions of a delayed matching task. *Neuroscience* **119**: 669-678, 2003.

Butler PD, Weiss JM, Stout JC, Nemeroff CB. Corticotrophin-releasing factor produces fear-enhancing and behavioral activating effects following infusion into the locus coeruleus. *J Neurosci* **10**: 176-183, 1990.

Butterweck V, Winterhoff H, Herkenham M. St John's wort, hypericin, and imipramine: a comparative analysis of mRNA levels in brain areas involved in HPA axis control following short-term and long-term administration in normal and stressed rats. *Mol Psychiatry* **6**: 547-564, 2001.

Cardenas VA, Du AT, Hardin D, Ezekiel F, Weber P, Jagust WJ, Chui HC, Schuff N, Weiner MW. Comparison of methods for measuring longitudinal brain change in cognitive impairment and dementia. *Neurobiol Aging* **24**: 537-544, 2003.

Casademont J, Miro O, Rodriguez-Santiago B, Viedma P, Blesa R, Cardellach F. Cholinesterase inhibitor rivastigmine enhances the mitochondrial electron transport chain in lymphocytes of patients with Alzheimer's disease. *J Neurol Sci* **206**: 23-26, 2003.

Chrousos GP. Stressors, stress, and neuroendocrine integration of the adaptive response. The 1997 Hans Selye Memorial Lecture. *Ann N Y Acad Sci* **851**: 311-335,1998.

Claustre Y, Rivy JP, Dennis T, Scatton B. Pharmacological studies on stress-induced increase in frontal cortical dopamine metabolism in the rat. *J Pharmacol Exptl Ther* **238**: 693-700, 1986.

Cole BJ, Robbins TW. Forebrain norepinephrine: role in controlled information processing in the rat. *Neuropsychopharmacol* **7**: 129-142, 1992.

Conti AC, Cryan JF, Dalvi A, Lucki I, Blendy JA. cAMP response element-binding protein is essential for the upregulation of brain-derived neurotrophic factor transcription, but not the behavioral or endocrine responses to antidepressant drugs. *J Neurosci* **22**: 3262-3268, 2002.

Coyle JT, Price DL, DeLong MR. Alzheimer's disease: a disorder of cortical cholinergic innervation. *Science* **219**: 1184-1190, 1983.

Cuadra G, Zurita A, Gioino G, Molina V. Influence of different antidepressant drugs on the effect of chronic variable stress on restraint-induced dopamine release in frontal cortex. *Neuropsychopharmacol* **25**: 384-394, 2001.

Czeh B, Michaelis T, Watanabe T, Frahm J, de Biurrun G, Van Kampen M, Bartolomucci A, Fuchs E. Stress-induced changes in cerebral metabolites, hippocampal volume, and cell proliferation are prevented by antidepressant treatment with tianeptine. *Proc Natl Acad Sci USA* **98**: 12796-12801, 2001.

Da Prada M, Zürcher G, Wüthrich I, Haefely WE. On tyramine, food, beverages and the reversible MAO inhibitor moclobemide. *J Neural Transm* **26 (Suppl)**: 31-56, 1988.

Danysz W, Parsons CG. The NMDA receptor antagonist memantine as a symptomatological and neuroprotective treatment for Alzheimer's disease: preclinical evidence. *Int J Geriatr Psychiatry* **18 (Suppl 1):** S23-32, 2003.

Datla KP, Curzon G. Behavioural and neurochemical evidence for the decrease of brain extracellular 5-HT by the antidepressant drug tianeptine. *Neuropharmacol* **32:** 839-845, 1993.

Davis M, Rainnie D, Cassell M. Neurotransmission in the rat amygdala related to fear and anxiety. *Trends Neurological Sci* **17:** 208-214, 1994.

Dazzi L, Ladu S, Spiga F, Vacca G, Rivano A, Pira L, Biggio G. Chronic treatment with imipramine or mirtazapine antagonizes stress- and FG7142-induced increase in cortical norepinephrine output in freely moving rats. *Synapse* **43:** 70-77, 2002a.

Dazzi L, Serra M, Spiga F, Pisu MG, Jentsch JD, Biggio G. Prevention of the stress-induced increase in frontal cortical dopamine efflux of freely moving rats by long-term treatment with antidepressant drugs. *Eur Neuropsychopharmacol* **11:** 343-349, 2001.

Dazzi L, Vignone V, Seu E, Ladu S, Vacca G, Biggio G. Inhibition by venlafaxine of the increase in norepinephrine output in rat prefrontal cortex elicited by acute stress or by the anxiogenic drug FG 7142. *J Psychopharmacol* **16:** 125-131, 2002b.

Deak T, Nguyen KT, Ehrlich A, Watkins LR, Spencer RL, Maier SF, Licinio J, Wong ML, Chrousos GP, Webster E, Gold PW. The impact of the nonpeptide corticotropin-releasing hormone antagonist antalarmin on behavioral and endocrine responses to stress *.Endocrinology* **140:** 79-86, 1999.

Delgado PL, Charney DS, Price LH, Aghajanian GK, Landis H, Heninger GR. Serotonin function and the mechanism of antidepressant action. Reversal of antidepressant-induced remission by rapid depletion of plasma tryptophan. *Arch Gen Psychiatry* **47:** 411–418, 1990.

Devanand DP, Pelton GH, Marston K, Camacho Y, Roose SP, Stern Y, Sackeim HA. Sertraline treatment of elderly patients with depression and cognitive impairment. *Int J Geriatr Psychiatry* **18:** 123-130, 2003.

Di Chiara G, Tanda G. Blunting of reactivity of dopamine transmission to palatable food: A biochemical marker of anhedonia in the CMS model? *Psychopharmacol* **112:** 398-402, 1997.

Doraiswamy PM, Krishnan KRR. Long-term effects of rivastigmine in moderately severe Alzheimer's disease. Does early initiation of therapy offer sustained benefits? *Prog Neuropsychopharmacol Behav Psychiat* **26:** 705-712, 2002.

Dowlatshani D, MacQueen GM, Wang JF, Young LT. Increased temporal cortex CREB concentrations and antidepressant treatment in major depression. *Lancet* **352:** 1754-1755,1998.

Drevets WC. Neuroimaging studies of mood disorders. *Biol Psychiatry* **48:** 813-829, 2000.

Dubrovsky B. Adrenal steroids and the physiopathology of a subset of depressive disorders. *Med Hypotheses* **36:** 300-305, 1991.

Duggan AW, Furmidge LJ. Probing the brain and spinal cord with neuropeptides in pathways related to pain and other functions *.Front Neuroendocrinol* **15:** 275-300, 1994.

Duman RS, Malberg J, Nakagawa S, D'Sa C. Neuronal plasticity and survival in mood disorders. *Biol Psychiatry* **48:** 732-739, 2000.

Ebmeier KP, Hunter R, Curran SM, Dougal NJ, Murray CL, Wyper DJ, Patterson J, Hanson MT, Siegfried K, Goodwin GM. Effects of a single dose of the acetylcholinesterase inhibitor velnacrine on recognition memory and regional cerebral blood flow in Alzheimer's disease. *Psychopharmacol* **108**:103-109, 1992.

Emson PC, Jessell T, Paxinos G, Cuello AC. Substance P in the amygdaloid complex, bed nucleus and stria terminalis of the rat brain. *Brain Res* **149**: 97-105, 1978.

Erkinjuntti T, Kurz A, Gauthier S, Bullock R, Lilienfeld S, Damaraju CRV. Efficacy of galantamine in probable vascular dementia and Alzheimer's disease combined with cerebrovascular disease: A randomised trial. *Lancet* **359**: 1283-1290, 2002.

Evers MM, Samuels SC, Lantz M, Khan K, Brickman AM, Marin D. The prevalence, diagnosis and treatment of depression in dementia patients in chronic care facilities in the last six months of life. *Int J Geriatr Psychiatry* **17**: 464-472, 2002.

Farlow M, Anand R, Messina J Jr, Hartman R, Veach JA. 52-week study of the efficacy of rivastigmine in patients with mild to moderately severe Alzheimer's disease. *Eur Neurol* **44**: 236-241, 2000.

Farlow M, Potkin S, Koumaras B, Veach J, Mirski D. Analysis of outcome in retrieved dropout patients in a rivastigmine vs placebo, 26-week, Alzheimer disease trial. *Arch Neurol.* **60**: 843-848, 2003.

Farlow MR, Hake A, Messina J, Hartman R, Veach J, Anand R. Response of patients with Alzheimer disease to rivastigmine treatment is predicted by the rate of disease progression. *Arch Neurol.* **58**: 417-422, 2001.

Feldman H, Gauthier S, Hecker J, Vellas B, Subbiah P, Whalen EA. 24-week, randomized, double-blind study of donepezil in moderate to severe Alzheimer's disease. *Neurology* **57**: 613-620, 2001.

Ferguson JM, Wesnes KA, Schwartz GE. Reboxetine versus paroxetine versus placebo: effects on cognitive functioning in depressed patients. *Int Clin Psychopharmacol* **18**: 9-14, 2003.

Finberg JP, Takeshima T, Johnston JM, Commissiong JW. Increased survival of dopaminergic neurons by rasagiline, a monoamine oxidase B inhibitor. *Neuroreport* **9**: 703-707. 1998.

Finlay JM, Zigmond MJ, Abercrombie ED. Increased dopamine and norepinephrine release in medial prefrontal cortex induced by acute and chronic stress: effects of diazepam. *Neurosci* **64**: 619–628, 1995.

Fontenot MB, Kaplan JR, Manuck SB, Arango V, Mann JJ. Long-term effects of chronic social stress on serotonergic indices in the prefrontal cortex of adult male cynomolgus macaques. *Brain Res* **705**:105-108,1995.

Foy MR, Stanton ME, Levine S, Thompson RF. Behavioral stress impairs long-term potentiation in rodent hippocampus. *Behav Neural Biol* **48**: 138-149, 1987.

Frackiewicz EJ, Sramek JJ, Cutler NR. Gender differences in depression and antidepressant pharmacokinetics and adverse events. *Ann Pharmacother* **34**: 80-88, 2000.

Frankiewicz T, Parsons CG. Memantine restores long term potentiation impaired by tonic N-methyl-D-aspartate (NMDA) receptor activation following reduction of $Mg2+$ In hippocampal slices. *Neuropharmacol* **38**: 1253-1259, 1999.

Freedman M, Rewilak D, Xerri T, Cohen S, Gordon AS, Shandling M, Logan AG. L-deprenyl in Alzheimer's disease: cognitive and behavioral effects. *Neurology* **50**: 660-668, 1998.

Fride E, Weinstock M. Alterations in behavioral and striatal dopamine asymmetries induced by prenatal stress. *Pharmacol Biochem Behav* **32**: 425-430, 1989.

Fujita M, Charney DS, Innis RB. Imaging serotonergic neurotransmission in depression: hippocampal pathophysiology may mirror global brain alteration. *Biol Psychiatry* **48**: 801-812, 2000.

Gambarana C, Ghiglieri O, De Montis MG. Desensitization of the D1 dopamine receptors in rats reproduces a model of escape deficit reverted by imipramine, fluoxetine and clomipramine. *Prog Neuropsychopharmacol Biol Psychiatry* **19**: 741–755, 1995a.

Gambarana C, Ghiglieri O, Taddei I, Tagliamonte A, De Montis MG. Imipramine and fluoxetine prevent the stress induced escape deficits in rats through a distinct mechanism of action. *Behav Pharmacol* **6**: 66–73, 1995b.

Gambarana C, Masi F, Tagliamonte A, Scheggi S, Ghiglieri O, De Montis MG. A chronic stress which impairs reactivity in rats also decreases dopaminergic transmission in the nucleus accumbens: A microdialysis study. *J Neurochem* **72**: 2039-2046, 1999.

Gareri P, De Fazio P, De Sarro G. Neuropharmacology of depression in aging and age-related diseases. *Ageing Res Revs* **1**: 113-134, 2002.

Gauthier S, Feldman H, Hecker J, Vellas B, Ames D, Subbiah P, Whalen E, Emir B. Donepezil MSAD Study Investigators Group. Efficacy of donepezil on behavioral symptoms in patients with moderate to severe Alzheimer's disease. *Int Psychogeriatrics* **14**: 389-404, 2002.

Geerlings MI, Bouter LM, Schoevers R, Beekman ATF, Jonker C, Deeg DJH, Van Tilburg W, Adèr HJ, Schmand B. Depression and risk of cognitive decline and Alzheimer's disease: Results of two prospective community-based studies in The Netherlands. *Brit J Psychiatry* **176**: 568-575, 2000.

Giacobini E. Do cholinesterase inhibitors have disease-modifying effects in Alzheimer's disease? *CNS Drugs* **15**: 85-91, 2001.

Goedert M, Jakes R Spillantini MG, Hasegawa M, Smith MJ, Crowther RA. Assembly of microtubule-associated protein tau into Alzheimer-like filaments induced by sulphated glycosaminoglycans. *Nature* **383**: 550-553, 1996.

Gold PW, Chrousos GP. The endocrinology of melancholic and atypical depression: relation to neurocircuitry and somatic consequences. *Proc Assoc Am Physicians* **111**: 22-34, 1999.

Gould E, Reeves AJ, Graziano MS, Gross CG. Neurogenesis in the neocortex of adult primates. *Science* **286**: 548-552, 1999.

Gould E, Tanapat P, McEwen BS, Flügge G, Fuchs E. Proliferation of granule cell precursors in the dentate gyrus of adult monkeys is diminished by stress. *Proc Natl Acad Sci USA* **95**: 3168-3171, 1998.

Gould E, Tanapat P, Rydel T, Hastings N. Regulation of hippocampal neurogenesis in adulthood. *Biol Psychiatry* **48**: 715-720, 2000.

Grappi S, Nanni G, Leggio B, Rauggi R, Scheggi S, Masi F, Gambarana C. The efficacy of reboxetine in preventing and reverting a condition of escape deficit in rats. *Biol Psychiatry* **53**: 890-898, 2003.

Green RC, Cupples LA, Kurz A, Auerbach S, Go R, Sadovnick D, Duara R, Kukull WA, Chui H, Edeki T, Griffith PA, Friedland RP, Bachman D, Farrer L. Depression as a risk factor for Alzheimer disease: the MIRAGE Study. *Arch Neurol* **60**:753-759, 2003.

Greenamyre JT. The role of glutamate in neurotransmission and in neurologic disease. *Arch Neurol* **43**: 1058-1063, 1986.

Greenwald BS, Kramer-Ginsberg E, Krishnan KRR, Ashtari M, Auerbach C, Patel M. Neuroanatomic localization of magnetic resonance imaging signal hyperintensities in geriatric depression. *Stroke* **29**: 613-617, 1998.

Griebel G, Perrault G, Soubrie P. Effects of SR48968, a selective non-peptide NK2 receptor antagonist on emotional processes in rodents *.Psychopharmacol* **158**: 241-251, 2001.

Habib KE, Weld K P, Rice KC, Pushkas J, Champoux M, Listwak S, Webster EL, Atkinson AJ, Schulkin J, Contoreggi C, Chrousos GP, McCann SM, Suomi SJ, Higley JD, Gold PW. Oral administration of a corticotropin-releasing hormone receptor antagonist significantly attenuates behavioral, neuroendocrine, and autonomic responses to stress in primates. *Proc Natl Acad Sci USA* **97**: 6079-6084, 2000.

Hafner H. Epidemiology of Alzheimer's disease. In: Maurer K, Riederer P, Beckmann H, editors. Alzheimer's Disease: Epidemiology, Neuropathology, Neurochemistry, and Clinics. Vienna: Springer-Verlag, 1990, pp. 23-39.

Harkins SW, Taylor JR, Mattay V, Regelson W. Tacrine treatment in Alzheimer's disease enhances cerebral blood flow and mental status and decreases caregiver suffering. *Ann N Y Acad Sci* **826**: 472-474, 1997.

Harrison PJ. The neuropathology of primary mood disorder. *Brain* **125**: 1428-1449, 2002.

Hartmann S, Mobius HJ. Tolerability of memantine in combination with cholinesterase inhibitors in dementia therapy. *Int Clin Psychopharmacol* **18**: 81-85, 2003.

Hassan AH, Patchev VK, Von Rosenstiel P, Holsboer F, Almeida OF. Plasticity of hippocampal corticosteroid receptors during aging in the rat. *FASEB J* **13**: 115-122, 1999.

Hayashi A, Nagaoka M, Yamada K, Ichitani Y, Miake Y, Okado N. Maternal stress induces synaptic loss and developmental disabilities of offspring. *Int J Devl Neurosci* **16**: 209-216, 1998.

Heilig M, Thorsell A. Brain neuropeptide Y (NPY) in stress and alcohol dependence. *Rev Neurosci* **13**: 85-94, 2002.

Heim C, Newport DJ, Heit S, Graham YP, Wilcox M, Bonsall R, Miller AH, Nemeroff CB. Pituitary-adrenal and autonomic responses to stress in women after sexual and physical abuse in childhood. *JAMA* **284**: 595-597, 2000.

Hebert C, Habimana A, Elie R, Reader TA. Effects of chronic antidepressant treatments on 5-HT and NA transporters in rat brain: an autoradiographic study. *Neurochem Int* **38**: 63-74, 2001.

Holsboer-Trachsler E, Stohler R, Hatzinger M. Repeated administration of the combined dexamethasone/hCRH stimulation test during treatment of depression. *Psychiatry Res* **38**: 163-171, 1991.

Huang W, Chen Y, Shohami E, Weinstock M. Neuroprotective effect of rasagiline, a selective MAO-B inhibitor, against closed head injury in the mouse. *Eur J Pharmacol* **366:** 127-135, 1999.

Jaiswal AK, Bhattacharya SK. Effects of gestational undernutrition, stress and diazepam treatment on spatial discrimination learning and retention in young rats. *Indian J Exp Biol* **31:** 353-359, 1993.

Kaneyuki H, Yokoo H, Tsuda A, Yoshida M, Mizuki Y, Yamada M, Tanaka M. Psychological stress increases dopamine turnover selectively in mesoprefrontal dopamine neurons in rats: Reversal by diazepam. *Brain Res* **557:** 154–161, 1991.

Knollema S, Aukema W, Hom H, Korf J, Horst GJT. L-Deprenyl reduces brain damage in rats exposed to transient hypoxia-ischemia. *Stroke* **26:** 1883-1887, 1995.

Kole MH, Swan L, Fuchs E. The antidepressant tianeptine persistently modulates glutamate receptor currents in the hippocampal CA3 commissural associational synapse in chronically stressed rats. *Eur J Neurosci* **16:** 807-816, 2002.

Kornstein SG, Schatzberg AF, Thase ME, Yonkers KA, McCullough JP, Keitner GI, Gelenberg AJ, Ryan CE, Hess AL, Harrison W, Davis SM, Keller MB. Gender differences in chronic major and double depression. *J Affect Disord* **60:** 1-11, 2000.

Kral VA, Emery OB. Long-term follow-up of depressive pseudodementia of the aged. *Can J Psychiatry* **34:** 445-446, 1989.

Lahtinen H, Koistinaho J, Kauppinen R, Haapalinna A, Keinanen R, Sivenius J. Selegiline treatment after transient global ischemia in gerbils enhances the survival of CA1 pyramidal cells in the hippocampus. *Brain Res* **757:** 260-267, 1997.

Lai MK, Tsang SW, Francis PT, Esiri MM, Keene J, Hope T, Chen CP. Reduced serotonin 5-HT1A receptor binding in the temporal cortex correlates with aggressive behavior in Alzheimer disease. *Brain Res* **974:** 82-87, 2003.

Leibowitz SF, Diaz S, Tempel D. Norepinephrine in the paraventricular nucleus stimulates corticosterone release. *Brain Res* **496:** 219-227, 1989.

Lemaire V, Koehl M, Le Moal M, Abrous DN. Prenatal stress produces learning deficits associated with an inhibition of neurogenesis in the hippocampus. *Proc Natl Acad Sci USA* **97:** 11032-11037, 2000.

Lenzi A, Maltinti E, Poggi E, Fabrizio L, Coli E. Effects of rivastigmine on cognitive function and quality of life in patients with schizophrenia. *Clin Neuropharmacol* **26:** 317-321, 2003.

Levy ML, Cummings JL, Fairbanks LA, Bravi D, Calvani M, Carta A. Longitudinal assessment of symptoms of depression, agitation, and psychosis in 181 patients with Alzheimer's disease. *Am J Psychiatry* **153:** 1438-1443, 1996.

Li S, Mallory M, Alford M, Tanaka S, Masliah E. Glutamate transporter alterations in Alzheimer disease are possibly associated with abnormal APP expression. *J Neuropathol Exp Neurol* **56:** 901-911, 1997.

Li Y-S, Meyer JS, Thornby J. Longitudinal follow-up of depressive symptoms among normal versus cognitively impaired elderly. *Int J Geriat Psychiat* **16:** 718-727, 2001.

Ljungdahl A, Hokfelt T, Nilsson G. Distribution of substance P-like immunoreactivity in the central nervous system of the rat. I. Cell bodies and nerve terminals. *Neuroscience* **3:** 861-943, 1978.

Maes M, Meltzer H. The serotonin hypothesis of major depression. In: Bloom FE, Kupfer DJ, editors. Psychophamacology: The Fourth Generation of Progress. New York: Raven Press, 1995, pp. 933-944.

Makino S, Hashimoto K, Gold PW. Multiple feedback mechanisms activating corticotropin-releasing hormone system in the brain during stress. *Pharmacol Biochem Behav* **73**: 147-158, 2002.

Malberg JE, Eisch AJ, Nestler EJ, Duman RS. Chronic antidepressant treatment increases neurogenesis in adult rat hippocampus. *J Neurosci* **20**: 9104-9110, 2000.

Manev H, Uz T, Smalheiser NR, Manev R. Antidepressants alter cell proliferation in the adult brain in vivo and in neural cultures in vitro. *Eur J Pharmacol* **411**: 67-70, 2001.

Mangiavacchi S, Masi F, Scheggi S, Leggio B, De Montis MG, Gambarana C. Long-term behavioral and neurochemical effects of chronic stress exposure in rats. *J Neurochem* **78**: 1-10, 2001.

Mann JJ, Aarons SF, Wilner PJ, Keilp JG, Sweeney JA, Pearlstein T, Frances AJ, Kocsis JH, Brown RP. A controlled study of the antidepressant efficacy and side effects of (-)-deprenyl. A selective monoamine oxidase inhibitor. *Arch Gen Psychiatry* **46**: 45-50, 1989.

Mann JJ, Stanley M, McBride PA, McEwen BS. Increased serotonin2 and beta-adrenergic receptor binding in the frontal cortices of suicide victims. *Arch Gen Psychiatry* **43**: 954-959, 1986.

Mantyh PW. Neurobiology of substance P and the NK1 receptor. *J Clin Psychiatry* **63 (suppl 11)**: 6-10, 2002.

Martin SJ, Grimwood PD, Morris RGM. Synaptic plasticity and memory: an evaluation of the hypothesis. *Ann Rev Neurosci* **23**: 649-711, 2000.

Maruyama W, Naoi M. Neuroprotection by (-)-deprenyl and related compounds. *Mech Ageing Dev* **111**: 189-200, 1999.

Maruyama W, Weinstock M, Youdim MBH, Nagai M, Naoi M. Anti-apoptotic action of the anti-Alzheimer drug, TV3326 [(N-propargyl)-(3R) –aminoindan-5-yl]-ethyl methyl carbamate, a novel cholinesterase-monoamine oxidase inhibitor. *Neurosci Letts* **341**: 233-236, 2003.

Maruyama W, Yamamoto T, Kitani K, Carrillo MC, Youdim MMH, Naoi M. Mechanism underlying anti-apoptotic activity of a (-) deprenyl-related propargylamine, rasagiline. *Mech. Aging Dev.* **116**:181-191, 2000.

Masliah E, Alford M, DeTeresa R, Mallory M, Hansen L. Deficient glutamate transport is associated with neurodegeneration in Alzheimer's disease. *Ann Neurol* **40**: 759-766, 1996.

Massicotte G, Bernard J, Ohayon M. Chronic effects of trimipramine, an antidepressant, on hippocampal synaptic plasticity. *Behav Neural Biol* **59**: 100-106, 1993.

Matthews KL, Chen CP, Esiri MM, Keene J, Minger SL, Francis PT. Noradrenergic changes, aggressive behavior, and cognition in patients with dementia. *Biol Psychiatry* **51**: 407-416, 2002.

Maura G, Marcoli M, Tortarolo M, Andrioli GC, Raiteri M. Glutamate release in human cerebral cortex and its modulation by 5-hydroxytryptamine acting at 5-HT_{1D} receptors *Br J Pharmac* **123**: 45-50, 1998.

McEwen BS. Stress and hippocampal plasticity. *Ann Rev Neurosci* **22:** 105-122, 1999.

McEwen BS, Conrad CD, Kuroda Y, Frankfurt M, Magarinos AM, McKittrick C. Prevention of stress-induced morphological and cognitive consequences. *Eur Neuropsychopharmacol* **7 (suppl 3):** S323-S328, 1997.

McKittrick CR, Magarinos AM, Blanchard DC, Blanchard RJ, McEwen BS, Sakai RR. Chronic social stress reduces dendritic arbors in CA3 of hippocampus and decreases binding to serotonin transporter sites. *Synapse* **36:** 85-94, 2000.

Meijer OC, Van Oosten RV, De Kloet ER. Elevated basal trough levels of corticosterone suppress hippocampal 5-hydroxytryptamine (1A) receptor expression in adrenally intact rats: implication for the pathogenesis of depression. *Neuroscience* **80:** 419-426, 1997.

Meldrum B, Garthwaite J. Excitatory amino acid neurotoxicity and neurodegenerative disease. *Trends Pharmacol Sci* **11:** 379-387, 1990.

Meneses A. Tianeptine: 5-HT uptake sites and $5-HT_{1-7}$ receptors modulate memory formation in an autoshaping Pavlovian/instrumental task. *Neurosci Biobehav Rev* **26:** 309-319, 2002.

Merikangas KR, Chakravarti A, Moldin SO, Araj H, Blangero JC, Burmeister M, Crabbe J Jr, Depaulo JR Jr, Foulks E, Freimer NB, Koretz DS, Lichtenstein W, Mignot E, Reiss AL, Risch NJ, Takahashi JS. Future of genetics of mood disorders research. *Biol Psychiatry* **52:** 457-477, 2002.

Mesulam MM. The systems-level organization of cholinergic innervation in the human cerebral cortex and its alterations in Alzheimer's disease. *Prog Brain Res* **109:** 285-297, 1996.

Michael-Titus AT, Bains S, Jeetle J, Whelpton R. Imipramine and phenelzine decrease glutamate overflow in the prefrontal cortex--a possible mechanism of neuroprotection in major depression? *Neuroscience* **100:** 681-684, 2000.

Miller HL, Delgado PL, Salomon RM, Berman R, Krystal JH, Heninger GR, Charney DS. Clinical and biochemical effects of catecholamine depletion on antidepressant-induced remission of depression. *Arch Gen Psychiatry* **53:** 117–128, 1996.

Mitchell AJ, Dening TR. Depression-related cognitive impairment: possibilities for its pharmacological treatment. *J Affective Dis* **36:** 79-87, 1996.

Mizoguchi K, Ishige A, Aburada M, Tabira T. Chronic stress attenuates glucocorticoid negative feedback: involvement of the prefrontal cortex and hippocampus. *Neuroscience* **119:** 887-897, 2003.

Mohs RC, Doody RS, Morris JC, Ieni JR, Rogers SL, Perdomo CA, Pratt RD. A 1-year, placebo-controlled preservation of function survival study of donepezil in AD patients. *Neurology* **57:** 481-488, 2001.

Mongeau R, Blier P, de Montigny C. The serotonergic and noradrenergic systems of the hippocampus: their interactions and the effects of antidepressant treatments. *Brain Res Rev* **23:** 145-195, 1997.

Montkowski A, Barden N, Wotjak C, Stec I, Ganster J, Meaney M, Engelmann M, Reul JM, Landgraf R, Holsboer F. Long-term antidepressant treatment reduces behavioural deficits in transgenic mice with impaired glucocorticoid receptor function. *J Neuroendocrinol* **7:** 841-845, 1995.

Morcuende S, Gadd CA, Peters M, Moss A, Harris EA, Sheasby A, Fisher AS, De Felipe C, Mantyh PW, Rupniak NM, Giese KP, Hunt SP. Increased neurogenesis and brain-derived neurotrophic factor in neurokinin-1 receptor gene knockout mice. *Eur J Neurosci* **18**: 1828-1836, 2003.

Moretti R, Torre P, Antonello RM, Cazzato G. Rivastigmine in subcortical vascular dementia: a comparison trial on efficacy and tolerability for 12 months follow-up. *Eur J Neurology* **8**: 361-362, 2001.

Murata T, Kimura H, Omori M, Kado H, Kosaka H, Iidaka T, Itoh H, Wada Y. MRI white matter hyperintensities, ^{1}H-MR spectroscopy and cognitive function in geriatric depression: a comparison of early- and late-onset cases. *Int J Geriatr Psychiatry* **16**:1129-1135, 2001.

Muscat R, Papp M, Willner P. Reversal of stress-induced anhedonia by atypical antidepressants, fluoxetine and maprotiline. *Psychopharmacology* **109**: 433-438, 1992.

Nebes RD, Pollock BG, Houck PR, Butters MA, Mulsant BH, Zmuda MD, Reynolds CF 3rd. Persistence of cognitive impairment in geriatric patients following antidepressant treatment: a randomized, double-blind clinical trial with nortriptyline and paroxetine. *J Psychiatr Res* **37**: 99-108, 2003.

Nemeroff CB, Widerlov E, Bissette G, Walleus H, Karlsson I, Eklund K, Kilts CD, Loosen PT, Vale W. Elevated concentrations of CSF corticotropin-releasing factor-like immunoreactivity in depressed patients. *Science* **226**: 1342-1344, 1984.

Neumaier JF, Petty F, Kramer GL, Szot P, Hamblin MW. Learned helplessness increases 5-hydroxytryptamine$_{1B}$ receptor mRNA levels in the rat dorsal raphe nucleus. *Biol Psychiatry* **41**: 668-674, 1997.

Nibuya M, Morinobu S, Duman RS. Regulation of BDNF and trkB mRNA in rat brain by chronic electroconvulsive seizure and antidepressant drug treatments. *J Neurosci* **15**: 7539-7547, 1995.

Nibuya M, Nestler EJ, Duman RS. Chronic antidepressant administration increases the expression of cAMP response element binding protein (CREB) in rat hippocampus. *J Neurosci* **16**: 2365-2372, 1996.

Nickel T, Sonntag A, Schill J, Zobel AW, Ackl N, Brunnauer A, Murck H, Ising M, Yassouridis A, Steiger A, Zihl J, Holsboer F. Clinical and neurobiological effects of tianeptine and paroxetine in major depression. *J Clin Psychopharmacol* **23**: 155-168, 2003.

Niittykoski M, Haapalinna A, Sirviö J. Selegiline reduces N-methyl-D-aspartic acid induced perturbation of neurotransmission but it leaves NMDA receptor dependent long-term potentiation intact in the hippocampus. *J Neural Transm* **110**: 1225-1240, 2003.

Nisenbaum LK, Zigmond MJ, Sved AF, Abercrombie ED. Prior exposure to chronic stress results in enhanced synthesis and release of hippocampal norepinephrine in response to a novel stressor. *J Neurosci* **11**: 1478-1484, 1991.

Nobili F, Koulibaly M, Vitali P, Migneco O, Mariani G, Ebmeier K, Pupi A, Robert PH, Rodriguez G, Darcourt J. Brain perfusion follow-up in Alzheimer's patients during treatment with acetylcholinesterase inhibitors. *J Nucl Med* **43**: 983-990, 2002.

Nowak G, Ordway GA, Paul IA. Alterations in the N-methyl-D-aspartate (NMDA) receptor complex in the frontal cortex of suicide victims. *Brain Res* **675**: 157-164, 1995.

Nowakowska E, Chodera A, Kus K, Nowak P, Szkilnik R. Reversal of stress-induced memory changes by moclobemide: the role of neurotransmitters. *Pol J Pharmacol* **53**: 227-233, 2001.

Nunomura A, Perry G, Aliev G, Hirai K, Takeda A, Balraj EK, Jones PK, Ghanbari H, Wataya T, Shimohama S, Chiba S, Atwood CS, Petersen RB, Smith MA. Oxidative damage is the earliest event in Alzheimer disease. *J Neuropathol Exptl Neurol* **60**: 759-767, 2001.

O'Conner JJ, Rowan MJ, Anwyl R. Use-dependent effects of acute and chronic treatment with imipramine and buspirone on excitatory synaptic transmission in the rat hippocampus in vivo. *Naunyn Schmiedebergs Arch Pharmacol* **348**: 158-163, 1993.

Oh C, Murray B, Bhattacharya N, Holland D, Tatton WG. (-)-Deprenyl alters the survival of adult murine facial motoneurons after axotomy: increases in vulnerable C57BL strain but decreases in motor neuron degeneration mutants. *Neurosci Res* **38**: 64-74, 1994.

Ohm TG, Munch S, Schonheit B, Zarski R, Nitsch R. Transneuronally altered dendritic processing of tangle-free neurons in Alzheimer's disease. *Acta Neuropathol* **103**: 437-443, 2002.

Ordway GA, Gambarana C, Tejani-Butt SM, Areso P, Hauptmann M, Frazer A. Preferential reduction in binding of ^{125}I-Iodopindolol to beta-1-adrenoceptors in the amygdala of rat after antidepressant treatments. *J Pharmacol Exptl Ther* **257**: 281-289, 1991.

Owens MJ, Nemeroff CB. Corticotropin-releasing factor antagonists in affective disorders. *Exp Opin Invest Drugs* **8**: 1849-1858, 1999.

Page ME, Detke MJ, Dalvi A, Kirby LG, Lucki I. Serotoninergic mediation of the effects of fluoxetine but not desipramine, in the rat forced swimming test. *Psychopharmacology* **147**: 162-167,1999.

Pancheri P, Delle-Chiaie R, Donnini M, Seripa S, Gambino C, Vicario E, Trillo L. Effects of moclobemide on depressive symptoms and cognitive performance in a geriatric population: a controlled comparative study versus imipramine. *Clin Neuropharmacol* **17 (suppl 1)**: S58-S73, 1994.

Pariente CM, Miller AH. Glucocorticoid receptors in major depression: relevance to pathophysiology and treatment. *Biol Psychiatry* **49**: 391-404, 2001.

Pepin MC, Pothier F, Barden N. Antidepressant drug action in a transgenic mouse model of the endocrine changes seen in depression. *Mol Pharmacol* **42**: 991-995, 1992.

Peselow ED, Corwin J, Fieve RR, Rotrosen J, Cooper TB. Disappearance of memory deficits in outpatient depressives responding to imipramine. *J Affect Disord* **21**: 173-183, 1991.

Plotsky PM, Cunningham ET Jr, Widmaier EP. Catecholaminergic modulation of corticotropin-releasing factor and adrenocorticotropin secretion. *Endoc Revs* **10**: 437-458,1989.

Plotsky PM, Meaney MJ. Early postnatal experience alters hypothalamic corticotropin-releasing factor (CRF) mRNA, median eminence CRF content and stress-induced release in adult rats. *Brain Res Mol Brain Res* **18**: 195-200, 1993.

Poltyrev T, Weinstock M. Gender difference in the prevention of hyperanxiety in adult prenatally-stressed rats by chronic treatment with amitriptyline. *Psychopharmacol* 2004, *in press*.

Poltyrev T, Youdim, MBH, Drigues N, Weinstock, M. Chronic treatment from adolescence with TV-3326, a brain-selective MAO-cholinesterase inhibitor, abolishes hyperanxiety in adult prenatally-stressed rats. *Neural Plasticity* 9: 106, 2002.

Popoli M, Gennarelli M, Racagni G. Modulation of synaptic plasticity by stress and antidepressants. *Bipolar Disord* 4: 166-182, 2002.

Raadsheer FC, Hoogendijk W J, Stam FC, Tilders FJ, Swaab DF. Increased numbers of corticotropin-releasing hormone expressing neurons in the hypothalamic paraventricular nucleus of depressed patients. *Clin Neuroendocrinol* 60: 436-444, 1994.

Raadsheer FC, Van Heerikhuize JJ, Lucassen PJ, Hoogendijk WJ, Tilders FJ, Swaab DF. Corticotropin-releasing hormone mRNA levels in the paraventricular nucleus of patients with Alzheimer's disease and depression. *Am J Psychiatry* 152: 1372-1376, 1995.

Rabey JM, Sagi I, Huberman M, Melamed E, Korczyn A, Giladi N, Inzelberg R, Djaldetti R, Klein C, Berecz G. Rasagiline mesylate, a new MAO-B inhibitor for the treatment of Parkinson's disease: a double-blind study as adjunctive therapy to levodopa. *Clin. Neuropharmacol* 23: 324-330, 2000.

Rajkowska G, Miguel-Hidalgo JJ, Wei J, Dilley G, Pittman SD, Meltzer HY, Overholser JC, Roth BL, Stockmeier CA. Morphometric evidence for neuronal and glial prefrontal cell pathology in major depression. *Biol Psychiatry* 45: 1085-1098, 1999.

Ranga K, Krishnan R. Clinical experience with substance P receptor (NK1) antagonists in depression. *J Clin Psychiatry* 63 (Suppl 11): 25-29, 2002.

Reisberg B, Doody R, Stoffler A, Schmitt F, Ferris S, Mobius HJ. Memantine Study Group. Memantine in moderate-to-severe Alzheimer's disease. *N Engl J Med* 348:1333-1341, 2003.

Roche M, Commons KG, Peoples A, Valentino RJ. Circuitry underlying regulation of the serotonergic system by swim stress. *J Neurosci* 23: 970-977, 2003.

Rogers MA, Bradshaw JL, Pantelis C, Phillips JG. Frontostriatal deficits in unipolar major depression. *Brain Res Bull* 47: 297-310, 1998.

Rombouts SA, Barkhof F, Van-Meel CS, Scheltens P.Alterations in brain activation during cholinergic enhancement with rivastigmine in Alzheimer's disease. *J Neurol Neurosurg Psychiatr* 73: 665-671, 2002.

Rösler M, Anand R, Cicin-Sain A, Gauthier S, Agid Y, Dal-Bianco P, Stahelin HB, Hartman R, Gharabawi M. Efficacy and safety of rivastigmine in patients with Alzheimer's disease: international randomised controlled trial. *Brit Med J* 318: 633-638,1999a.

Rösler M, Retz W, Retz-Junginger P, Dennler HJ. Effects of two-year treatment with the cholinesterase inhibitor rivastigmine on behavioural symptoms in Alzheimer's disease. *Behav Neurol* 11: 211-216, 1999b.

Rupniak NM. New insights into the antidepressant actions of substance P (NK1 receptor) antagonists. *Can J Physiol Pharmacol* 80: 489-494, 2002.

Salmon E, Gregoire MC, Delfiore G, Lemaire C, Degueldre C, Franck G, Comar D. Combined study of cerebral glucose metabolism and [^{11}C] methionine accumulation in probable Alzheimer's disease using positron emission tomography. *J Cereb Blood Flow Metab* 16: 309-408, 1996.

Samuel W, Caligiuri M, Galasko D, Lacro J, Marini M, McClure FS, Warren K, Jeste DV. Better cognitive and psychopathologic response to donepezil in patients prospectively diagnosed as dementia with Lewy bodies: a preliminary study. *Int J Geriatric Psychiatry* **15**: 794-802, 2000.

Santarelli L, Gobbi G, Debs PC, Sibille ET, Blier P, Hen R, Heath MJ. Genetic and pharmacological disruption of neurokinin 1 receptor function decreases anxiety-related behaviors and increases serotonergic function. *Proc Natl Acad Sci* **98**: 1912-1917, 2001.

Sapolsky RM. Glucocorticoids and hippocampal atrophy in neuropsychiatric disorders. *Arch Gen Psychiatry* **57**: 925-935, 2000.

Saura J, Luque JM, Cesura AM, Da Prada M, Chan-Palay V, Huber G, Loffler J, Richards JG. Increased monoamine oxidase B activity in plaque-associated astrocytes of Alzheimer brains revealed by quantitative radioautography. *Neuroscience* **62**: 15-30, 1994.

Schildkraut JJ. The catecholamine hypothesis of affective disorders: A review of supporting evidence. *Am J Psychiatry* **122**: 509–522, 1965.

Sheline YI. Hippocampal atrophy in major depression: a result of depression-induced neurotoxicity? *Mol Psychiatry* **1**: 298–299, 1996.

Shoham S, Bejar C, Kovalev E, Weinstock M. Intracerebroventricular injection of streptozotocin causes neurotoxicity to myelin that contributes to spatial memory deficits in rats. *Exp Neurol* 2004, *in press*.

Shors TJ, Seib TB, Levine S, Thompson RF. Inescapable versus escapable shock modulates long-term potentiation in the rat hippocampus. *Science* **244**: 224-226, 1989.

Shoulson I. DATATOP: a decade of neuroprotective inquiry. Parkinson study group. Deprenyl and tocopherol antioxidative therapy of Parkinsonism. *Ann Neurol* **44 (Suppl 1)**: S160-S166, 1998.

Schulz R, Antonin KH, Hoffmann E, Jedrychowski M, Nilsson E, Schick C, Bieck PR. Tyramine kinetics and pressor sensitivity during monoamine oxidase inhibition by selegiline. *Clin Pharmacol Ther* **46**: 528-536, 1989.

Skolnick P. Antidepressants for the new millennium. *Eur J Pharmacol* **375**: 31-40, 1999.

Small GW, Ercoli LM, Silverman DH, Huang SC, Komo S, Bookheimer SY, Lavretsky H, Miller K, Siddarth PM, Rasgon NL, Mazziotta JC, Saxena S, Wu HM, Mega MS, Cummings JL, Saunders AM, Pericak-Vance MA, Roses AD, Barrio JR, Phelps ME. Cerebral metabolic and cognitive decline in persons at genetic risk for Alzheimer's disease. *Proc Natl Acad Sci* **97**: 6037-6042, 2000.

Smith MA, Makino S, Kvetnansky R, Post RM. Stress and glucocorticoids affect the expression of brain-derived neurotrophic factor and neurotrophin-3 mRNAs in the hippocampus. *J Neurosci* **15**: 1768-1777, 1995.

Steckler T, Rammes G, Sauvage M, Van Gaalen MM, Weis C, Zieglgansberger W, Holsboer F. Effects of the monoamine oxidase A inhibitor moclobemide on hippocampal plasticity in GR-impaired transgenic mice. *J Psychiatr Res* **35**: 29-42, 2001.

Steinberg R, Alonso R, Griebel G, Bert L, Jung M, Oury-Donat F, Poncelet M, Gueudet C, Desvignes C, Le Fur G, Soubrié P. Selective blockade of neurokinin-2 receptors produces antidepressant-like effects associated with reduced corticotropin-releasing factor function. *J Pharmacol Exptl Ther* **299**: 449–458, 2001.

Stewart CA, Reid IC. Repeated ECS and fluoxetine administration have equivalent effects on hippocampal synaptic plasticity. *Psychopharmacology* **148**: 217-223, 2000.

Stewart CA, Reid IC. Antidepressant mechanisms: functional and molecular correlates of excitatory amino acid neurotransmission. *Mol Psychiatry* **7 (suppl 1):** S15-S22, 2002.

Stone EA, Platt JE. Brain adrenergic receptors and resistance to stress. *Brain Res* **237:** 405-414, 1982.

Stone EA, Slucky AV, Platt JE, Trullas R. Reduction of the cyclic adenosine 3',5'-monophosphate response to catecholamines in rat brain slices after repeated restraint stress. *J Pharmacol Exptl Ther* **233:** 382-388, 1985.

Stoudemire A, Hill CD, Morris R, Martino-Saltzman D, Lewison B. Long-term affective and cognitive outcome in depressed older adults. *Am J Psychiatry* **150:** 896-900, 1993.

Stout SC, Owens MJ, Nemeroff CB. Regulation of corticotropin-releasing factor neuronal systems and hypothalamic-pituitary-adrenal axis activity by stress and chronic antidepressant treatment. *J Pharmacol Exp Ther* **300:** 1085-1092, 2002.

Stryjer R, Strous RD, Bar F, Werber E, Shaked G, Buhiri Y, Kotler M, Weizman A, Rabey JM. Beneficial effect of donepezil augmentation for the management of comorbid schizophrenia and dementia. *Clin Neuropharmacol* **26:**12-17, 2003.

Tam SY, Roth RH. Selective increase in dopamine metabolism in the prefrontal cortex by the anxiogenic beta-carboline FG 7142. *Biochem Pharmac* **34:** 1595-1598, 1985.

Teri L, Reifler BV, Veith RC, Barnes R, White E, McLean P, Raskind M. Imipramine in the treatment of depressed Alzheimer's patients: impact on cognition. *J Gerontol* **46:** P372-P377, 1991.

Tsukada H, Takiuchi T, Ando I, Shizuno H, Nakanishi S, Ouchi Y. Regulation of cerebral blood fow response to somatosensory stimulation through cholinergic system: a PET study in unanesthetized monkey brain. *Brain Res* **749:** 10-17, 1997.

Vakili K, Pillay SS, Lafer B, Fava M, Renshaw PF, Bonello-Cintron CM, Yurgelun-Todd DA. Hippocampal volume in primary unipolar major depression: a magnetic resonance imaging study. *Biol Psychiatry* **47:** 1087-1090, 2000.

Van Bockstaele EJ, Colago EE, Valentino RJ. Corticotropin- releasing factor-containing axon terminals synapse onto catecholamine dendrites and may presynaptically modulate other afferents in the rostral pole of the nucleus locus coeruleus in the rat brain. *J Comp Neurol* **364:** 523-534, 1996.

Van der Hart MG, Czeh B, De Biurrun G, Michaelis T, Watanabe T, Natt O, Frahm J, Fuchs E. Substance P receptor antagonist and clomipramine prevent stress-induced alterations in cerebral metabolites, cytogenesis in the dentate gyrus and hippocampal volume. *Mol Psychiatry* **7:** 933-941, 2002.

Van Oekelen D, Luyten WH, Leysen JE. 5-HT$_{2A}$ and 5-HT$_{2C}$ receptors and their atypical regulation properties. *Life Sci* **72:** 2429-2449, 2003.

Van-Laar, MW, Volkerts ER, Verbaten MN, Trooster S, Van-Megen HJ, Kenemans JL. Differential effects of amitriptyline, nefazodone and paroxetine on performance and brain indices of visual selective attention and working memory. P*sychopharmacology* **162:** 351-363, 2002.

Vaucher E, Aumont N, Pearson D, Rowe W, Poirier J, Kar S. Amyloid beta peptide levels and its effects on hippocampal acetylcholine release in aged, cognitively-impaired and -unimpaired rats. *J Chem Neuroanat* **21:** 323-329, 2001.

Vazquez DM. Stress and the developing limbic-hypothalamic-pituitary-adrenal axis. *Psychoneuroendocrinol* **23**: 663-700, 1998.

Vazquez DM, Eskandari R, Phelka A, Lopez JF. Impact of maternal deprivation on brain corticotropin-releasing hormone circuits: prevention of CRH receptor-2 mRNA changes by desipramine treatment. *Neuropsychopharmacol* **28**: 898-909, 2003.

Venneri A, Shanks MF, Staff RT, Pestell SJ, Forbes KE, Gemmell HG, Murray AD. Cerebral blood flow and cognitive responses to rivastigmine treatment in Alzheimer's disease. *Neuroreport* **13**: 83-87, 2002.

Von Frijtag JC, Reijmers LG, Van der Harst JE, Leus IE, Van den Bos R, Spruijt BM. Defeat followed by individual housing results in long-term impaired reward- and cognition-related behaviours in rats. *Brain Behav Res* **117**: 137-146, 2000.

Von Frijtag JC, Van den Bos R, Spruijt BM. Imipramine restores the long-term impairment of appetitive behavior in socially stressed rats. *Psychopharmacology* **162**: 232-238, 2002.

Waggie KS, Kahle PJ, Tolwani RJ. Neurons and mechanisms of neuronal death in neurodegenerative diseases: a brief review. *Lab Animal Science* **49**: 358-362, 1999.

Walton MR, Dragunow M. Is CREB a key to neuronal survival? *Trends Neurosci* **23**: 48-53, 2000.

Ward HE, Johnson EA, Salm AK, Birkle DL. Effects of prenatal stress on defensive withdrawal behavior and corticotropin releasing factor systems in rat brain. *Physiol Behav* **70**: 359-366, 2000.

Weinstock M. Does prenatal stress impair coping and regulation of the hypothalamic-pituitary-adrenal axis? *Neurosci Biobehav Revs* **21**: 1-10, 1997.

Weinstock M. Alterations induced by gestational stress in brain morphology and behaviour of the offspring. *Prog Neurobiol* **65**: 427-451, 2001.

Weinstock M, Bejar C, Wang R-H, Poltyrev T, Gross A, Finberg JPM, Youdim MBH. TV3326, a novel neuroprotective drug with cholinesterase and monoamine oxidase inhibitory activities for the treatment of Alzheimer's disease. *J Neural Transm* **60 (suppl)**:157-169, 2000a.

Weinstock M, Goren T, Youdim MBH. Development of a novel neuroprotective drug (TV3326) for the treatment of Alzheimer's disease with cholinesterase and monoamine oxidase inhibitory activities. *Drug Dev Res* **50**: 216-222, 2000b.

Weinstock M, Gorodetsky E, Poltyrev T, Gross A, Sagi Y, Youdim MBH. A novel cholinesterase and brain-selective monoamine oxidase inhibitor for the treatment of dementia co-morbid with depression and Parkinson's disease. *Prog Neuro Psychopharmacol Biol Psychiatry* **27**: 555-561, 2003.

Weinstock M, Gorodetsky E, Wang R-H, Gross A, Weinreb O, Youdim MBH. Limited potentiation of blood pressure response to oral tyramine by brain-selective monoamine oxidase A-B inhibitor, TV-3326 in conscious rabbits. *Neuropharmacology* **43**: 999-1005, 2002a.

Weinstock M, Kirschenbaum-Slager N, Lazarovici P, Bejar C, Youdim MBH, Shoham S. Neuroprotective effects of novel cholinesterase inhibitors derived from rasagiline as potential anti-Alzheimer drugs. *Ann NY Acad Sci* **939**: 148-161, 2001.

Weinstock M, Poltyrev T, Bejar C, Youdim MBH. Effect of TV3326, a novel monoamine-oxidase-cholinesterase inhibitor, in rat models of anxiety and depression. *Psychopharmacology* **160**:318-324, 2002b.

Weiss JM, Goodman PA, Losito BG, Corrigan S, Charry JM, Bailey WH. Behavioral depression produced by an uncontrollable stressor: Relationship to norepinephrine, dopamine and serotonin levels in various regions of the rat brain. *Brain Res Rev* **3**: 167-205,1981.

Wesnes KA, McKeith IG, Ferrara R, Emre M, Del Ser T, Spano PF, Cicin-Sain A, Anand R, Spiegel R. Effects of rivastigmine on cognitive function in dementia with lewy bodies: a randomised placebo-controlled international study using the cognitive drug research computerised assessment system. *Dement Geriatr Cogn Disord* **13**: 183-192, 2002.

Westrin A, Ekman R, Traskman-Bendz L. Alterations of corticotropin releasing hormone (CRH) and neuropeptide Y (NPY) plasma levels in mood disorder patients with a recent suicide attempt. *Eur Neuropsychopharmacol* **9**: 205-211,1999.

Willner P, Muscat R, Papp M. Chronic mild stress-induced anhedonia: a realistic animal model of depression. *Neurosci Biobehav Rev* **16**: 525-534, 1992.

Wissink S, Meijer O, Pearce D, Van Der Burg B, Van Der Saag PT. Regulation of the rat serotonin-1A receptor gene by corticosteroids. *J Biol Chem* **275**: 1321-1326, 2000.

Wong ML, Kling MA, Munson PJ, Listwak S, Licinio J, Prolo P, Karp B, McCutcheon IE, Geracioti TD Jr, DeBellis MD, Rice KC, Goldstein DS, Veldhuis JD, Chrousos GP, Oldfield EH, McCann SM, Gold PW. Pronounced and sustained central hyper-noradrenergic function in major depression with melancholic features: relation to hypercortisolism and corticotropin-releasing hormone. *Proc Natl Acad Sci USA* **97**: 325-330, 2000a.

Wong TP, Marchese G, Casu MA, Ribeiro da Silva A, Cuello AC, De Koninck Y. Loss of presynaptic and postsynaptic structures is accompanied by compensatory increase in action potential-dependent synaptic input to layer V neocortical pyramidal neurons in aged rats. *J Neurosci* **20**: 8596-8606, 2000b

Xu L, Anwyl R, Rowan MJ. Behavioural stress facilitates the induction of long-term depression in the hippocampus. *Nature* **387**: 497-500, 1997.

Xu L, Holscher C, Anwyl R, Rowan MJ. Glucocorticoid receptor and protein/RNA synthesis-dependent mechanisms underlie the control of synaptic plasticity by stress. *Proc Natl Acad Sci USA* **95**: 3204-3208,1998.

Yau, JLW, Hibberd C, Noble J, Seckl JR.The effect of chronic fluoxetine treatment on brain corticosteroid receptor mRNA expression and spatial memory in young and aged rats. *Mol Brain Res* **106**: 117-123, 2002.

Yogev-Falach M, Amit T, Bar-Am O, Weinstock M, Youdim MBH. The involvement of mitogen-activated protein (MAP) kinase in the regulation of amyloid precursor protein processing by novel cholinesterase inhibitors derived from rasagiline. *FASEB* **16**: 1674-1676, 2002.

Yoritaka A, Hattori N, Uchida K, Tanaka M, Stadtman ER, Mizuno Y. Immunohisto-chemical detection of 4-hydroxynonenal protein adducts in Parkinson disease. *Proc Natl Acad Sci* **93**: 2696-2701, 1996.

Youdim MBH, Weinstock M. Molecular basis of neuroprotective activities of rasagline and the anti-Alzheimer drug, TV3326, [(*N*-propargyl-(3*R*)aminoindan-5-YL)-ethyl methyl carbamate] *Cell Mol Biol* **21**: 555-573, 2002.

Zink M, Sartorius A, Lederbogen F, Henn FA. Electroconvulsive therapy in a patient receiving rivastigmine. *J Electroconvulsive Ther* **3**: 162-164, 2002.

Zobel AW, Nickel T, Kunzel HE, Ackl N, Sonntag A, Ising M, Holsboer F. Effects of the high-affinity corticotropin-releasing hormone receptor 1 antagonist 121919 in major depression: the first 20 patients treated. *J Psychiatr Res* **34**:171-181, 2000.

Index

B

C

D

E

F